Atlas of Endometrial Histopathology

Gisela Dallenbach-Hellweg • Dietmar Schmidt
Friederike Dallenbach

Atlas of Endometrial Histopathology

Third Edition

Springer

Prof. Dr. Gisela Dallenbach-Hellweg
Ludolf-Krehl-Str. 57
69120 Heidelberg
Germany
G.Dallenbach@t-online.de

Prof. Dr. Dr. h.c. Dietmar Schmidt
Institut für Pathologie
Referenzzentrum für Gynäkopathologie
A 2, 2
68159 Mannheim
Germany
schmidt@gyn-patho.de

Dr. Friederike Dallenbach
Institut für Pathologie
Konsultations-und Referenzzentrum
für Lymphomdiagnostik
und Hämatopathologie
Universitätsklinikum Ulm
Albert-Einstein-Allee 11
89081 Ulm
Germany
friederike.dallenbach@uniklinik-ulm.de

ISBN 978-3-662-50644-8 ISBN 978-3-642-01541-0 (eBook)

DOI 10.1007/978-3-642-01541-0

Springer Heidelberg Dordrecht London New York

Cover design: eStudio Calamar, Figueres/Berlin

Printed on acid-free paper

Springer is part of Springer Science+Business Media (www.springer.com)

Preface to the Third Edition

This new edition differs from the preceding ones in that there has been extensive revision of most chapters. Recent advances in research gained by immunohistochemical, molecular biological, and cytogenetic methods are included, as far as they are applicable for daily diagnostic work. The chapter on neoplasms, in particular, has been greatly expanded in accordance with the new WHO International Histological Classification of genital tract tumors, covering all pertinent differential diagnostic aspects. The chapter on malignant lymphomas and hematopoetic neoplasms involving the endometrium is a new contribution to this edition (F.D., Ulm). We have revised the chapter on gestational diseases, incorporating recent advances in the differential diagnosis of gestational trophoblastic tumors. New discoveries and experiences in correlating structure and function in infertility and in hormone replacement therapy of peri- and postmenopausal patients are also included. Many new microphotographs have been added to illustrate the advances in tumor research and in immunohistochemical detection methods. We have updated the list of references including recent relevant publications.

To the correspondents and consultants who have contributed valuable observations and suggestions, bringing thereby to our attention omissions in the second edition, we acknowledge our cordial thanks. We thank Dr. Wolfram Klapper, Director of the Lymphom Register of the University of Kiel, for case material for making the microphotographic illustrations of lymphomas. The staff of Springer-Verlag has earned our gratitude for their skill in preparing this new edition.

Heidelberg, Mannheim, Ulm
November 2009

Gisela Dallenbach-Hellweg
Dietmar Schmidt
Friederike Dallenbach

Contents

Introduction to the First Edition

1

The cyclic changes in the function and histology of the endometrium and the rapidity with which they take place complicate the histopathologic diagnosis. Disease states of varying intensities which superimpose themselves on these fluctuating functional changes often produce complex admixtures of the functional state and the damage wrought by the pathologic processes.

The pathologist's functional and morphologic diagnoses should represent the result of constant cooperation with the attending gynecologist. The prime purpose of this atlas is to help the pathologist to find, classify, and diagnose differentially the changes he sees under his microscope. We have kept the text brief. It provides a short description of the pathology of the disease, summarizes and differentiates the possible causes, and explains the clinical importance of the condition and thus how to treat it. Accordingly, this book's approach to diseases is the opposite to that of a textbook, which systematically presents the histopathology of the endometrium according to etiology. This atlas proceeds from the histologic changes and relates these to the possible cause. It follows, as it were, the line of thought which the diagnostic pathologist uses, sparing him the search through different chapters on etiology in a textbook of comparable histologic states. In addition, it obviates the need to duplicate pictures of similar structural changes caused by different diseases.

The atlas is restricted to the endometrium. Neighboring parts of the uterus are included only where we considered them important in differential diagnoses. We have not included electron microscopic pictures, since they can be dispensed with in routine diagnostic studies.

This book is intended for all pathologists, to aid them in their routine diagnostic work and to explain as clearly as possible just how comprehensive, complex, and important the histopathology of the endometrium has become in the last few years. The book is also meant for the clinician, to help guide him through the broad spectrum of possibilities of histopathologic diagnosis of the endometrium, especially in functional disturbances. If this atlas, through its sharp distinction of histopathologic states, helps to improve dialogue between pathologists and clinicians so that optimal therapy of the patients can be provided, then it has fulfilled its purpose.

Gisela Dallenbach-Hellweg and *Hemming Poulsen*
Mannheim and Copenhagen
May 1984

G. Dallenbach-Hellweg et al., *Atlas of Endometrial Histopathology*,
DOI: 10.1007/978-3-642-01541-0_1, © Springer-Verlag Berlin Heidelberg 2010

Technical Remarks 2

2.1 Procedures for Obtaining Endometrial Tissue

A *complete curettage* is the ideal method for optimal diagnostic evaluation of the endometrium. A *fractionated curettage* has additional advantages; it helps to localize the site and extent of malignancy and assists in evaluating endocervical changes that develop during hormonal therapy. For functional diagnosis in infertile patients, *endometrial biopsies* will usually suffice if properly taken with a single-stroke biopsy from the uterine fundus, and they offer the advantage that they can be repeated within the same menstrual cycle. Interpreting biopsies taken by brush or aspiration may prove quite difficult and inaccurate, except for advanced carcinomas.

2.2 Selection of the Proper Time for Curettage

In order to obtain optimal diagnostic results, the time for curettage must be carefully selected. In *infertile patients,* differential diagnosis of the various causes of sterility is best made shortly before the onset of menstruation. Only at this late time can the failure in endometrial differentiation be completely surveyed. In *menorrhagia* possibly due to irregular shedding, the best time for curettage is 5–10 days after the onset of menstruation, in order to recognize remnants of nonlysed mucosa. In *metrorrhagia,* curettage is best done without delay when much of the endometrium is still available for examination. With *amenorrhea* in a patient of reproductive age, pregnancy must be excluded before curettage is performed.

Clinical information is equally important to the pathologist, mainly about the patient's age, menstrual history, any hormone therapy, contraceptive device, endocrinologic disorders, and size and cavity of the uterus, including sonographic and/or hysteroscopic reports.

G. Dallenbach-Hellweg et al., *Atlas of Endometrial Histopathology*,
DOI: 10.1007/978-3-642-01541-0_2, © Springer-Verlag Berlin Heidelberg 2010

2.3
Preparation of the Endometrial Specimen

For *fixation*, a 4% neutral solution of formaldehyde is commonly used and is ideal for most of the diagnostic procedures involved in endometrial examination. *Routine staining* of all specimens should include hematoxylin-eosin (H & E) and a connective tissue stain, for instance van Gieson's solution. The latter is particularly important for recognizing endometrial polyps, or portions of them, and hyalinized placental villi. An additional periodic acid-Schiff (PAS) reaction may be helpful in detecting small amounts of glycogen or mucopolysaccharides in glandular epithelial cells. A reticulin impregnation can be useful for verifying tissue lysis or for distinguishing between various types of tumors. These four staining methods suffice for most questions arising in routine examination of the endometrial biopsy.

For subclassification of endometrial carcinomas, sarcomas, carcinosarcomas and other nonepithelial and nonmesenchymal tumors such as neuroectodermal tumors or lymphomas, *immunohistochemical stainings* may be helpful or needed. Among these, monoclonal antibodies against various cytokeratins, vimentin and carcinoembryonic antigen (CEA) are the most important for adenocarcinomas. In addition, immunostainings for the estrogen and progesterone receptor might be desired by the clinicans as a prerequisite for adjuvant hormonal treatment. In case of neuroendocrine differentiation of a carcinoma, chromogranin A, synaptophysin and CD56 are useful. Tumors of neuroectodermal origin (tumors of the PNET-group) typically express vimentin, CD99, NSE, Fli-1, and may partially express CD57, S-100, and neuroendocrine markers. Malignant lymphomas of the endometrium are preferentially B cell lymphomas (see p. 196 ff). Therefore, markers for lymphatic differentiation antigens such us CD3, CD5, CD10, CD11c, CD20, CD23, CD30, CD75 in combination with markers for BCL-2, BCL-6, Cyclin D1, Mum-1, IgM, IgD and immunoglobulin light chains should be applied. To clarify the dignity of a lymphatic proliferation, a molecular pathological clonality analysis with the polymerase chain reaction (PCR method) might be indicated. For all questional reactive processes and neoplastic lesions in the endometrium, the proliferation marker Ki-67 (MIB-1 antibody) and p53 should be applied to clarify the dignity and the clinical behavior. For the distinction between mucinous adenocarcinomas of the endocervix and those of the endometrium p16 may be a helpful additional marker (see p. 163).

2.4
Interpretation of Endometrial Specimens

Since the endometrial biopsy may contain admixtures of small pieces from various endometrial layers, its interpretation is more difficult than that of intact endometrium received with a surgically removed uterus. Only the functional layer is of diagnostic value in the recognition of functional disturbances. On the other hand, early adenomatous or carcinomatous changes may best be detected in the basal layer. The isthmus mucosa is unsuited for functional diagnosis; it may give a false impression of atrophy or functional deficiency (for differential diagnoses, see p. 43). Regions of necrosis in curettings may have various causes; they should always be reported. Myomatous proliferations may indicate the presence of submucous leiomyomas as the cause of functional bleeding. If the endometrial biopsy contains only endocervical mucosa, the gynecologist may not have reached the endometrial cavity for various reasons, e.g., stenosis of the isthmus or endocervical canal. If fragments of tissue not occurring in the uterine cavity are found in the endometrial biopsy, e.g., fatty tissue, this finding should raise strong suspicions, if not being indicative, of a perforation of the uterine wall and should therefore always be reported (for further details, see Dallenbach-Hellweg 1987).

Artificial changes that should not be misinterpreted may be produced, e.g. when endometrial glands are squeezed by handling the curettage fragments and their lining epithelium intussuscepts to lie within the glandular lumen. Severe freezing artifacts occur when endometrial tissue in formalin solution is allowed to freeze slowly, as may happen when it is sent by mail in winter (Fig. 2.1).

In addition to a histopathologic diagnosis, the pathologist should always try to answer all questions raised by the gynecologist. In postmenopausal patients, there are generally two main reasons for the gynecologist to perform a curettage: either postmenopausal bleeding or a suspicious sonogram. Accordingly, he should explain why the patient was bleeding (e.g., polyps, hyperplasia, spotting from vascular breakage of atrophic vessels, or focal differences in receptor content). If the gynecologist has performed the curettage because of a suspicious sonogram with thickened endometrium and the endometrial specimen obtained is very small, it may not be representative of the lesion. The pathologist should discuss the discrepancy with the gynecologist and encourage him to repeat the curettage if the sonographic lesion is still present.

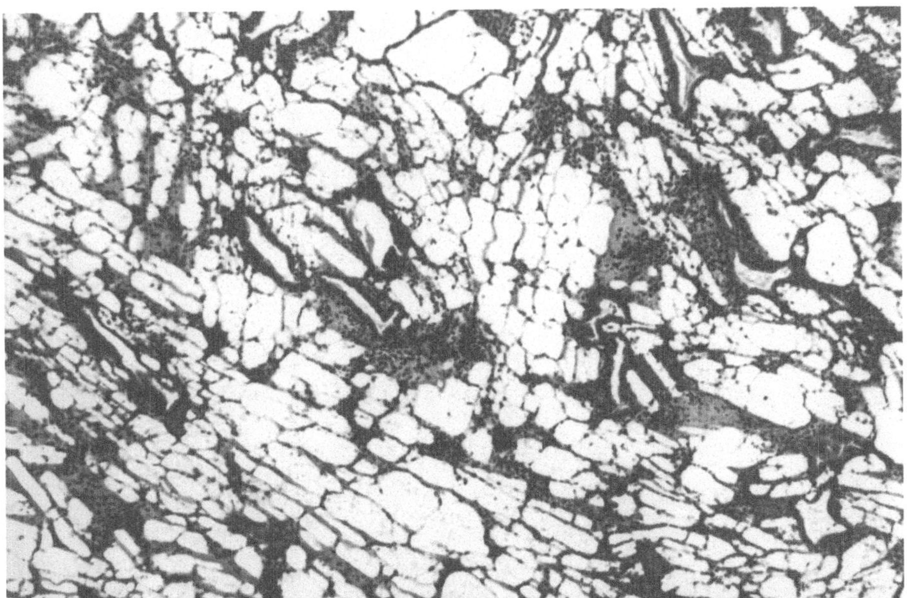

Fig. 2.1 Freezing artifact of the endometrium. Irregular empty spaces produced by ice crystals separate glands and push stromal cells aside. These spaces have no cellular lining (from Dallenbach-Hellweg 1987)

Normal Endometrium 3

Before puberty, the endometrium is resting. The first cycles at the onset of puberty are anovulatory, resulting in deficient or irregular proliferation (see p. 63).

3.1 Normal Menstrual Cycle

The normal menstrual cycle consists of the proliferative and secretory phases, menstruation, and regeneration.

3.1.1 Proliferative Phase

The proliferative phase usually lasts 14 days, but under physiologic conditions may fluctuate between 10 and 20 days. It is therefore impossible to distinguish each day during this phase. Consequently, it is subdivided only into the early, middle, and late proliferative phases. For clinical purposes this subdivision suffices, since the relevant functional changes become evident only in the secretory phase.

Early Proliferative Phase

In the early proliferative phase (Figs. 3.1–3.3), the endometrium is low with sparse, narrow, and straight glands evenly distributed in a loose stroma of spindle-shaped cells. The glandular epithelial cells are low columnar cells; they contain small, rounded, or oval-shaped chromatin-dense nuclei in a sparse cytoplasm. The stromal cells are poorly differentiated and of equal size with small, dense nuclei in a scanty cytoplasm. Nucleoli are inconspicuous and mitoses are very rare. The cells are surrounded by a firm reticulin network. Spiral arterioles are undeveloped. The surface epithelium is flat and still regenerating.

G. Dallenbach-Hellweg et al., *Atlas of Endometrial Histopathology*,
DOI: 10.1007/978-3-642-01541-0_3, © Springer-Verlag Berlin Heidelberg 2010

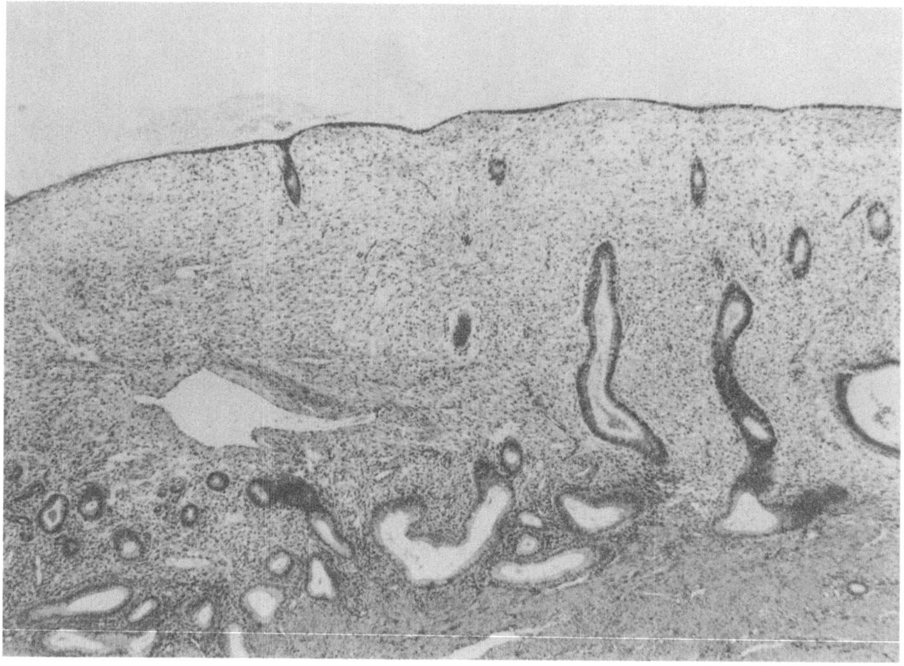

Fig. 3.1 Early proliferative phase. H & E, ×25

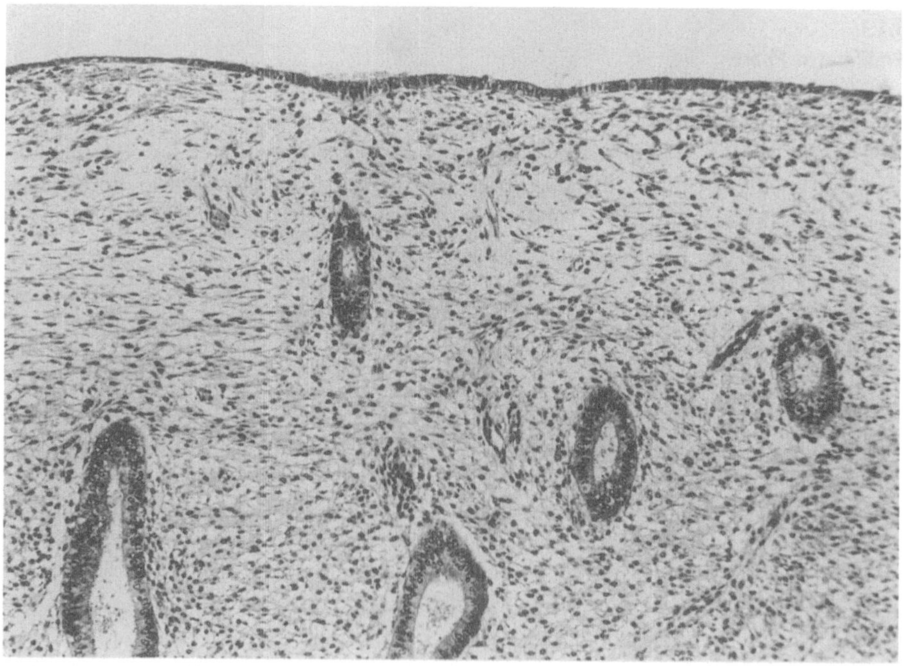

Fig. 3.2 Early proliferative phase. H & E, ×100

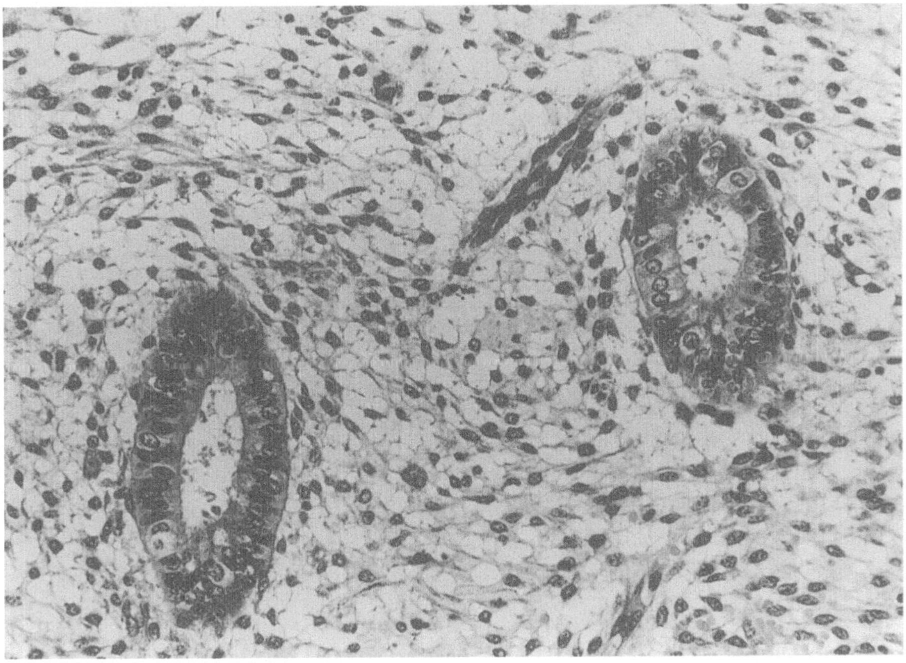

Fig. 3.3 Early proliferative phase. H & E, ×350

Clinical Possibilities. (a) fourth to seventh day of a normal menstrual cycle; (b) anovulatory cycle with follicular insufficiency; (c) deficient proliferation, if the patient is beyond the seventh day of her cycle, or is postmenopausal, with continuing, but deficient estrogen production or replacement therapy.

Distinction is possible only by precise statement of the day of the menstrual cycle and by recording (in anovulatory cycles) the basal body temperature curve. Distinction on morphologic grounds alone is not possible.

Midproliferative Phase

In the midproliferative phase (Figs. 3.4, 3.5), there is beginning tortuosity of glands due to their increase in length, which exceeds the growth in height of the endometrium. The glandular epithelial cells are tall columnar cells and contain slightly enlarged oval-shaped, chromatin-rich nuclei in a dense, sparse cytoplasm rich in RNA. Nucleoli are prominent, and mitoses frequent. The spindle-shaped stromal cells are still poorly differentiated, but rich in DNA and RNA with occasional mitoses and separated by interstitial edema (Harkin 1956). Spiral arterioles are not seen. The surface epithelium has increased in height and is now low columnar.

Clinical Possibilities. (a) Eighth to 11th day of a normal menstrual cycle; (b) anovulatory cycle.

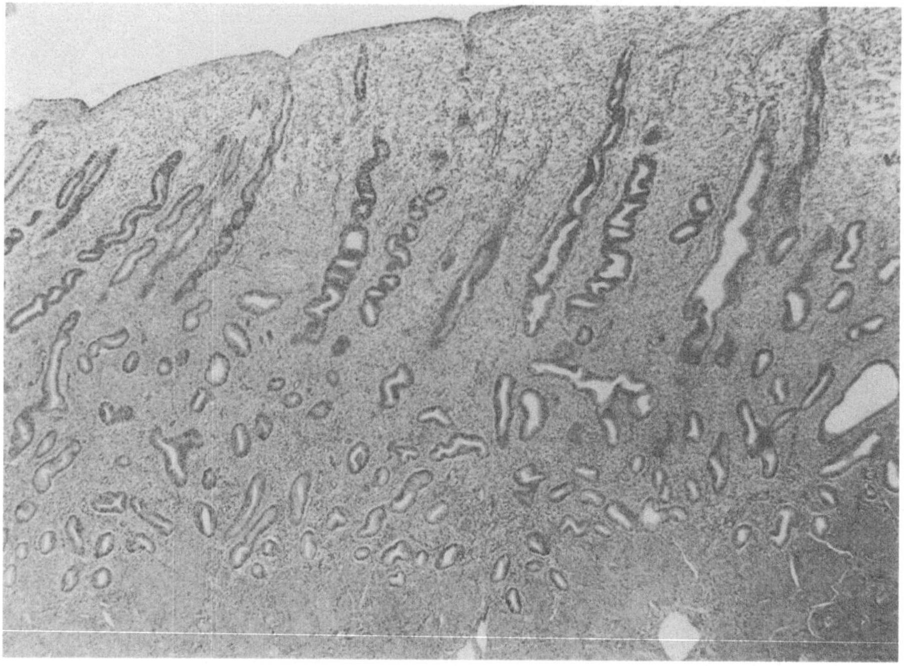

Fig. 3.4 Midproliferative phase. H & E, ×25

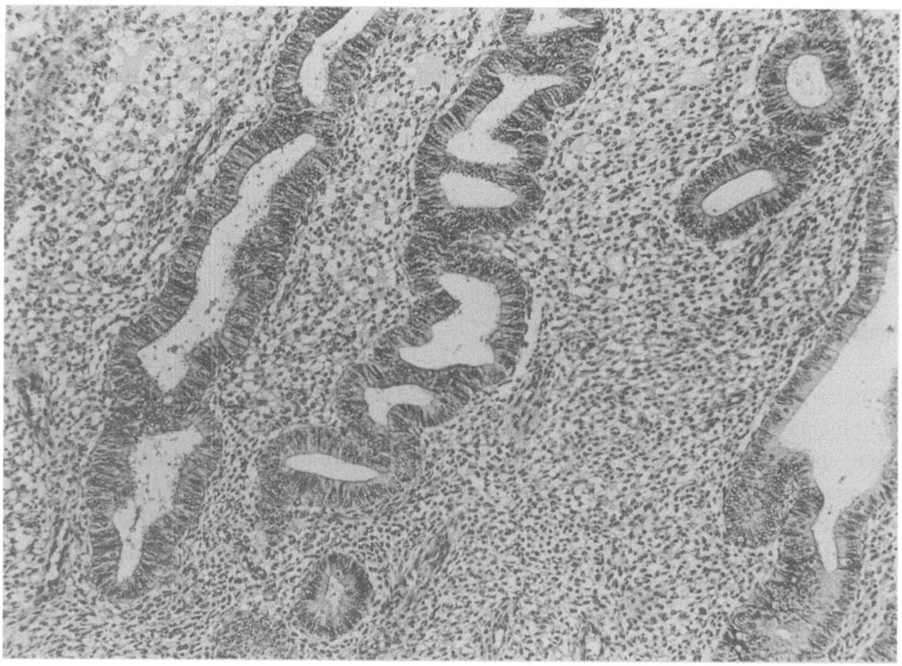

Fig. 3.5 Midproliferative phase. H & E, ×100

Distinction is possible only by precise statement of the day of the menstrual cycle and by recording (in anovulatory cycles) the basal body temperature curve.

Late Proliferative Phase

In the late proliferative phase (Figs. 3.6, 3.7), there is marked tortuosity of glands, which are lined by tall columnar epithelial cells piled up against one another with their nuclei at different levels, giving a pseudostratified appearance. The nuclei are enlarged still further, rich in DNA, and more elongated or oval shaped. Nucleoli are quite prominent, and mitoses are frequent. The cytoplasm is still sparse and poorly differentiated, but rich in RNA. The stromal cells are further enlarged and contain increased amounts of DNA and RNA. Stromal mitoses are frequent. The cells are still of uniform size and without signs of differentiation. The stromal edema has subsided. The reticulin network is dense. Spiral arterioles are still absent. The general height may be slightly lower than that of the midproliferative phase due to decrease of edema. The surface epithelium is distinctly columnar.

Clinical Possibilities. (a) Twelfth–14th day of a normal menstrual cycle; (b) anovulatory cycle with follicular persistence.

Distinction is possible only by precise statement of the day of the menstrual cycle and by recording (in anovulatory cycles) the basal body temperature curve.

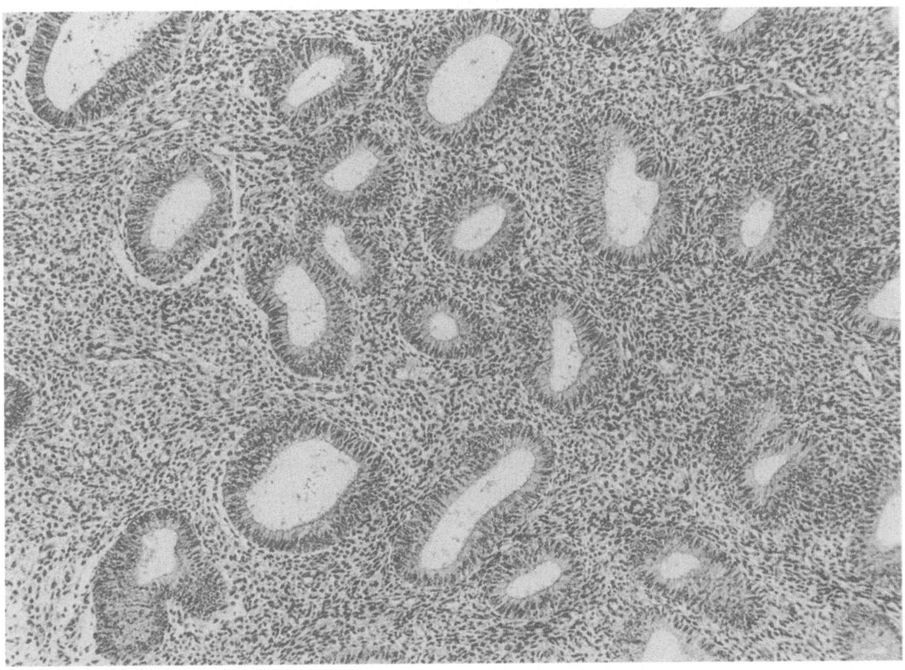

Fig. 3.6 Late proliferative phase. H & E, ×100

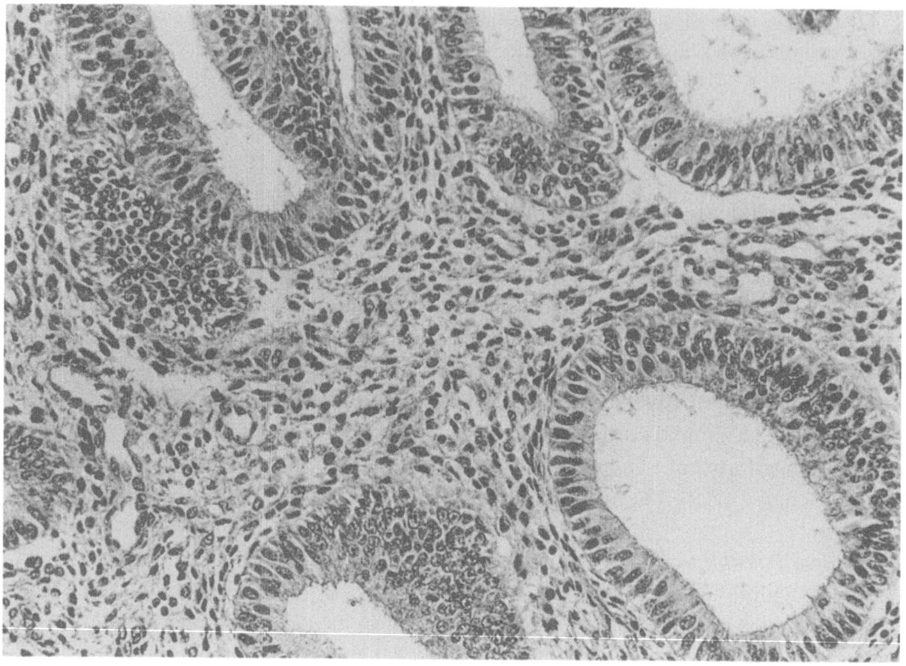

Fig. 3.7 Late proliferative phase. H & E, ×250

3.1.2 Secretory Phase

In the presence of a normally developing and involuting corpus luteum, the secretory phase lasts precisely 14 days (±1 day; Rock and Hertig 1944). If the deviation from this limit is more than 2 days, a functional disturbance should be diagnosed. The daily changes induced in the endometrium by the influence of progesterone enable us to date the endometrium (Noyes et al. 1950; Moricard 1954; Philippe et al. 1965; Dallenbach and Dallenbach-Hellweg 1968; see Fig. 3.8). Because the glandular epithelium reacts more quickly to the influence of progesterone than do the stromal cells, histologic dating is based mainly on the changes of the glandular epithelium during the first week of the secretory phase and on the changes in the stromal cells during the second week. The histologic signs induced in the endometrium by hormones are never uniform. Differences are related to various factors, such as local blood supply, cellular nutrition, and various metabolic factors, e.g., receptors for estrogen and progesterone. For dating the endometrium, those regions showing the most advanced changes are relevant.

The *first day after ovulation* is morphologically mute and therefore designated as interphase because it takes 36–48 h before changes induced by the progesterone secretion can be detected with certainty under the light microscope. Sporadic vacuoles appear in some of the glandular cells even immediately before ovulation, but are unreliable as definite signs of ovulation.

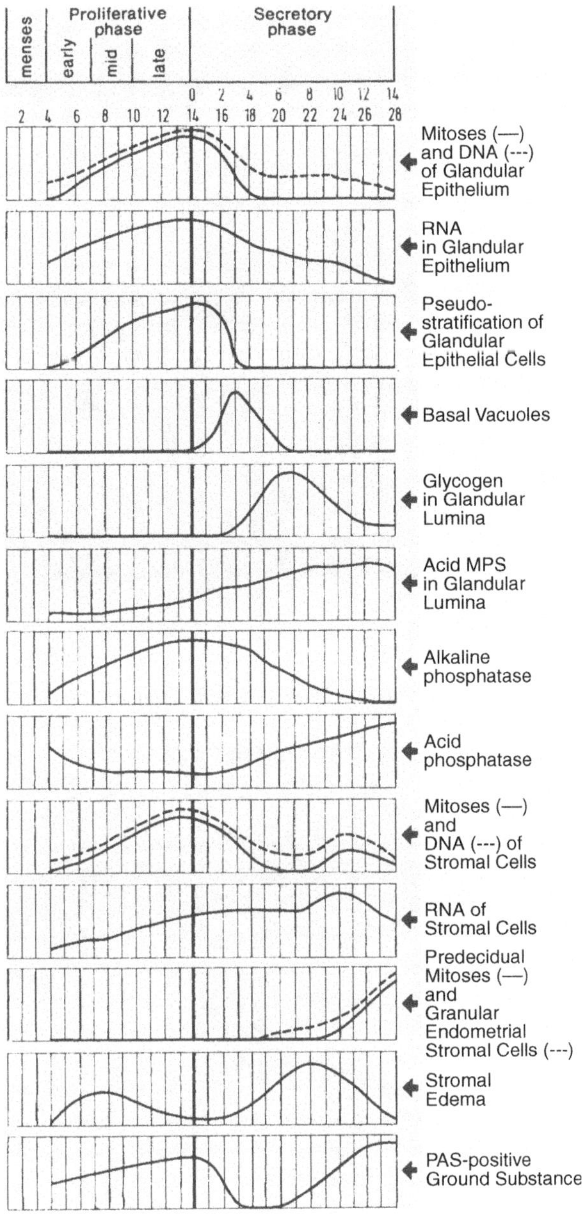

Fig. 3.8 Morphologic criteria important in dating the endometrial cycle (from Dallenbach-Hellweg 1987)

On the *second day after ovulation* (Figs. 3.9, 3.10) numerous basal glycogen vacuoles have appeared in the glandular epithelium (at least in 50% of the glandular cells). They have pushed the nucleus towards the lumen. At their formation the previously pseudostratified appearance of the nuclei disappears; the nuclei again form a single row. They are still

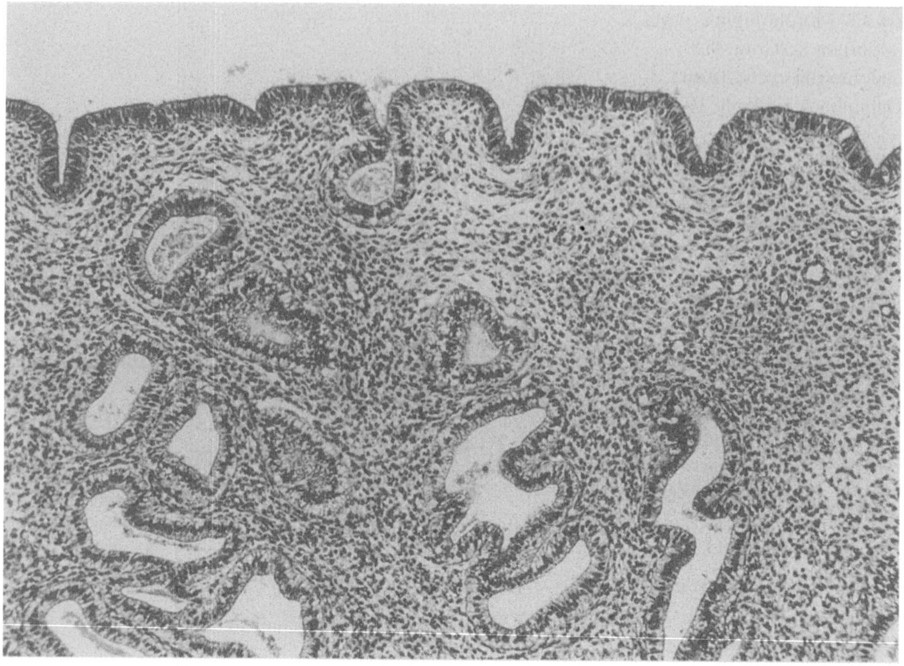

Fig. 3.9 Second day after ovulation. H & E, ×100

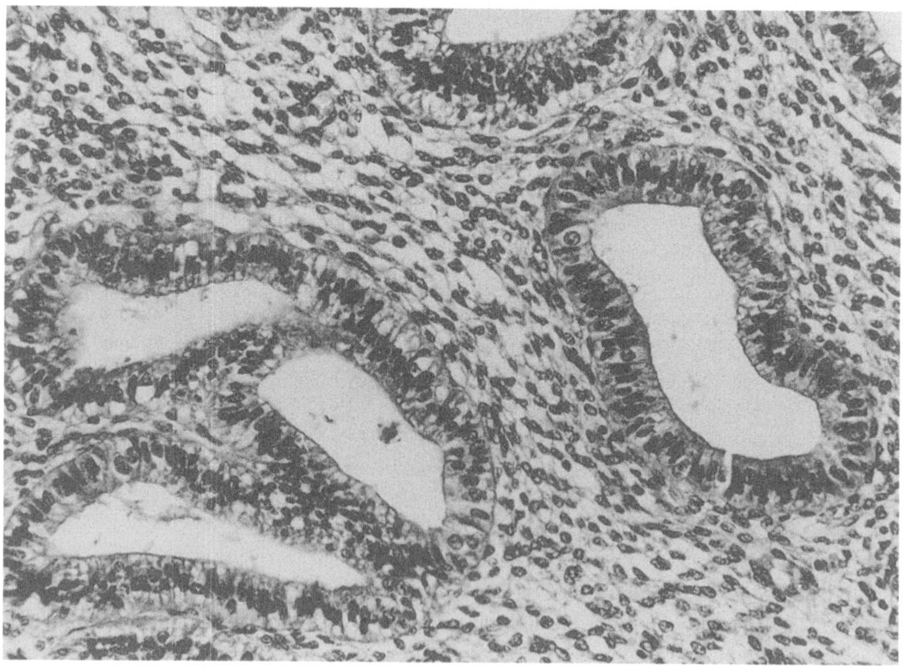

Fig. 3.10 Second day after ovulation. H & E, ×250

oval shaped and chromatin dense. With this new arrangement of the nuclei, the glands become increasingly tortuous and enlarge their surfaces at the glandular lumen. Basal vacuoles, however, fail to appear in the superficial portions of the gland where it merges with the surface epithelium (Fig. 3.9). The surface epithelium of the endometrium remains tall, with no signs of basal secretion. No remarkable changes can be detected in the stroma when compared with those of the late proliferative phase.

Based on morphology, ovulation can be confirmed when distinct basal vacuoles have appeared in most of the glandular epithelial cells.

The *third day after ovulation* (Figs. 3.11, 3.12) shows enlarged basal vacuoles now occupying all the glandular epithelial cells. This secretion has pushed all the nuclei toward the apical end of the cell, where they form a uniform row around the lumen. The nuclei remain dense and rich in chromatin, and only a few mitoses are seen. The cytoplasm still contains abundant RNA.

On the *fourth day after ovulation* (Figs. 3.13–3.15) the nuclei of the glandular epithelial cells have become distinctly rounded and less chromatin dense. A few of them start to return to the base of their cells, while tiny amounts of glycogen move towards the lumen.

A small rim of mucopolysaccharides can be observed at the luminal margin of the epithelial cells, but only with special stains (Fig. 3.15). This rim is characteristic of the fourth day after ovulation.

On the *fifth day after ovulation* (Fig. 3.16) the majority of the nuclei in the glandular epithelial cells have returned to the base of their cells and are distinctly rounded. The glycogen has moved or is moving towards the lumen of the cells on both sides of the nucleus,

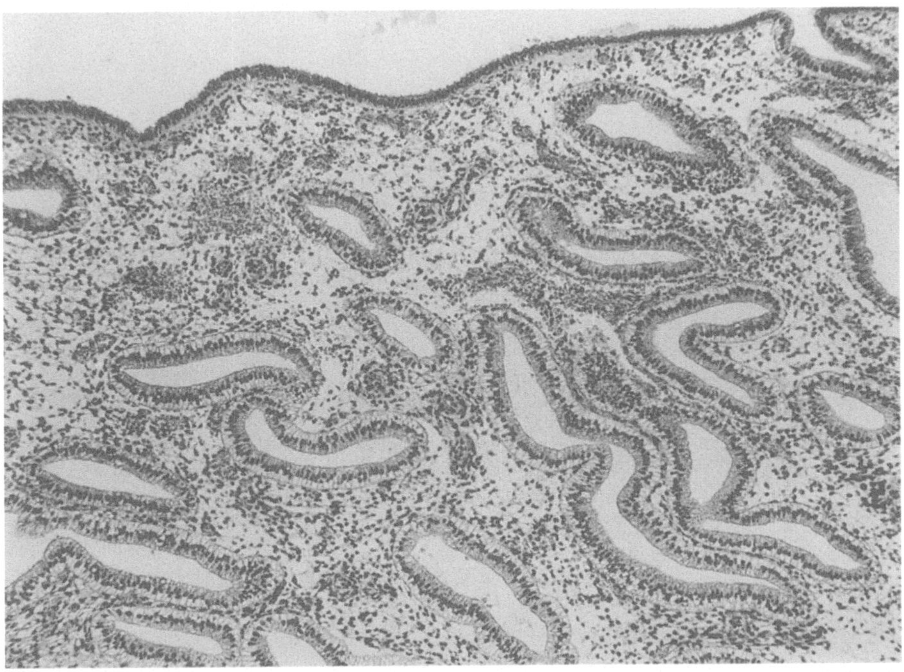

Fig. 3.11 Third day after ovulation. H & E, ×100

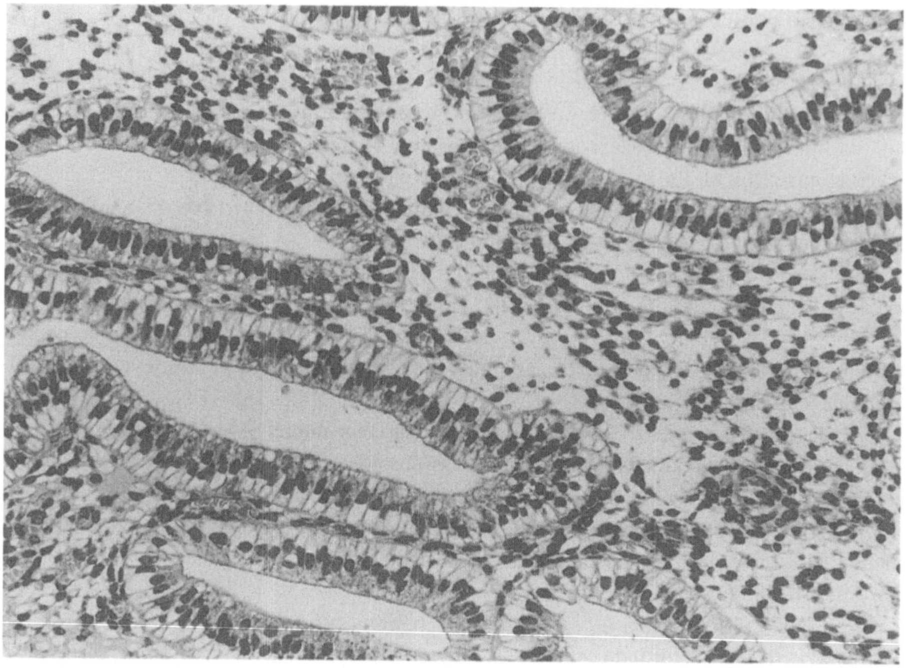

Fig. 3.12 Third day after ovulation. H & E, ×250

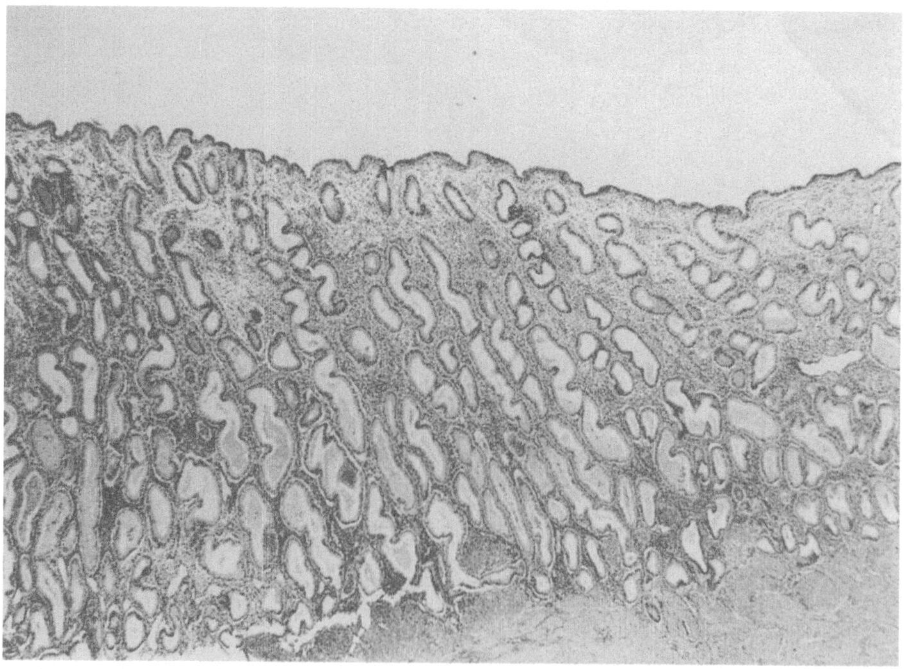

Fig. 3.13 Fourth day after ovulation. H & E, ×25

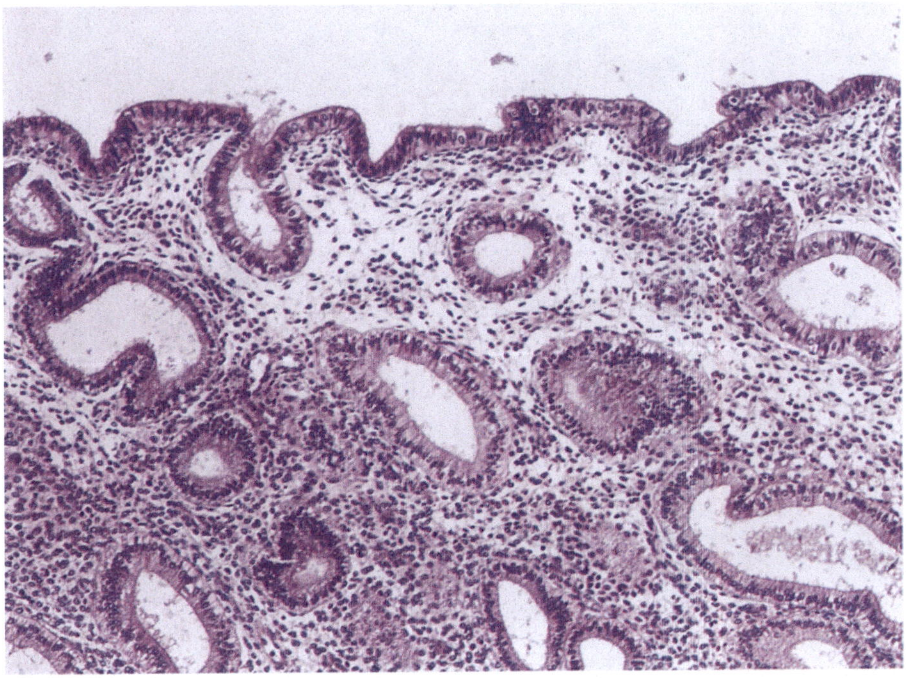

Fig. 3.14 Fourth day after ovulation. H & E, ×100

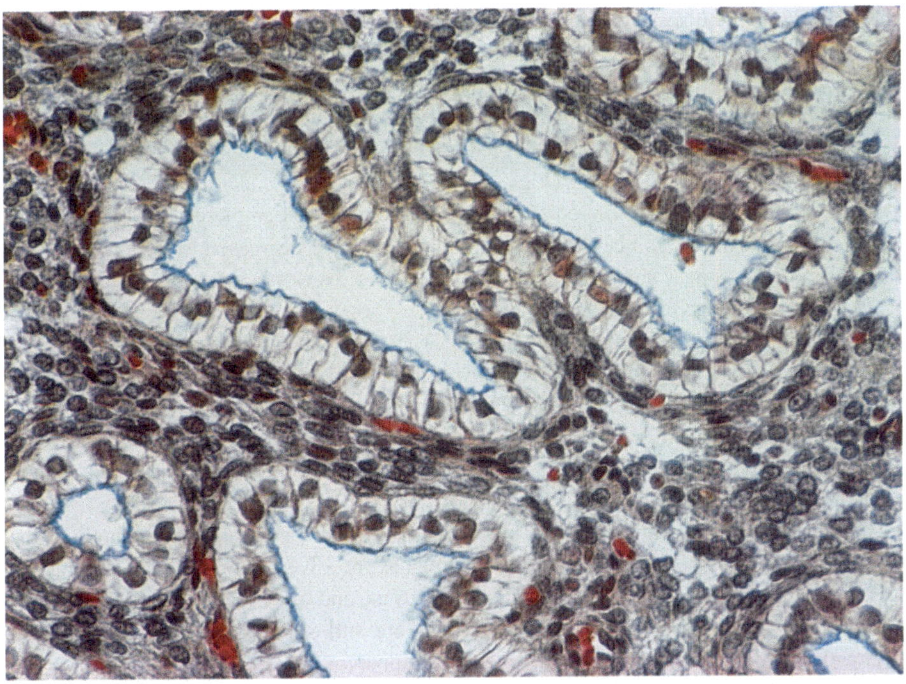

Fig. 3.15 Fourth day after ovulation. Pentachrome reaction, ×350

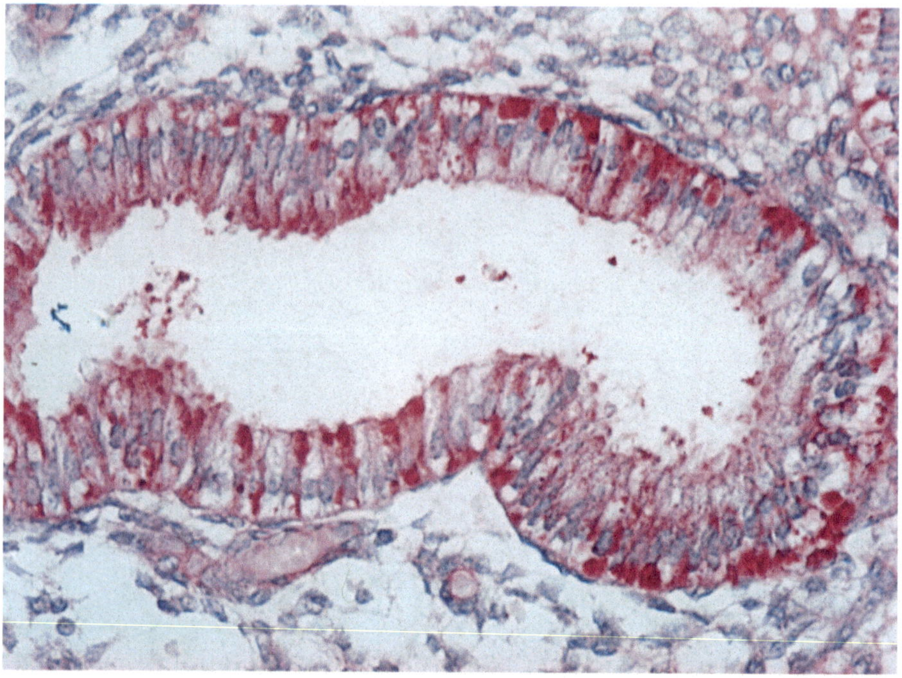

Fig. 3.16 Fifth day after ovulation. Periodic acid-Schiff (PAS) reaction, ×350

and secretion can be seen beginning as tiny globular caps at the free margin of the cells. The movement of the glycogen can best be followed with a PAS stain. Since the nuclei are now vesicular and pale upon staining, they can be easily distinguished from the dense, elongated, basally located nuclei of the cells before the glycogen vacuoles appeared. The nucleoli have now become greatly enlarged.

The *sixth day after ovulation* (Figs. 3.17, 3.18) shows a dilatation of the glandular lumina produced by the continued secretion of glycogen. All epithelial nuclei have now returned to the base of the cells. The glandular cells have decreased in height and their luminal margins appear shredded and hazy due to the excessive apocrine secretion. The RNA content of the cytoplasm is decreased.

On the *seventh day after ovulation* (Figs. 3.19–3.21) the dilated glandular lumen is filled with glycogen, which is partly dissolved in H & E-stained preparations, giving the lumen a false, empty appearance. As a sign of active secretion, the apical ends of the glandular cells appear frayed. No new glycogen is secreted from the cell base. The first stromal reaction after ovulation has occurred and becomes apparent on this day; there is a patchy reaccumulation of stromal edema.

On the *eighth day after ovulation* (Figs. 3.22–3.24) there is virtually no change in the glandular epithelium compared with the preceding day; however, stromal edema has reached its maximum for the secretory phase. It is now diffuse and quite intense, with the stromal cells widely separated from one another. These are still spindle shaped, but somewhat enlarged. Their differentiation becomes even more apparent from this day on (Fig. 3.24). The overall height of the endometrium has increased.

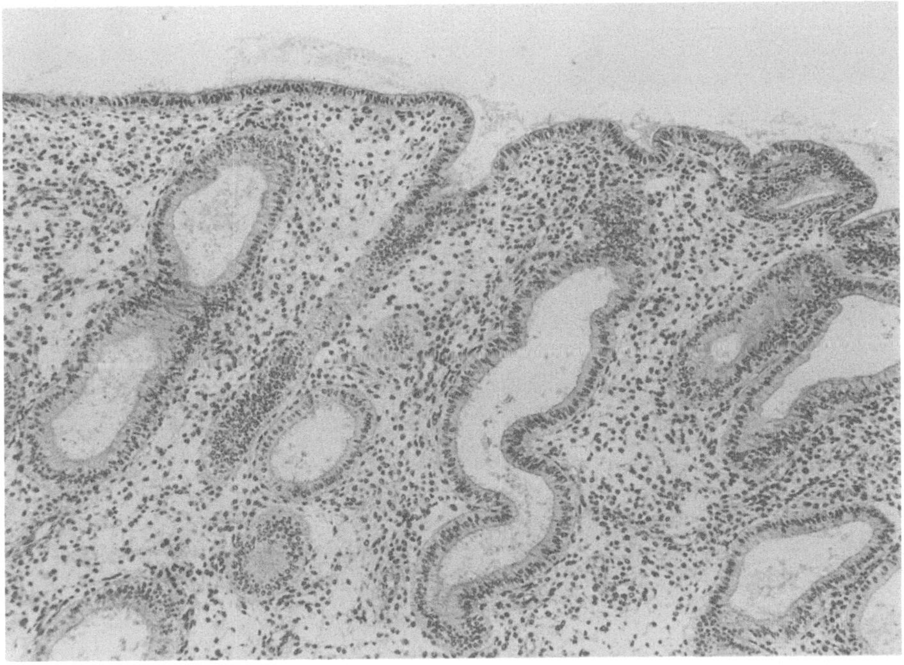

Fig. 3.17 Sixth day after ovulation. H & E, ×100

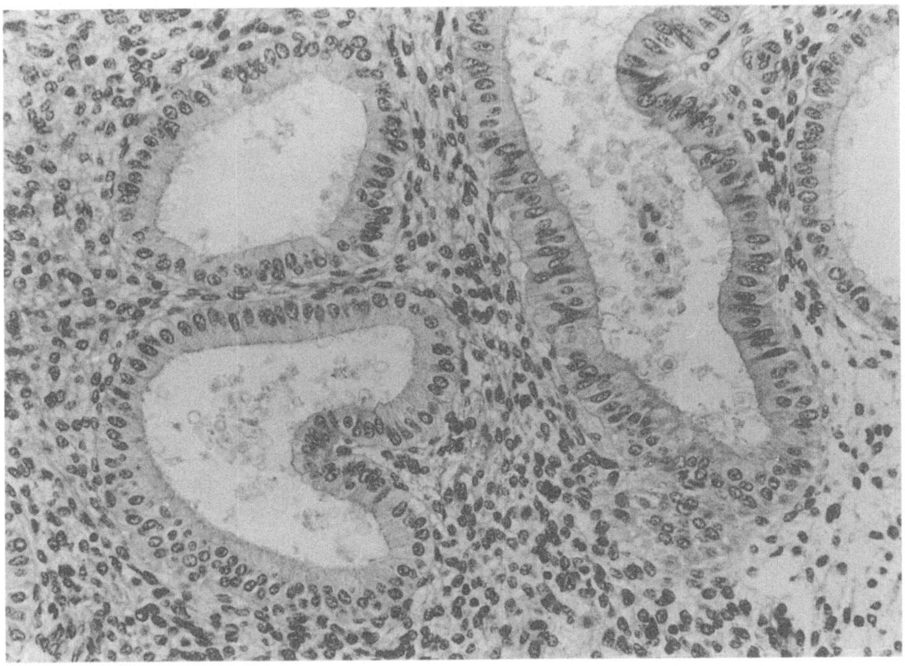

Fig. 3.18 Sixth day after ovulation. H & E, ×250

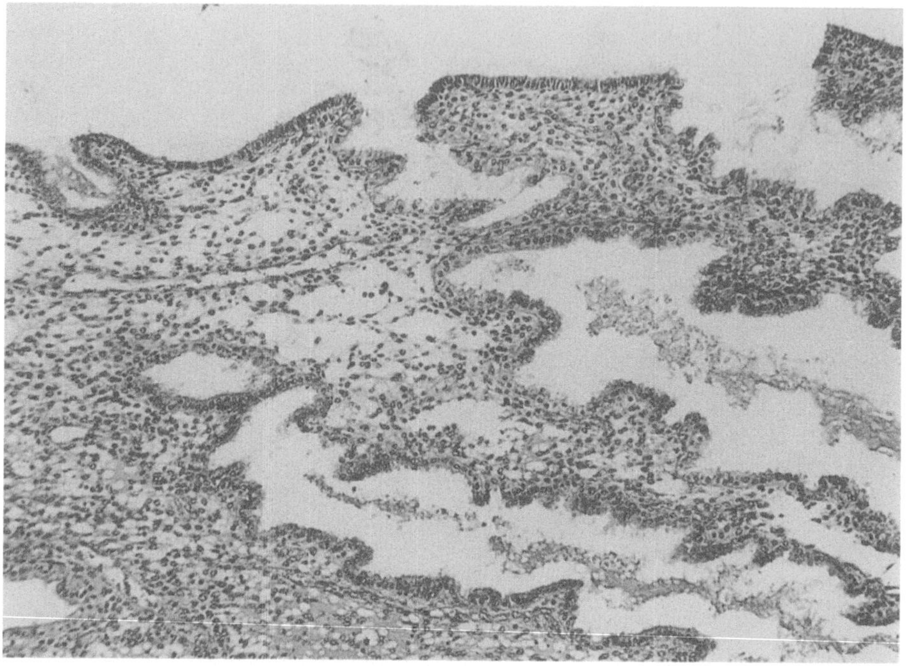

Fig. 3.19 Seventh day after ovulation. H & E, ×100

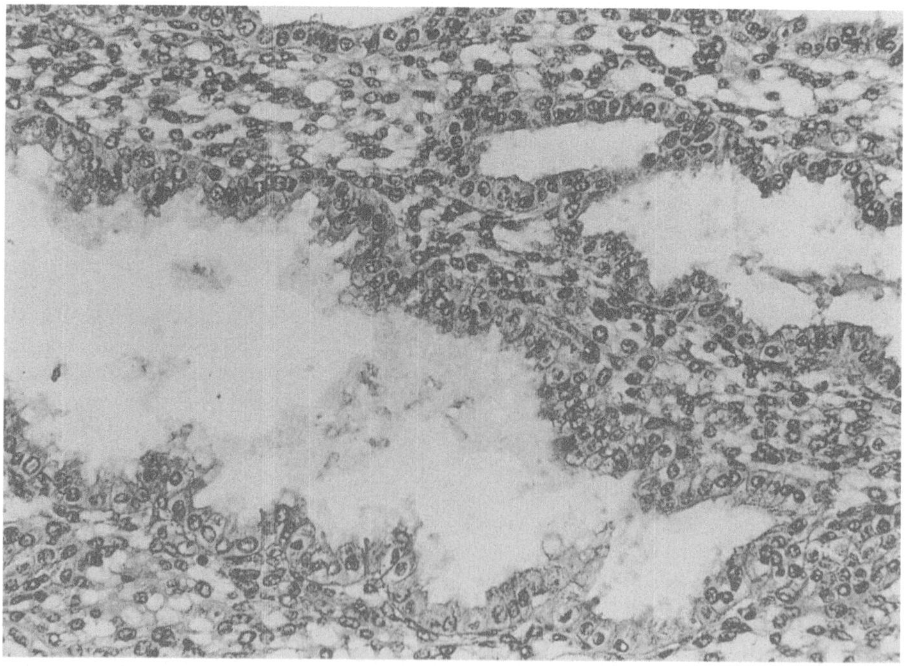

Fig. 3.20 Seventh day after ovulation. H & E, ×250

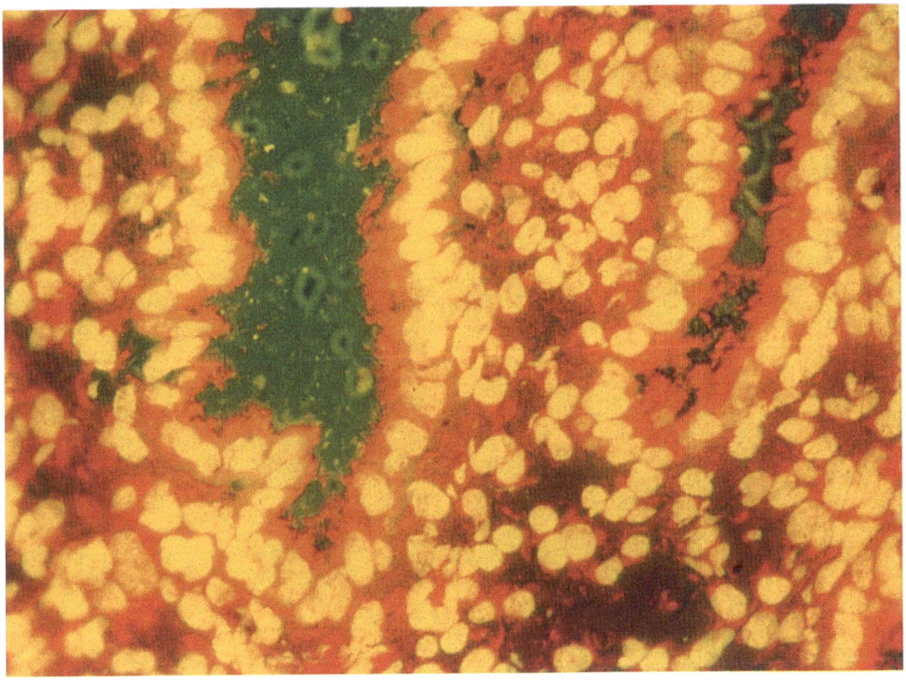

Fig. 3.21 Seventh day after ovulation. The glandular lumen is filled with green-staining glycogen. Acridine orange fluorochromation, ×350

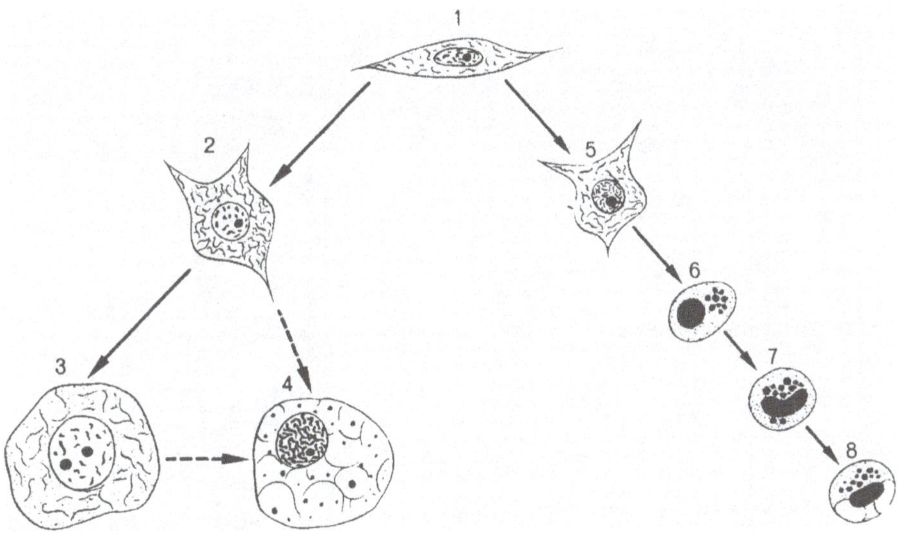

Fig. 3.22 Endometrial stromal differentiation (from Dallenbach-Hellweg 1987). 1, Poorly differentiated stromal cell; 2, stromal cell becoming larger and more globular; 3, decidual cell; 4, foamy decidual cell laden with metachromatic granules; 5, stromal cell becoming smaller and more rounded; 6–8, various stages in the development of granular endometrial stromal cells

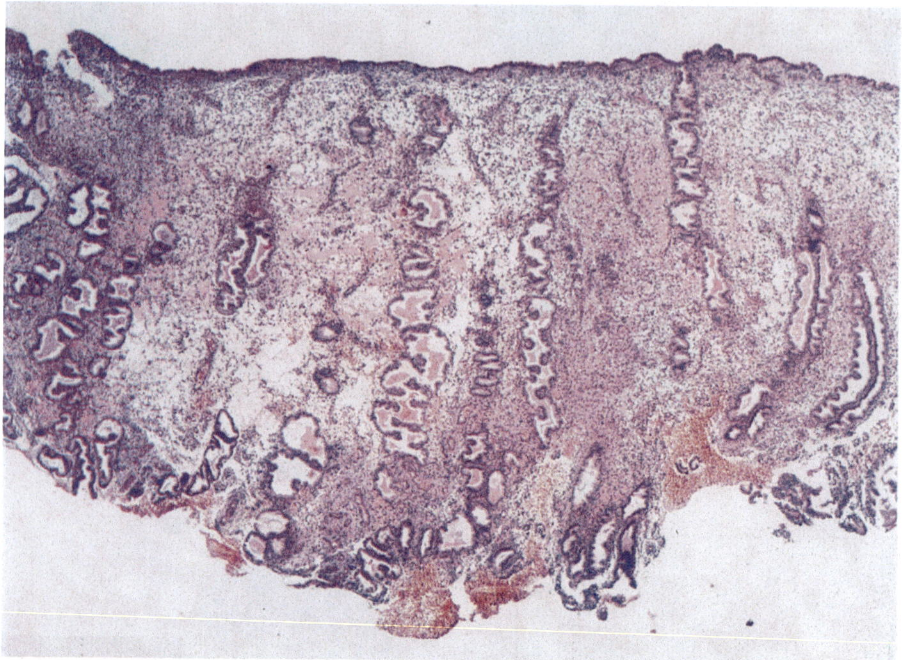

Fig. 3.23 Eighth day after ovulation. H & E, ×25

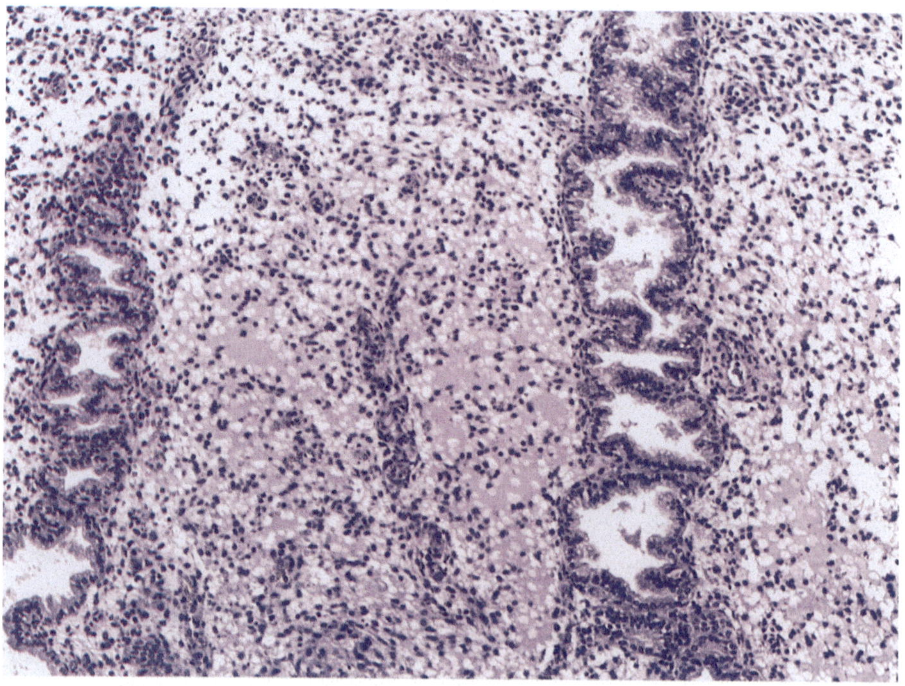

Fig. 3.24 Eighth day after ovulation. H & E, ×100

On the *ninth day after ovulation* (Figs. 3.25–3.27) the stromal edema has slightly subsided, but is still distinct. Groups of spiral arterioles are now prominent. The stromal cells surrounding these spiral arterioles grow larger and more rounded. Their nuclei enlarge and appear less chromatin dense. Their cytoplasm is increased in amount and in RNA content. The stromal cells which are further away from the arterioles remain only slightly enlarged. Glandular secretion has ceased, but remnants of secreted substance may be found in the glandular lumina.

On the *tenth day after ovulation* (Figs. 3.28–3.32) two distinct layers of the endometrium can be distinguished under low magnification: the upper compact layer, consisting mainly of stromal cells, and the lower spongious layer, containing distended tortuous glands with serrated edges, empty glandular epithelial cells, and remnants of inspissated secretion in the wide glandular lumina. The stromal cells around the spiral arterioles have developed into either predecidual cells with large, round, clear nuclei and abundant cytoplasm, or granular stromal cells with dense, indentated, or kidney-shaped nuclei and phloxinophilic granules in their cytoplasm (Hamperl 1954; Hellweg 1954; Fig. 3.32, see also Fig. 3.22), which in addition is rich in RNA. These two types of differentiated stromal cells are present in almost equal numbers. This differentiation has only taken place adjacent to the arterial blood supply, whereas regions further away have as yet not participated. At this time, a sheet-like predecidual change develops in the compact layer of the endometrium.

The *11th day after ovulation* (Figs. 3.33–3.35) shows a complete predecidual and granular change of the stromal cells in the compact layer, with no remaining undifferentiated stromal cells. The surface epithelium has gradually become lower over the previous few days and now appears cuboidal with slightly rounded nuclei.

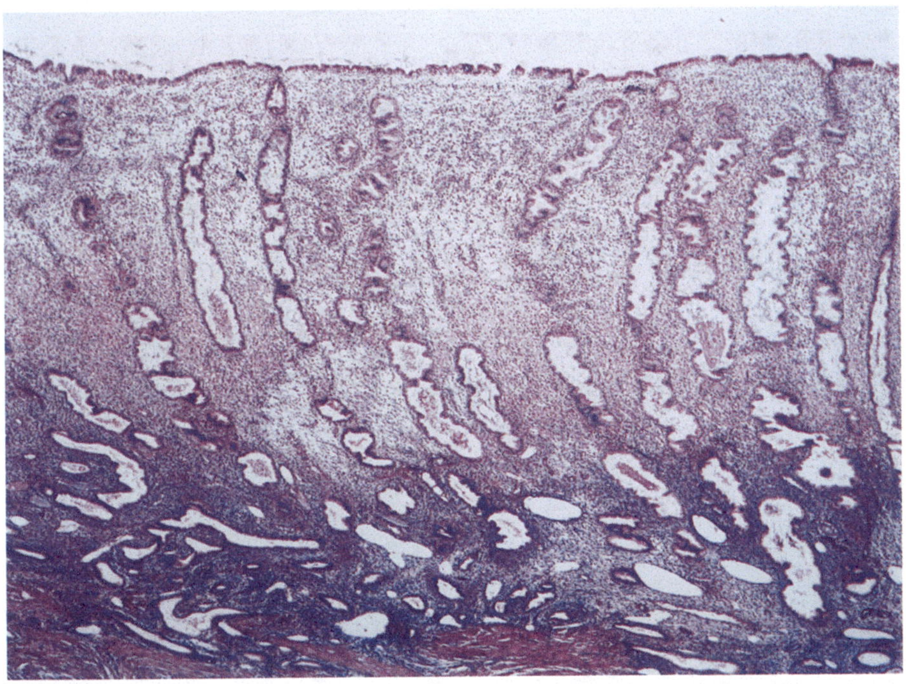

Fig. 3.25 Ninth day after ovulation. H & E, ×25

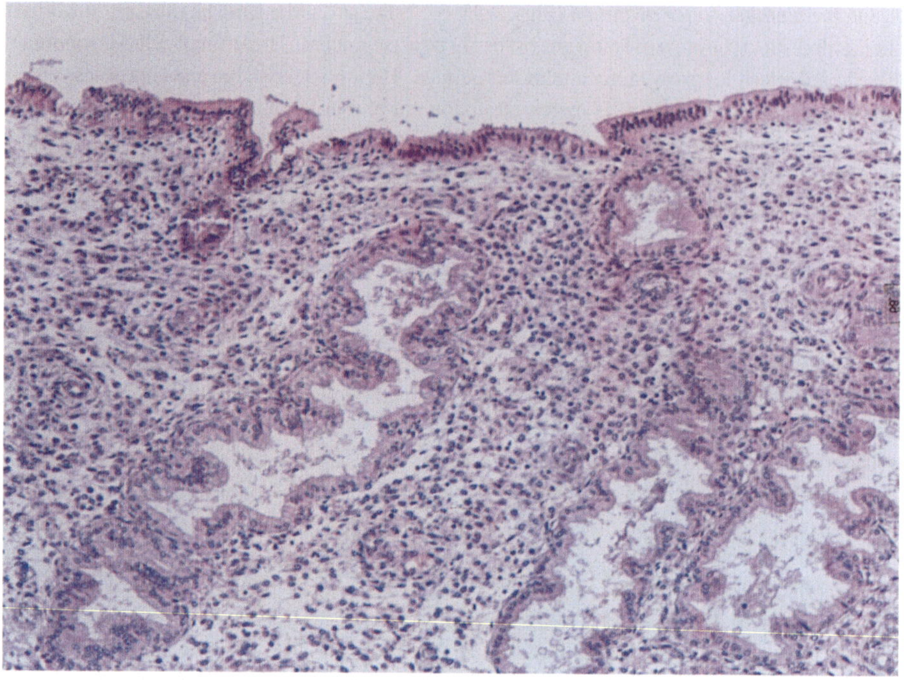

Fig. 3.26 Ninth day after ovulation. H & E, ×100

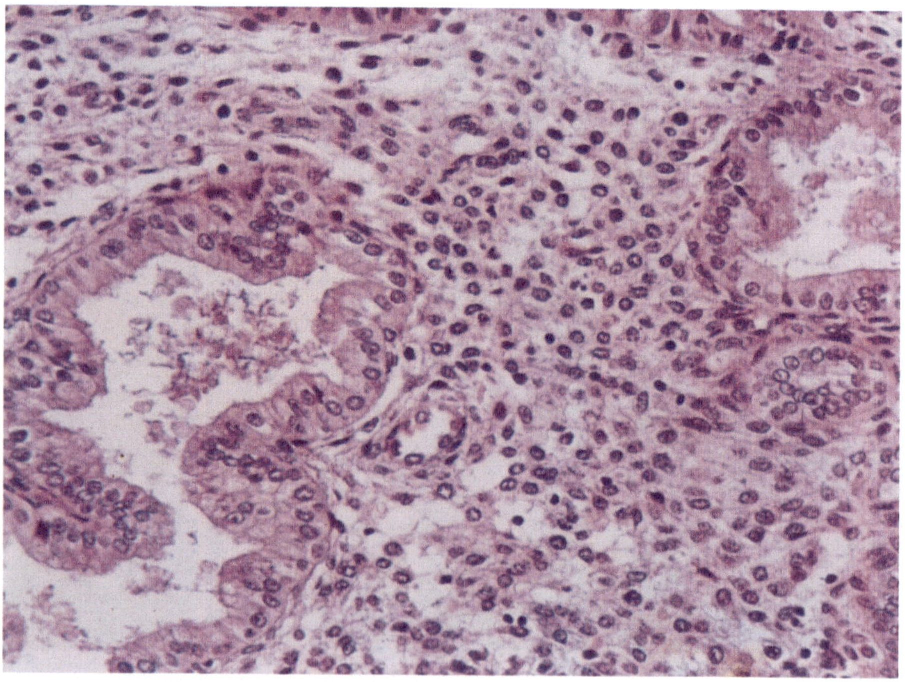

Fig. 3.27 Ninth day after ovulation. H & E, ×250

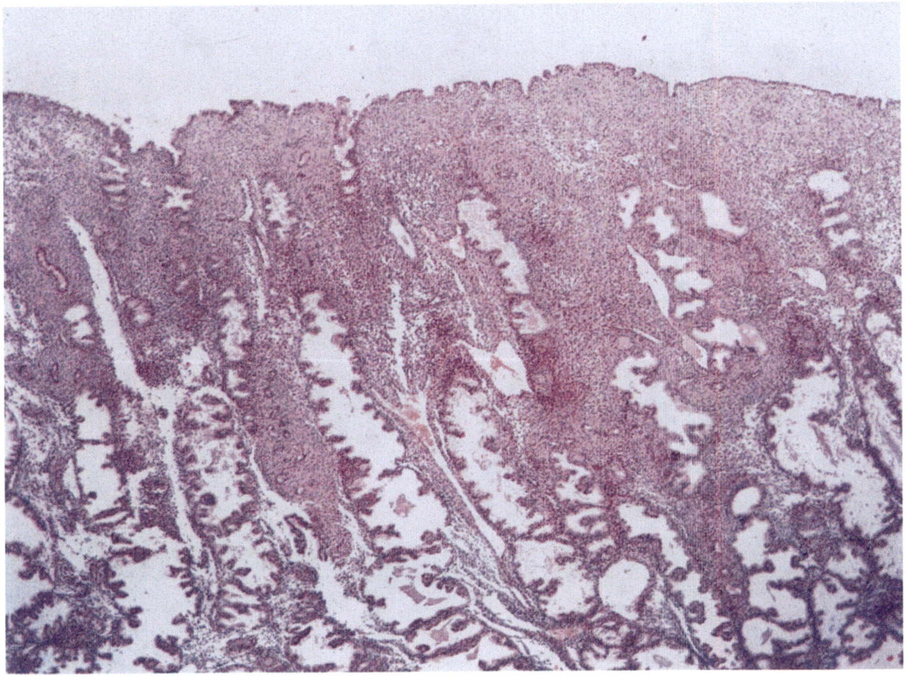

Fig. 3.28 Tenth day after ovulation. H & E, ×25

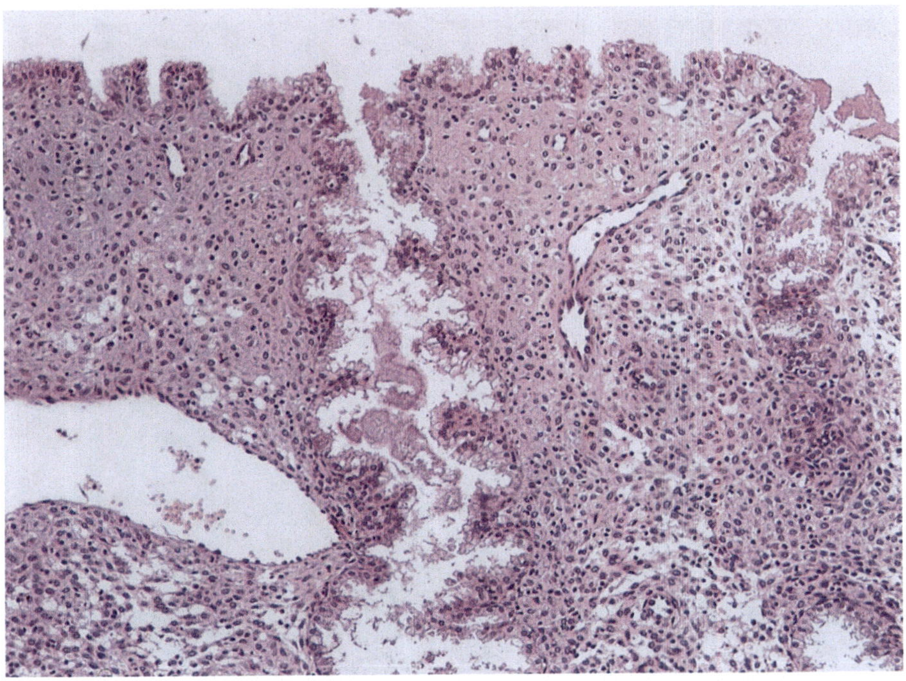

Fig. 3.29 Tenth day after ovulation. H & E, ×100

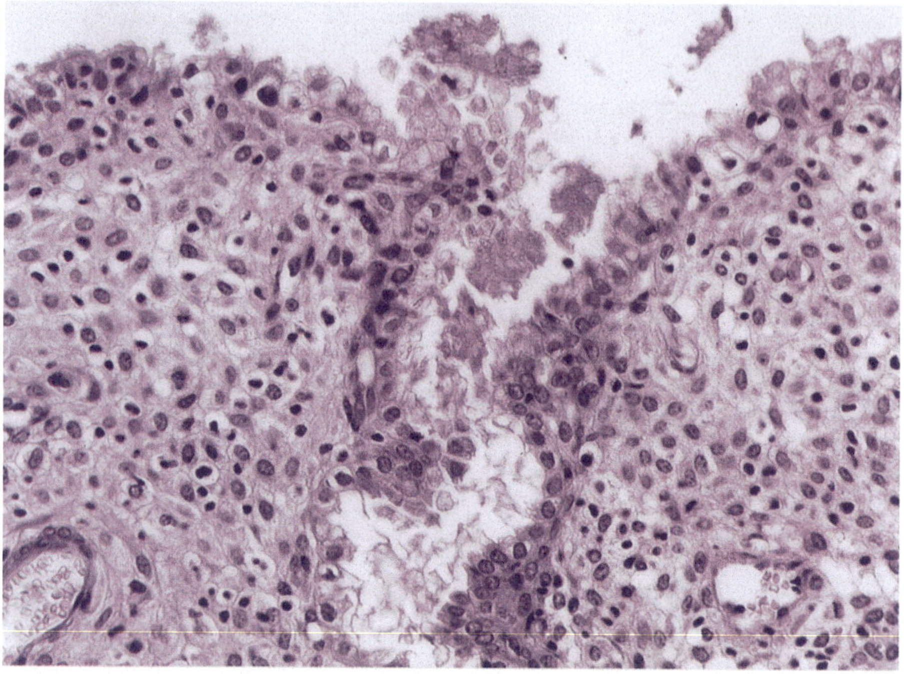

Fig. 3.30 Tenth day after ovulation. H & E, ×250

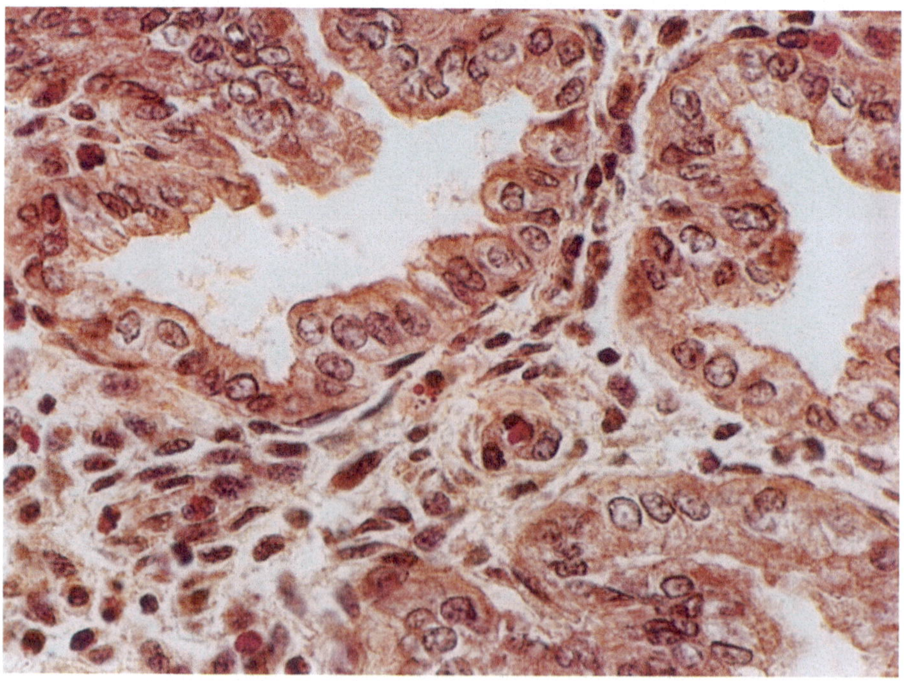

Fig. 3.31 Tenth day after ovulation. Phloxine-tartrazin stain, ×350

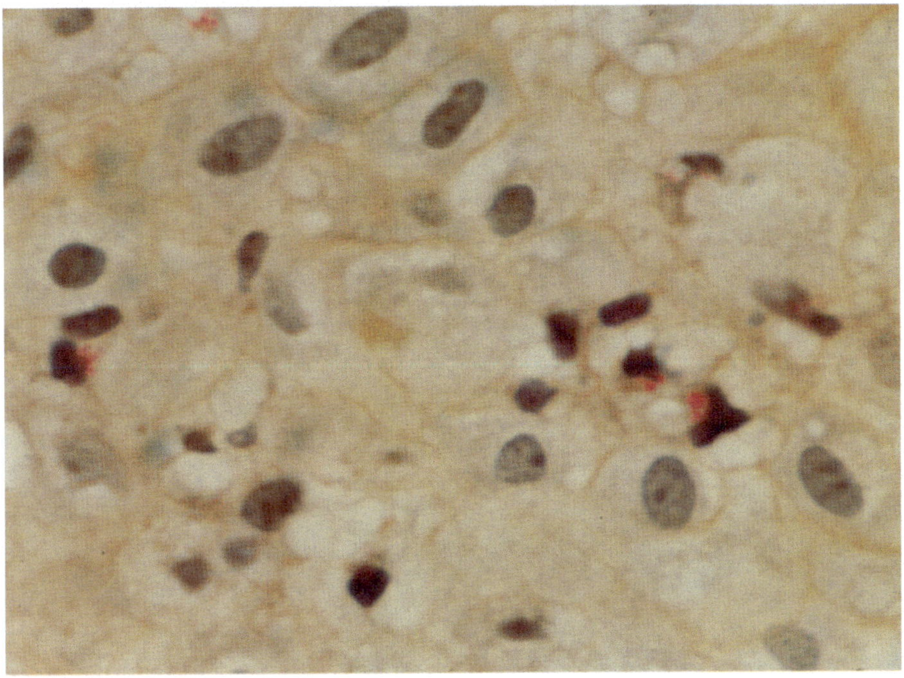

Fig. 3.32 Tenth day after ovulation, high magnification of the upper compact layer. Phloxine-tartrazin stain, ×1000

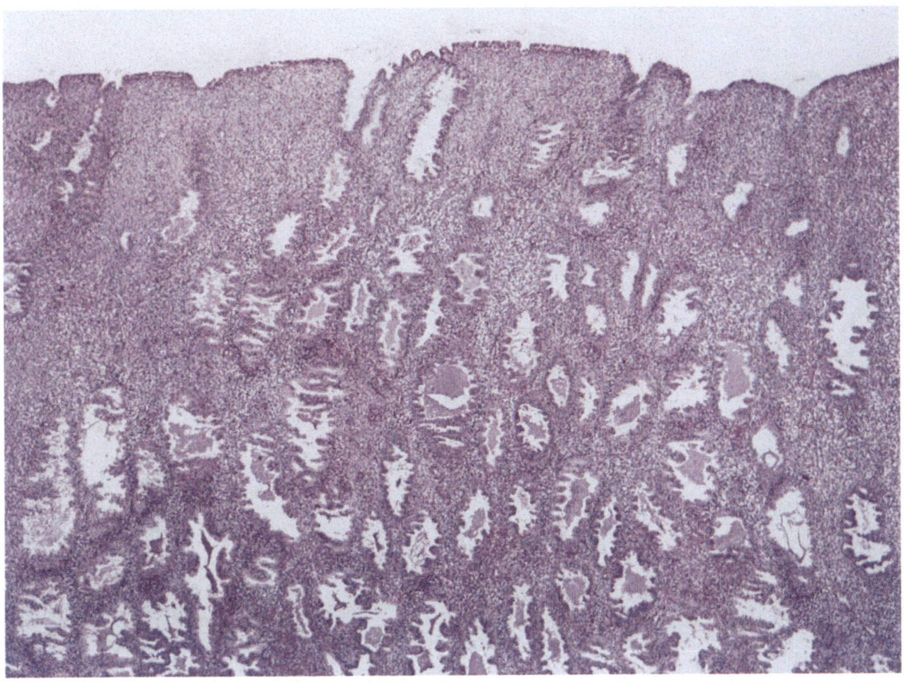

Fig. 3.33 Eleventh day after ovulation. H & E, ×25

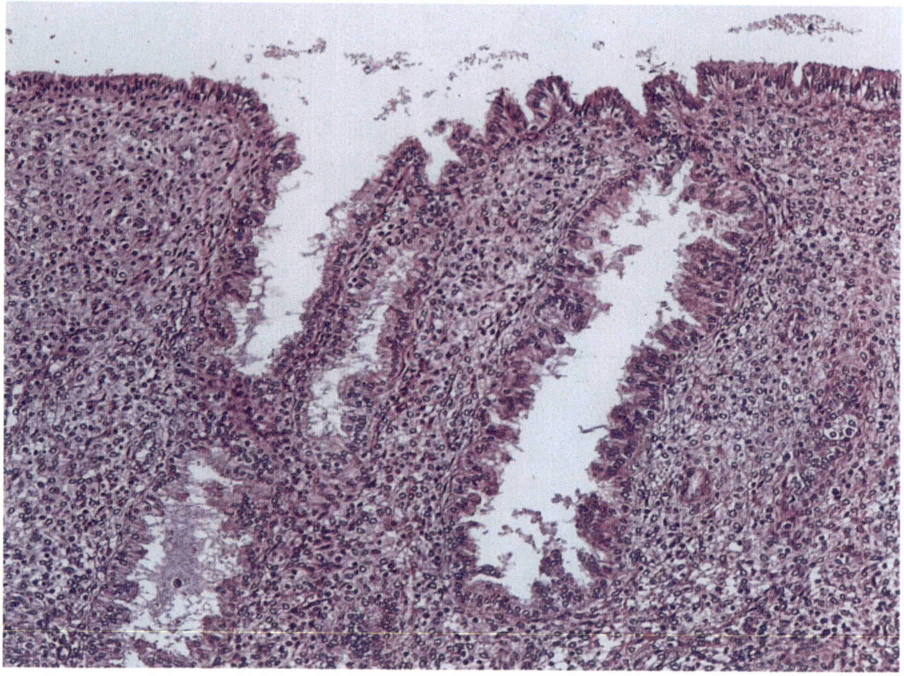

Fig. 3.34 Eleventh day after ovulation. H & E, ×100

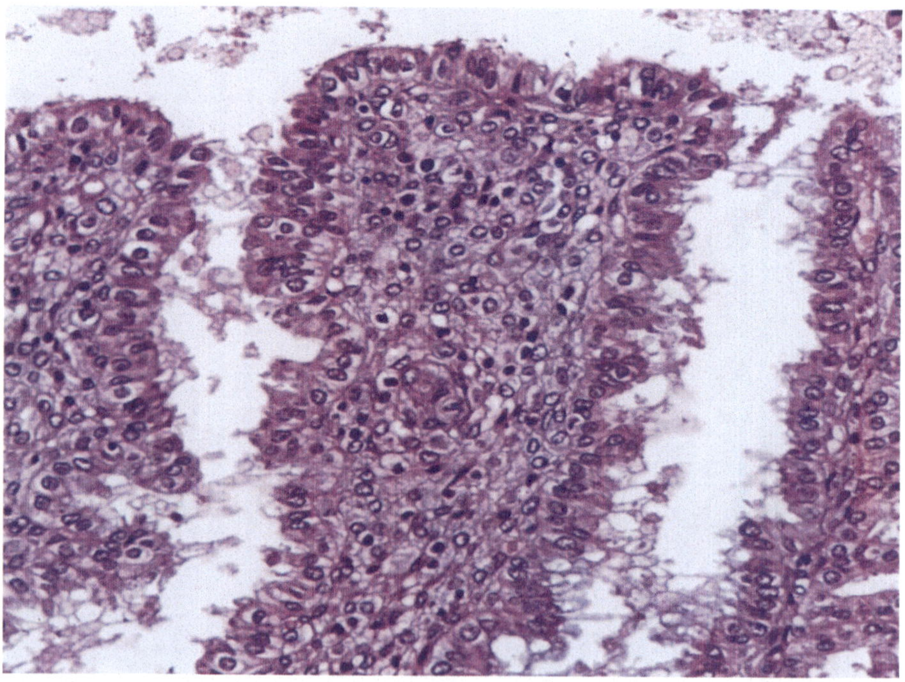

Fig. 3.35 Eleventh day after ovulation. H & E, ×250

On the *12th day after ovulation* (Figs. 3.36, 3.37) there is the beginning of a decrease in the general height of the endometrium, with shrinkage and collapse of the glands, while the stroma loses its edema, becomes dense, and remains well differentiated.

The *13th day after ovulation* (Figs. 3.38–3.40) shows extensive shrinkage in the overall height of the endometrium. The collapsed glands present a saw-toothed appearance. The predecidual stroma is now very dense. The RNA content in the glandular epithelial cells has diminished, whereas the stromal cells still contain large amounts of RNA.

The *14th day after ovulation* (Figs. 3.41–3.43) shows a very marked delineation between the upper compact layer and the lower spongious layer of the endometrium (Fig. 3.41). The glandular lumina in the compact layer are narrow and the lining epithelium is low, cuboidal, and appears inactive (Fig. 3.42), whereas the lumina of the glands in the spongious layer are still saw-toothed and lined by empty epithelial cells with a clear cytoplasm now almost devoid of RNA (Fig. 3.43). The glandular cell nuclei reveal a marked decrease in their DNA content. The beginning of dissociation of the stromal cells becomes apparent in the compact layer, particularly close to the surface epithelium and around the spiral arterioles, due to the beginning of reticulin fiber dissolution. This is caused by secretion of relaxin, which sets in immediately before menstruation (Dallenbach and Dallenbach-Hellweg 1964). The granular endometrial stromal cells, which have lost their granules, can be recognized at this late stage of dissolution only by their characteristic lobulated nuclei and their vacuolated cytoplasm. The surface epithelium is low and appears inactive.

Relaxin supports not only the physiological mucosal shedding during menstruation, but also the implantation of the blastocyst in many ways, mainly by locally controlled

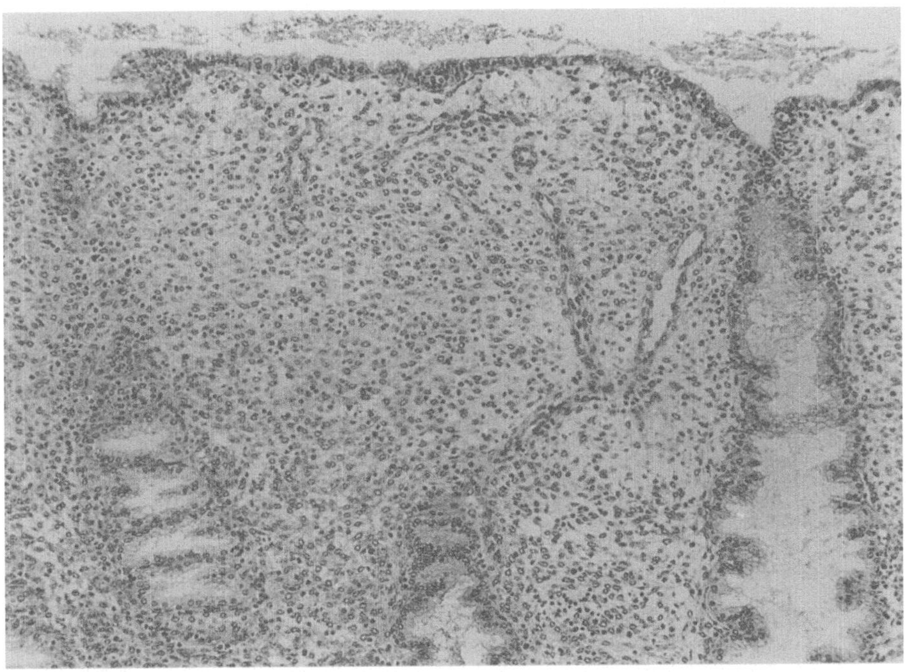

Fig. 3.36 Twelfth day after ovulation. H & E, ×100

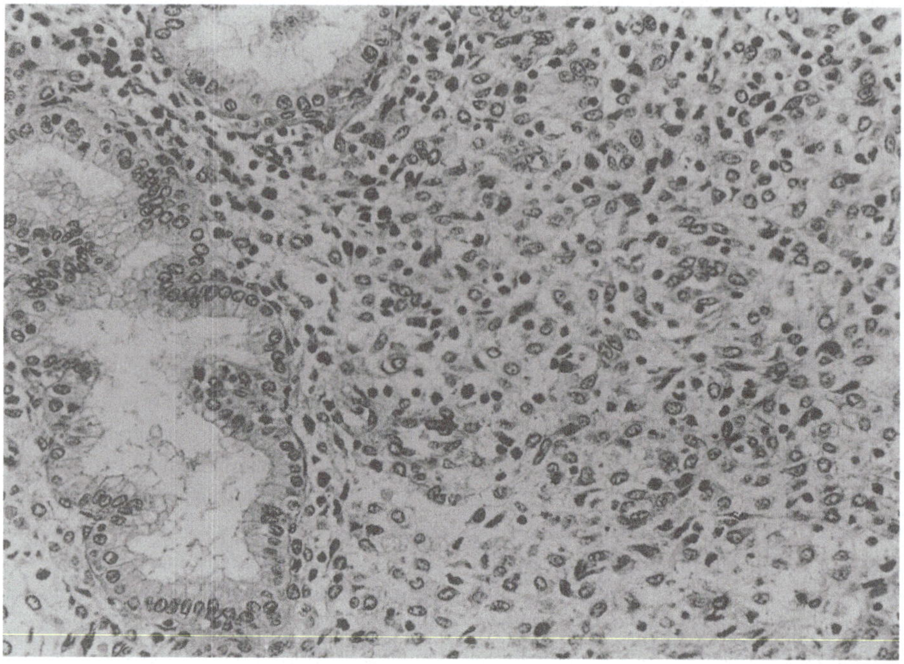

Fig. 3.37 Twelfth day after ovulation. H & E, ×250

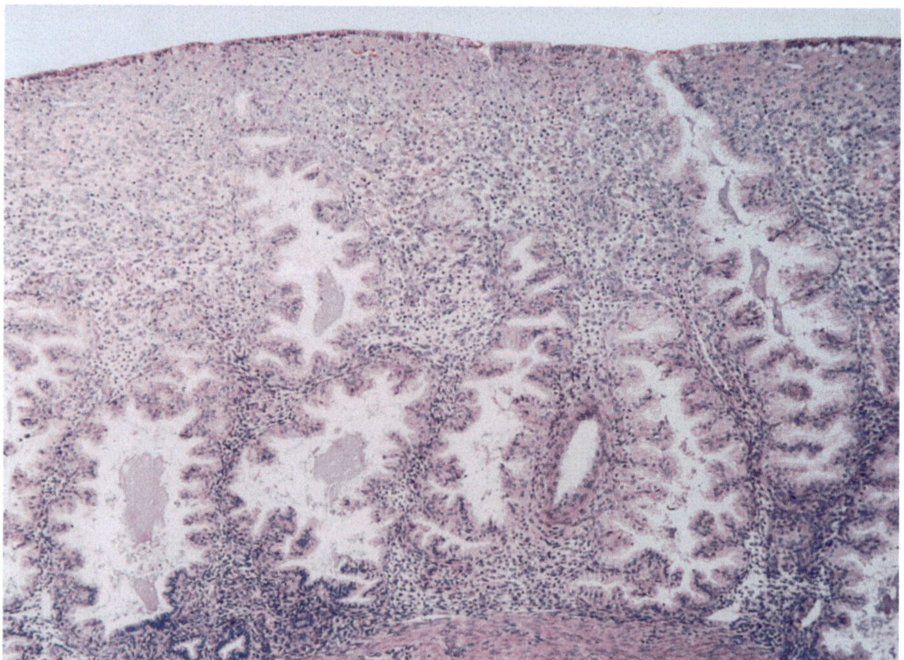

Fig. 3.38 Thirteenth day after ovulation. H & E, ×25

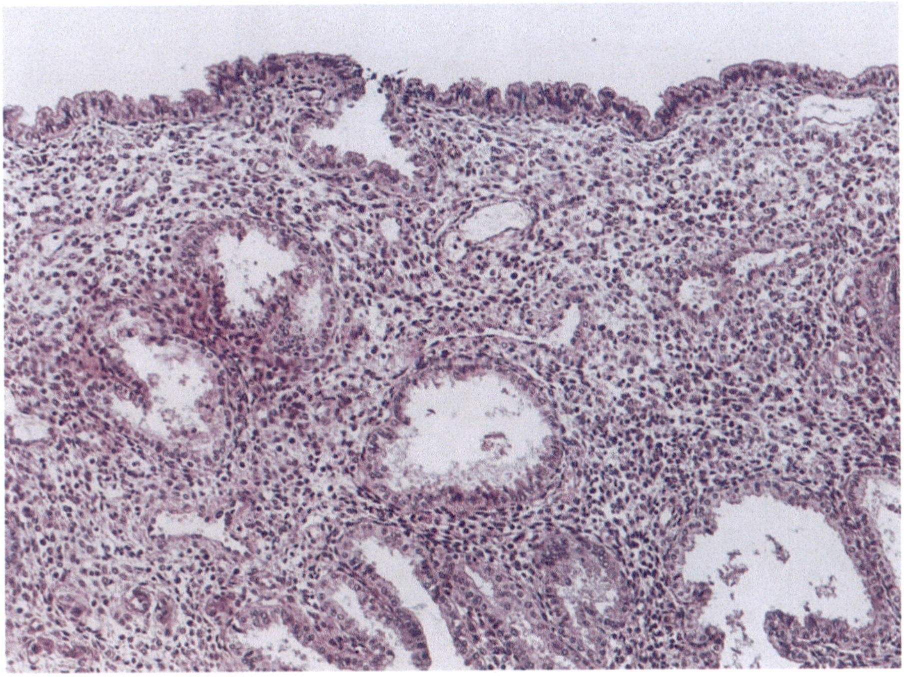

Fig. 3.39 Thirteenth day after ovulation. H & E, ×100

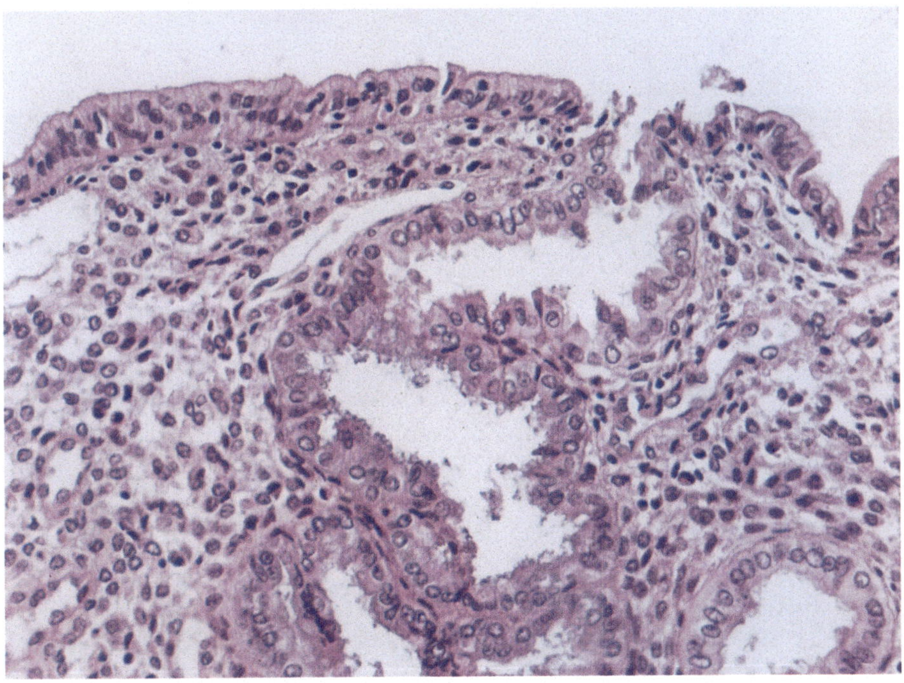

Fig. 3.40 Thirteenth day after ovulation. H & E, ×250

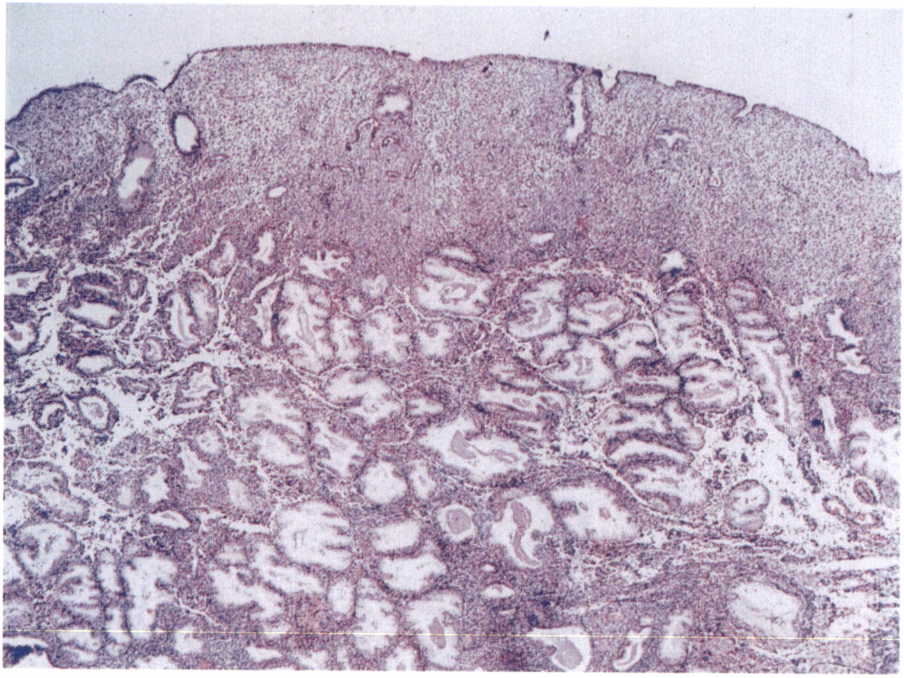

Fig. 3.41 Fourteenth day after ovulation. H & E, ×25

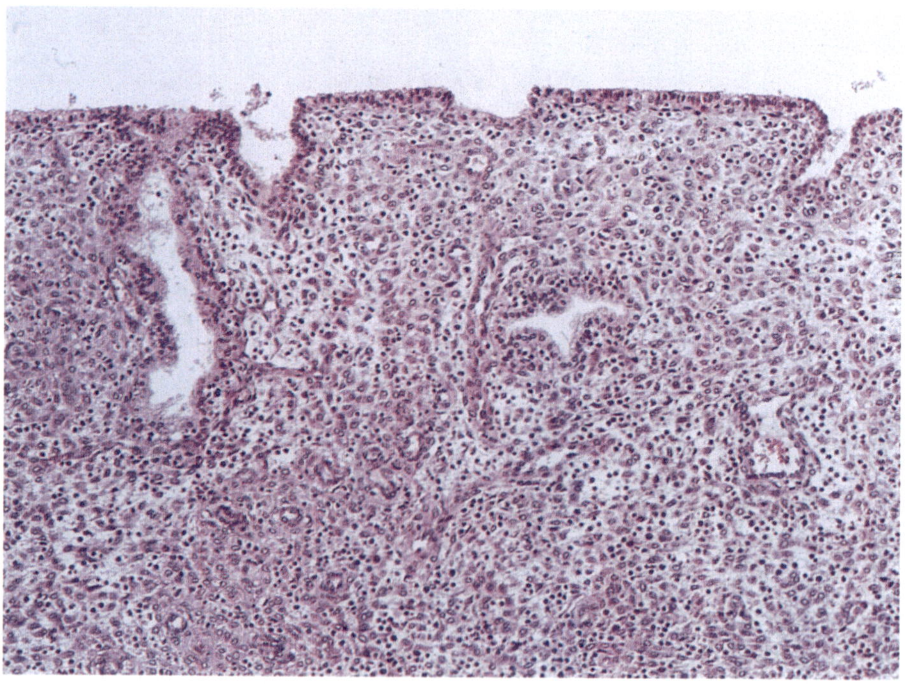

Fig. 3.42 Fourteenth day after ovulation, upper compact layer. H & E, ×100

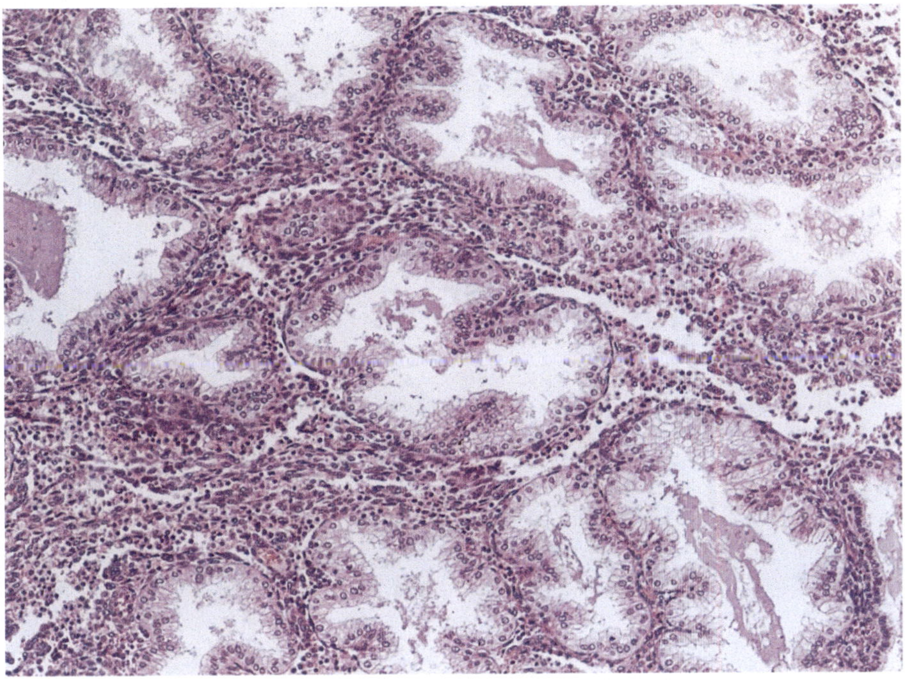

Fig. 3.43 Fourteenth day after ovulation, lower spongious layer. H & E, ×100

dissolution of reticulum fibers at the implantation site and at the area of timely correct decidual shedding and separation of the placenta post partum. In addition, dilatation of spiral arterioles and endothelial proliferation observed in the human and in monkeys most likely help to control the blood supply to the decidua and the blastocyst. (Dallenbach-Hellweg et al. 1966).

Relaxin and its receptor RXFP1 have been located biochemically and histochemically in the human decidua and in predecidual endometrium (Dallenbach and Dallenbach-Hellweg 1964; Bigazzi et al. 1980; Bryant-Greenwood 1991; Lippert et al 1993; Dallenbach-Hellweg and Dallenbach 1993) and also in monkeys (Dallenbach-Hellweg et al. 1966; Einspanier et al.2009) and in murine blastocysts (Baston-Büst et al. 2007). Immunohistochemically, relaxin is localized in the granules of the granular endometrial stromal cells, which, according to ultrastructural studies (Cardell et al. 1969) appear to be the main site of production, storage and release (Fig. 3.44). Focally, part of the glandular epithelial cells are also positive for the relaxin receptor (Einspanier et al. 2009). As soon as dissolution of the decidua sets in during spontaneous or induced abortion, most of the granula have been released, and a diffuse positive reaction for relaxin can be seen in the decidual cells (Fig. 3.45). Further studies are needed to clarify the detailed connections of these observations (FE Dallenbach et al., in preparation).

The granular endometrial stromal cells can be clearly distinguished ultrastructurally (Cardell et al. 1969) und immunohistochemically from neighboring polymorphonuclear granulocytes, lymphocytes and monocytoid cells (Press and King 1986) by their negative reaction with leukocyte common antigen (LCA), CD3, CD15 and CD68. They can be distinguished from lymphoid tissue (Morris et al. 1985) and from immunologically competent

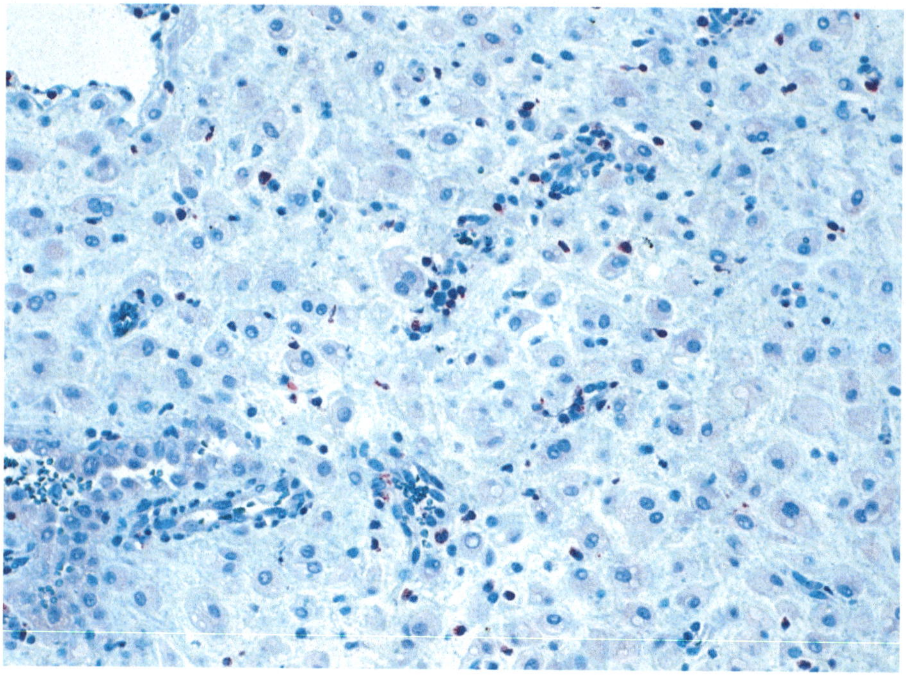

Fig. 3.44 Decidua of early pregnancy in beginning dissolution. Granular endometrial stromal cells with granules positive for relaxin receptor RXFP1. Immunohistochemical reaction with RXFP1

lymphocytes (Kamat and Isaaksen 1987), which infiltrate the endometrium during various phases of the menstrual cycle (Fig. 3.46) and in the postmenopausal endometrium. All markers for T- and B-Lymphocytes (CD 3, CD 5, CD 10, CD 20, CD 79a), for monocytes, macrophages and mast cells are constantly negative on the granular endometrial stromal cells (FE Dallenbach, in preparation). The granules of the endometrial stromal cells are distinctly positive with the phloxine-tartrazin stain (Fig. 3.32).

In summary, there are different types of T lymphocytes, mast cells, and polymorphonuclear granulocytes in the normal premenstrual endometrium and in the decidua with varying functions. They can be differentiated immunohistochemically, whereas their differentiation in routine H & E stains is virtually impossible. All these cells occurring in the normal, noninfectious endometrium cannot be correlated with inflammatory reactions, but have various physiologic functions. Even the development of lymphoid follicles in the endometrial stroma is a physiologic phenomenon.

Clinical Possibilities for the Entire Secretory Phase. (a) Normal secretory phase, if it corresponds to the day of the menstrual cycle; (b) deficient secretory phase with coordinated true delay, if the day of the menstrual cycle is 3–10 days further advanced than the histologic differentiation; and (c) normal secretory phase in amenorrhea due to silent menstruation (Philippe et al. 1966).

Distinction is possible only by precise statement of the day of the menstrual cycle and/or recording of the basal body temperature curve.

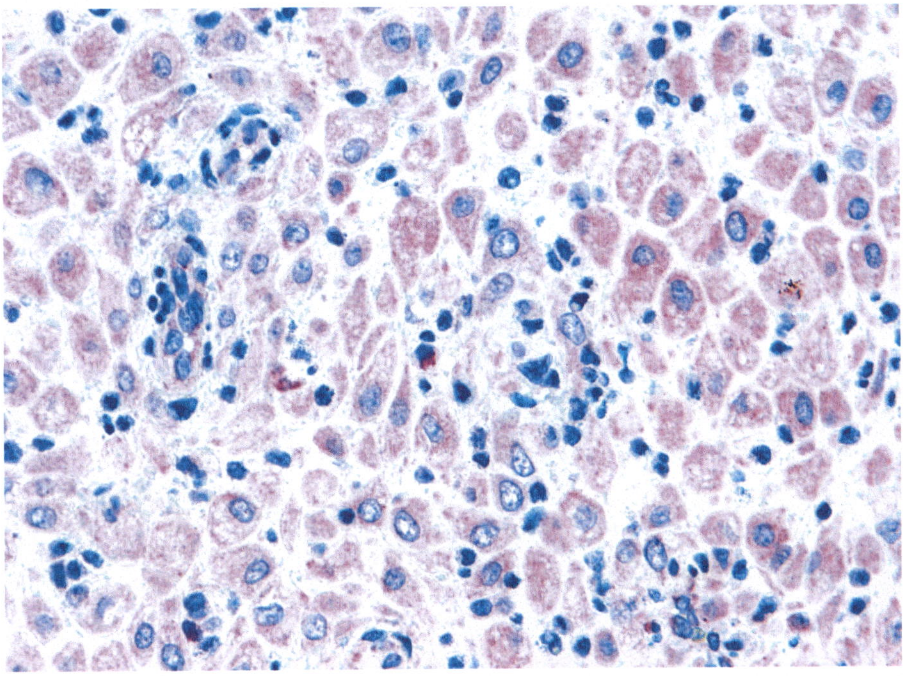

Fig. 3.45 Decidua of early intrauterine abortion. Regression and dissociation of decidual cells with diffuse staining for relaxin receptor. In the center a few endometrial stromal cells with preserved red granules. Immunohistochemical reaction with RXFP1

3.1.3 Menstruation

The *first day of menstruation* (Figs. 3.47–3.49) is characterized by dissociation of glands and stroma and by hemorrhage into the superficial layer. The extent of dissociation and bleeding corresponds to the area of the compact layer, which contains granular endometrial stromal cells. The dissociated cells still show their predecidual change, the granular stromal cells have lost their relaxin granules, and the surface epithelium is still intact (Fig. 3.48). The collapsed glands may contain sparse remnants of previous secretion. From their structure it is possible, even after the onset of menstruation, to diagnose whether ovulation has taken place. The lower portion of the endometrium shows no disintegration of stroma and glands, but only shrinkage (Fig. 3.49). The remaining intact portions participate in the restoration of the endometrium during the next cycle (Sengel and Stoebner 1970).

The *second day of menstruation* (Figs. 3.50–3.52) shows extensive disintegration and demarcation of those portions of the endometrium which are shed, while the more basal portions remain intact. Scattered degenerating stromal cells and remnants of glandular epithelium lie admixed in unclotted blood and aggregates of polymorphonuclear cells (Flowers and Wilborn 1978).

Clinical Possibilities for Both Days. Normal menstruation.

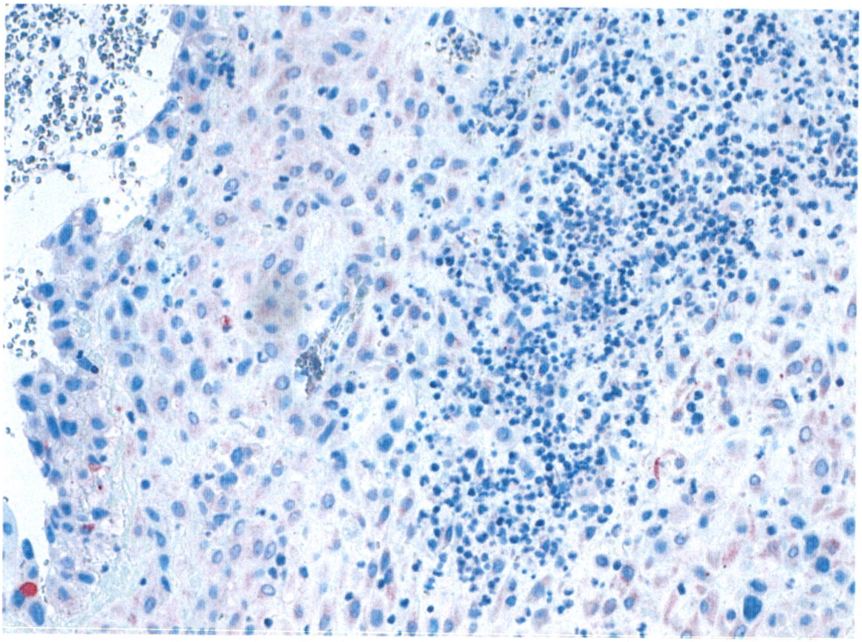

Fig. 3.46 Decidua in regression after intrauterine abortion. Decidual cells spindle-shaped, loose with faint positive staining. A few granular endometrial stromal cells still containing positive granules between decidual cells and in the glandular epithelium. On the right an area of inflammatory cells which are negative for relaxin. Immunohistochemical reaction with RXFP1

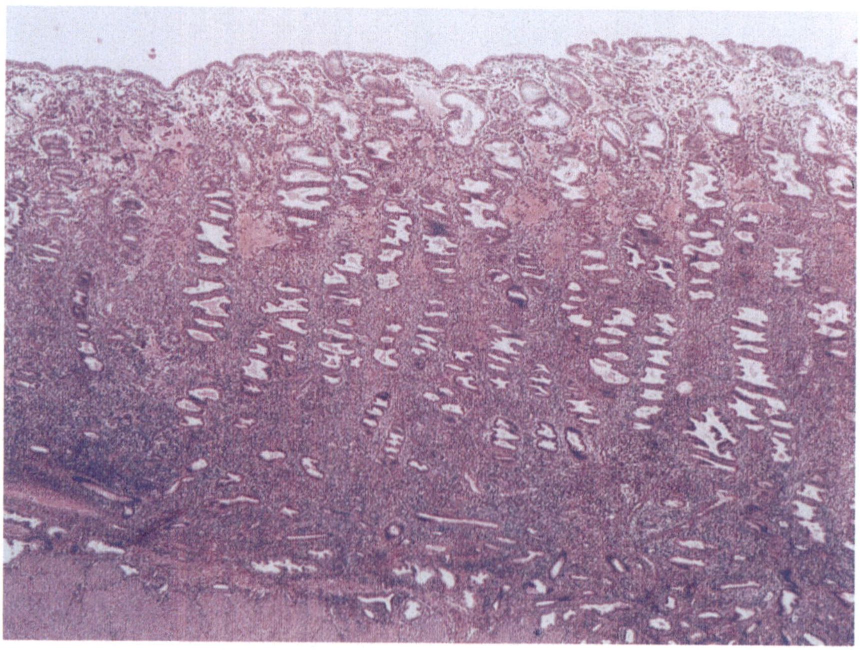

Fig. 3.47 Menstruation, first day. H & E, ×25

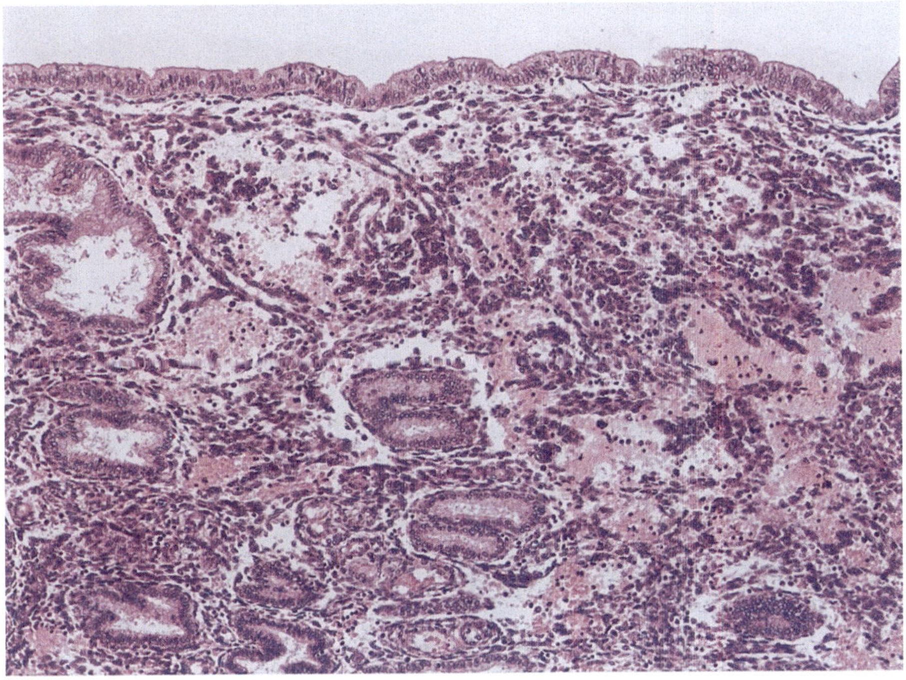

Fig. 3.48 Menstruation, first day. H & E, ×100

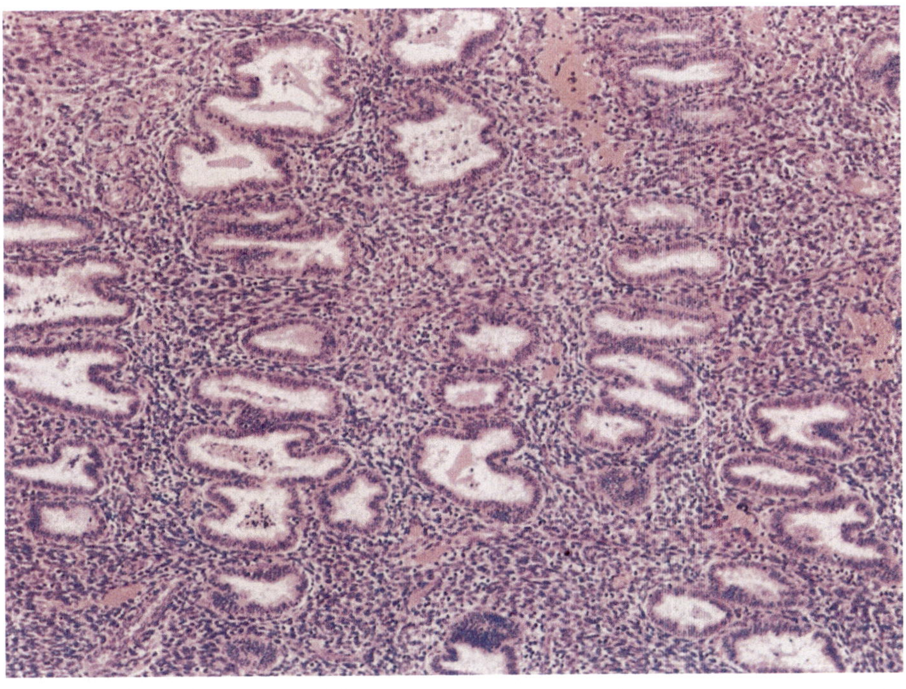

Fig. 3.49 Menstruation, first day. H & E, ×100

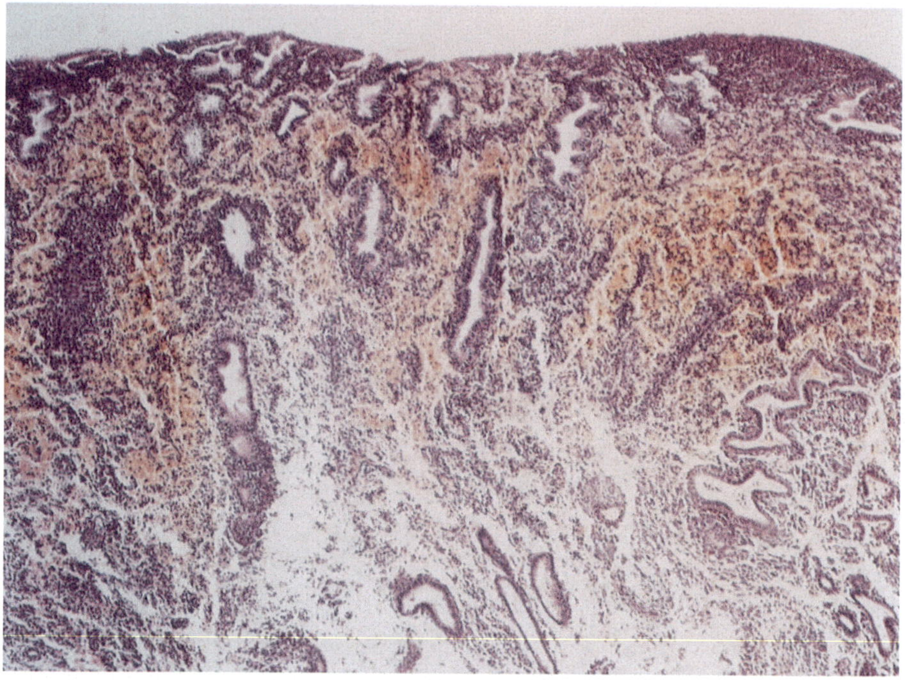

Fig. 3.50 Menstruation, second day. H & E, ×25

3.1.4 Regeneration

During regeneration (Figs. 3.53, 3.54), the endometrium is very low and consists mainly of the basal remnants of glands and stroma which are partly reepithelialized, while neighboring areas are still denuded (Nogales et al. 1969, 1978). Stromal cells take a minor part in the regeneration. In the epithelial cells, the nuclear DNA and cytoplasmic RNA are again increasing, but mitoses are still absent (Ferenczy 1976).

Clinical Possibilities. Regeneration after normal menstruation, anovulatory cycle or ovulatory functional disturbances, or after curettage. Except for regeneration after curettage, distinction is not possible at this early stage. When a functional diagnosis is desired by the clinician, the curettage should be repeated later in the cycle, preferably during the late secretory phase.

3.2 Physiologic Variations in the Climacterium

3.2.1 Proliferative Phase

The proliferative phase (Fig. 3.55) shows variations in the width of some glands, although most of the glands are still normal in size, shape, and arrangement. The height of the glandular epithelium may vary somewhat.

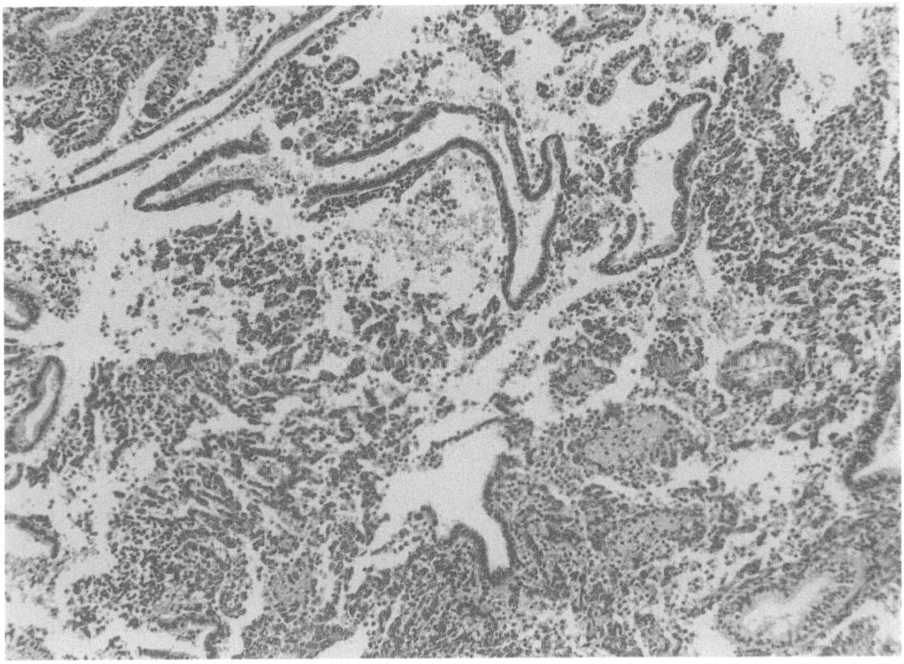

Fig. 3.51 Menstruation, second day. H & E, ×100

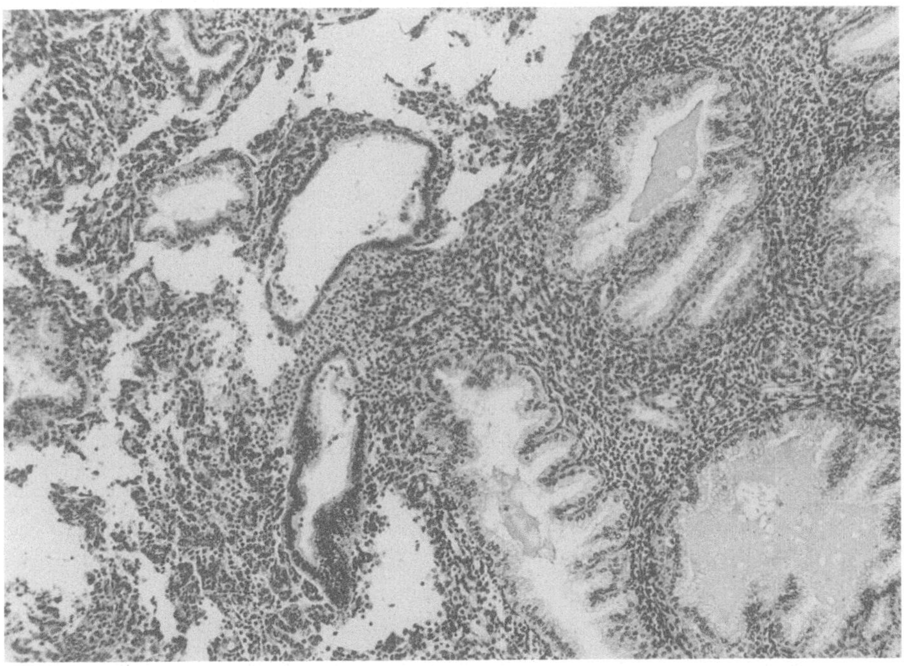

Fig. 3.52 Menstruation, second day. H & E, ×100

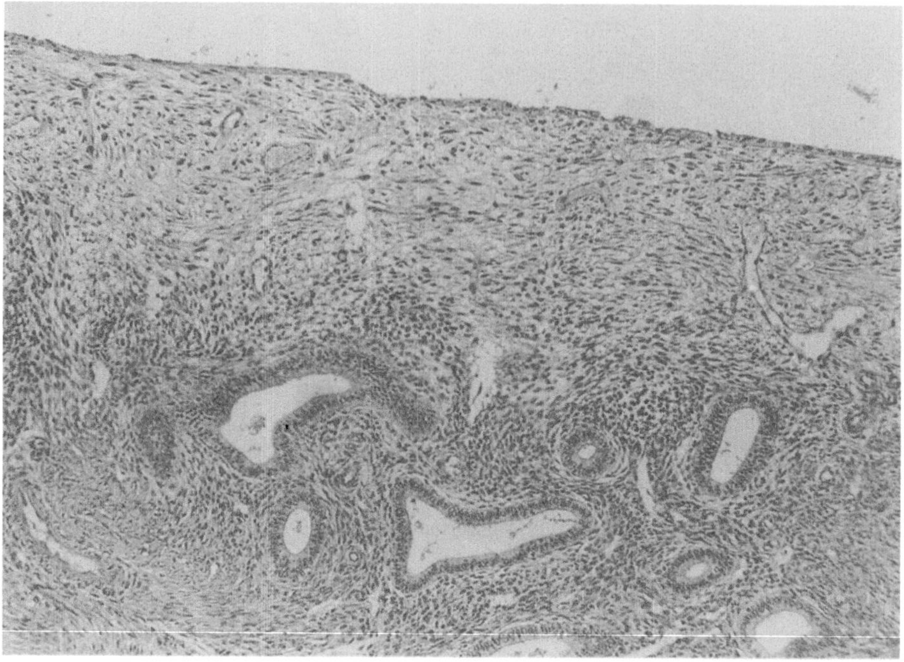

Fig. 3.53 Regeneration. H & E, ×100

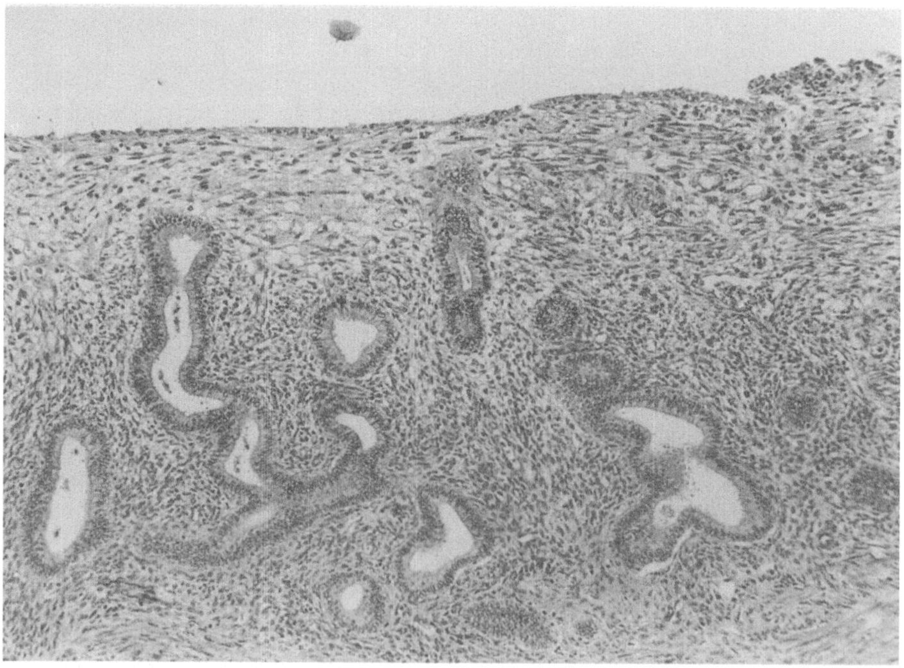

Fig. 3.54 Regeneration. H & E, ×100

Clinical possibilities: see below.

3.2.2 Secretory Phase

The secretory phase (Fig. 3.56) shows slight underdevelopment of some of the glands; these are poorly convoluted and lined by a low, cuboidal, rather inactive epithelium with dense, small nuclei, whereas the epithelium of neighboring glands is normally differentiated according to the day of the cycle. The general height of the endometrium varies slightly from one region to another. In the lower layers, the stroma may be poorly differentiated.

Clinical Possibilities. (a) Proliferative or secretory phase with climacteric variations; (b) a very early stage of irregular proliferation or deficient or irregular secretion if the patient is below age 40.

Distinction is possible by the age of the patient and the menstrual history.

3.3 Normal Postmenopausal Endometrium

After the decline of ovarian function, the unresponding endometrium atrophies, whereby the glands that existed before the menopause retain their shapes.

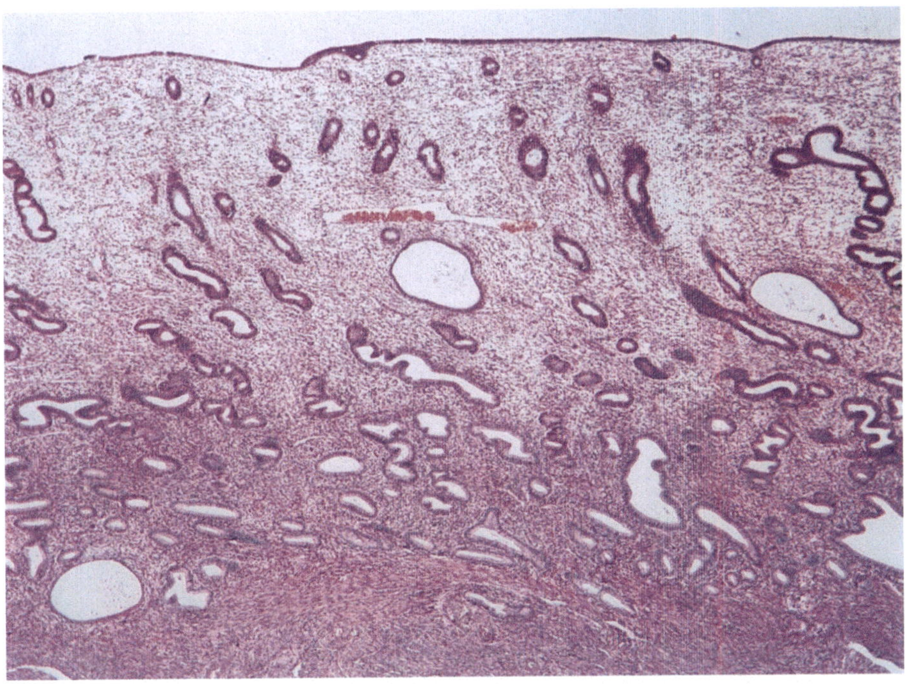

Fig. 3.55 Physiologic variation of the proliferative phase in the climacterium. H & E, ×25

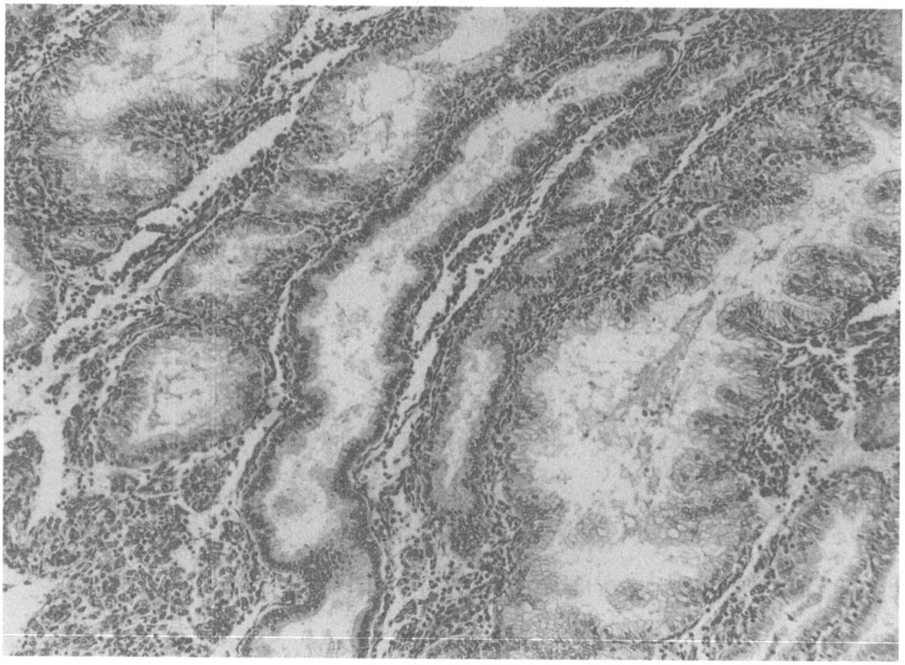

Fig. 3.56 Physiologic variation of the secretory phase in the climacterium. H & E, ×100

If the last cycle ends with deficient proliferation or secretion, simple atrophy will develop with sparse, narrow glands lined by atrophic epithelium within a dense, fibrous stroma. If an irregular proliferation or a simple (glandular cystic) hyperplasia precedes the fall in estrogen secretion, then a cystic atrophy results. If the decline in hormonal function is protracted, a spectrum of incomplete to complete atrophy will result. If a focal hyperplasia precedes the menopause, then after it both simple and cystic atrophy will be found.

3.4 Isthmus Mucosa

The isthmus mucosa (Figs. 3.57, 3.58) is located between the endocervix and endometrium and is uniformly flat, consisting of slender, often horizontally directed, slit-like glands surrounded by a dense, fibrous stroma of small, spindle-shaped cells (Fig. 3.57). The surface and glandular epithelium is low, cuboidal, and inactive. It does not participate in cyclic changes of either the endocervical or the endometrial type. Occasionally in the isthmus some glands of the endocervical type can be found lined by tall, columnar, mucus-secreting epithelium among inactive glands of the endometrial type. The endocervical type of glands may occasionally be cystically dilated (Fig. 3.57).

Morphologic Differential Diagnosis. (a) Basal endometrium: the glands of the basal layer branch more, show various degrees of proliferative changes, and their supporting stroma is more irregular since the collagen fibers anchorning the basalis to the myometrium extend in all directions; (b) endometrial atrophy: the glands of the atrophic endometrium are much smaller and their epithelial lining is flat; they are surrounded by a dense stroma of small cells devoid of distinctive fibers; and (c) deficient proliferation: whereas the glands of the isthmus mucosa may be similar to those of deficient proliferation, the general height of the isthmus mucosa is much lower, and the tangential arrangement of the isthmus glands differs from the perpendicular course of the proliferating glands in deficient proliferation.

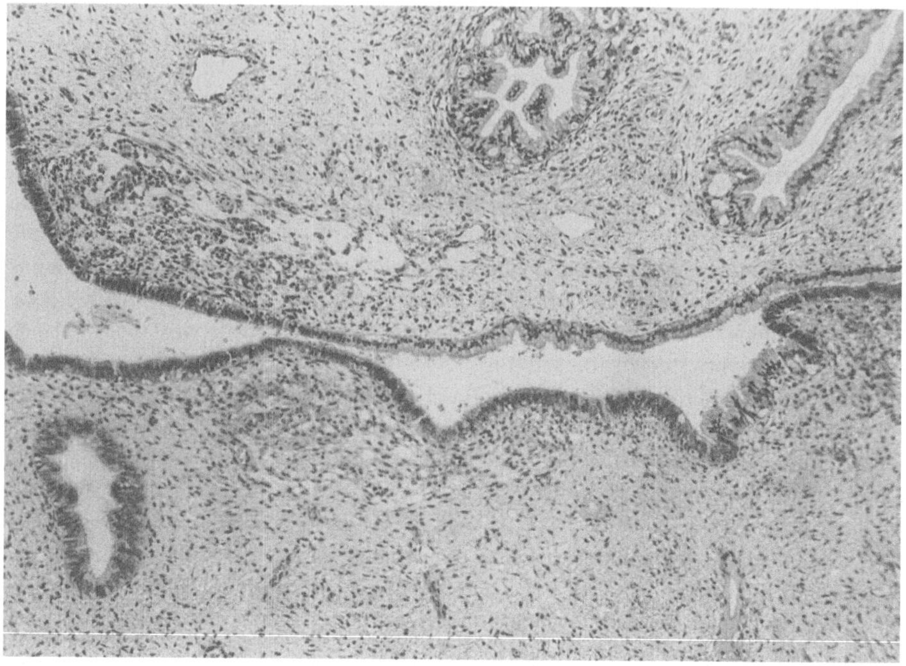

Fig. 3.57 Isthmus mucosa, H & E, ×100

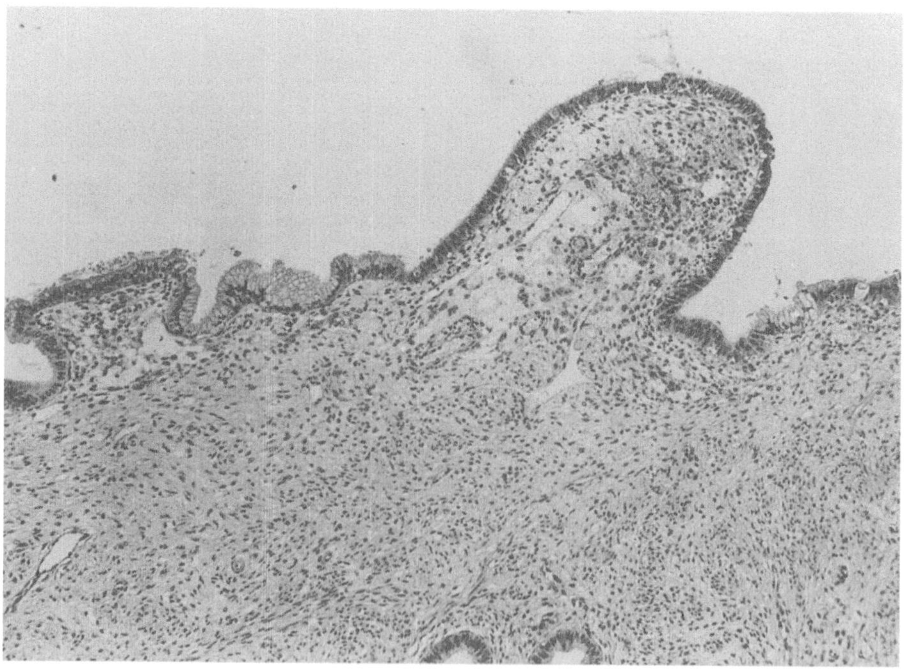

Fig. 3.58 Isthmus mucosa, H & E, ×100

Metaplastic Changes 4

The endometrial epithelium may be replaced focally, seldom diffusely, by any other epithelium of Müllerian type. The same holds true for the endometrial stromal cells.

4.1 Epithelial Metaplasia

4.1.1 Squamous Metaplasia and Ichthyosis

Squamous Metaplasia. Nodules of squamous epithelium arise from the glandular epithelium of irregularly proliferating or cystically dilated hyperplastic glands. Such nodules may develop focally or diffusely and may be found in all endometrial layers (see Fig. 6.35). All transitional stages are encountered, from a few small nodules to extensive metaplasia, which may also involve the surface epithelium (ichthyosis). When the surface epithelium becomes involved (Fig. 4.1), there is no sharp line of distinction between extensive squamous metaplasia and ichthyosis.

The squamous epithelium may be well differentiated, resembling either mature or metaplastic squamous epithelium of the ectocervix, or be immature as morules with scant cytoplasm and poorly delineated cytoplasmic borders, as seen in reserve cell hyperplasia of the endocervical glands.

Ichthyosis. In senile atrophy, the surface epithelium alone may undergo metaplasia, which is then called ichthyosis (Baggish and Woodruff 1967; Heckeroth and Ziegler 1986). Such a sheet-like surface metaplasia may be smooth (Fig. 4.2), or papillary, normally stratified and mature, occasionally covered with keratinized cells or may show loss of stratification with cellular irregularity, depolarization, and enlargement of nuclei with occasional mitoses, thus representing epithelial dysplasia (Fig. 4.3). The underlying endometrium is usually very low consisting only of small, spindle-shaped stromal cells without glands or containing a very few atrophic glandular remnants. The stroma may contain chronic inflammatory infiltrates comprising mainly lymphocytes and plasma cells (Fig. 4.3).

Morphologic Differential Diagnosis. Foci or nodules of squamous metaplasia can be found in simple, complex or atypical hyperplasia and in well differentiated endometrial

G. Dallenbach-Hellweg et al., *Atlas of Endometrial Histopathology*,
DOI: 10.1007/978-3-642-01541-0_4, © Springer-Verlag Berlin Heidelberg 2010

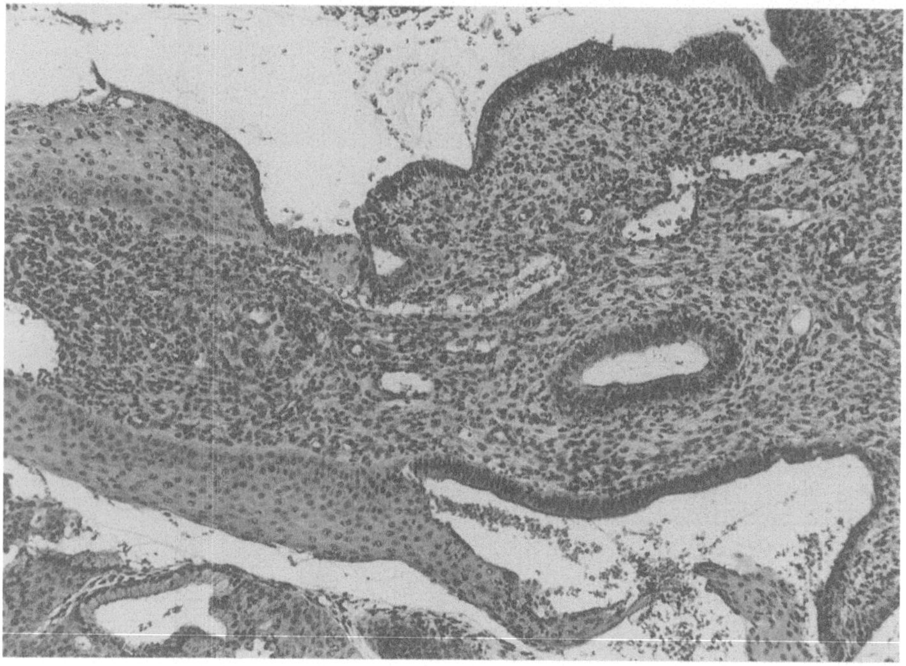

Fig. 4.1 Ichthyosis uteri. H & E, ×100

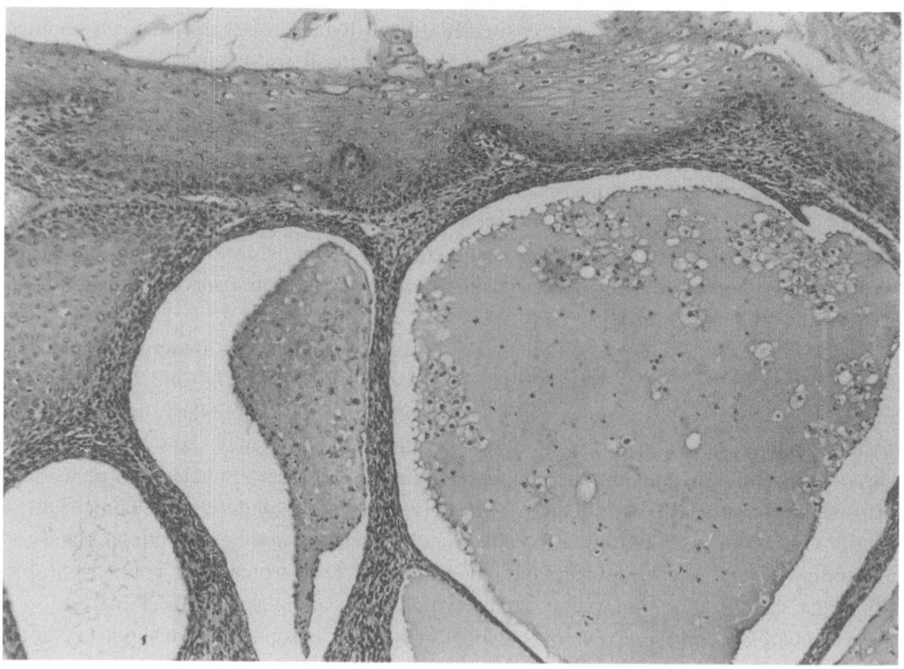

Fig. 4.2 Ichthyosis uteri. H & E, ×100

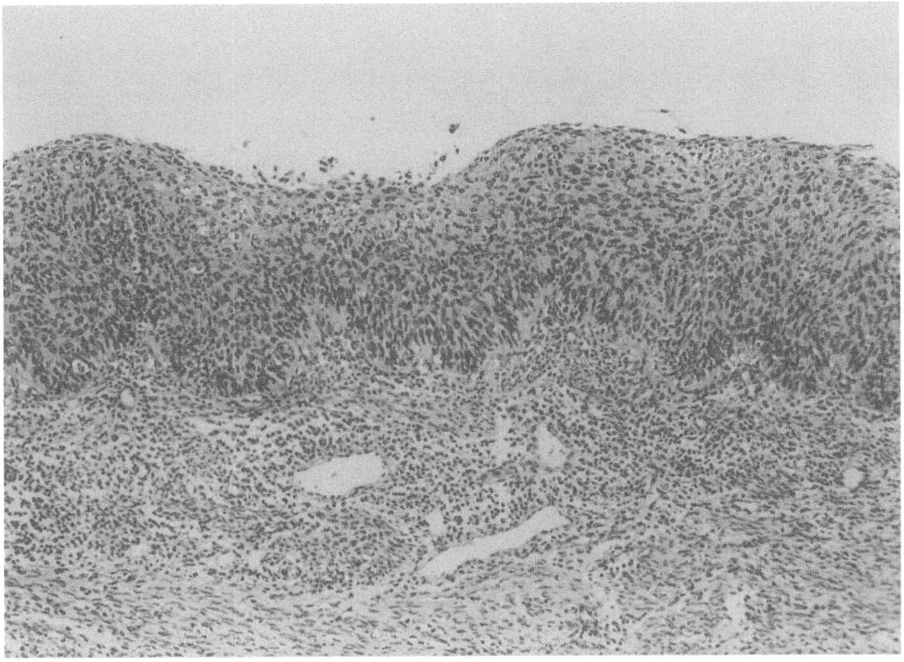

Fig. 4.3 Ichthyosis uteri with epithelial dysplasia, overlying atrophic endometritis. H & E, ×100

adenocarcinoma with squamous differentiation. Sheets of squamous epithelium found as components of curettings are always suspicious of carcinoma, regardless of their stage of differentiation. Well differentiated stratified squamous epithelium may occasionally line the uterine cavity and grow over a mucoepidermoid adenocarcinoma in a postmenopausal woman. On the other hand, an ichthyosis over a senile atrophic endometritis may become dysplastic without underlying malignancy. Therefore, a thorough fractionated curettage is always required to determine the origin of ichthyosis.

Clinical Possibilities. (a) Individual reaction to long-standing endogenous or exogenous unopposed hyperestrogenism; (b) heterotopic metaplasia of Müllerian origin; (c) reactive squamous cell metaplasia that covers the defect following intrauterine device (IUD) or senile ulcerative endometritis; and (d) superficial portion of a well differentiated mucoepidermoid or squamous cell carcinoma.

4.1.2 Mucinous Metaplasia

In mucinous metaplasia (also called endocervical metaplasia; Fig. 4.4), small neighboring groups or larger areas of glands within a proliferating or resting endometrium are found lined by high, columnar mucinous epithelium of the mature endocervical type with small, dense nuclei at the cellular base. The abundant cytoplasm of the cells is pale in H & E

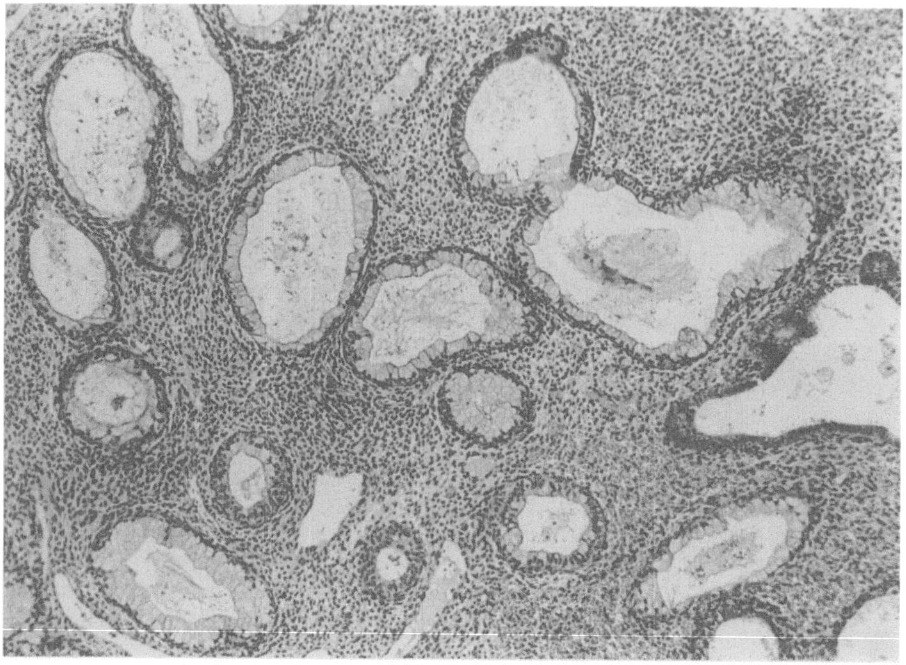

Fig. 4.4 Mucinous metaplasia, H & E, ×100

stains and strongly positive with the PAS reaction. These groups of glands are usually located close to the basal layer and are not shed with menstruation. The surrounding endometrial glands are resting or atrophic or are occasionally cystically dilated. The stroma is evenly spindle celled, large celled or predecidualized. The metaplastic glands show an arrangement similar to normal glands, but may occasionally be crowded or convoluted. In rare instances, the mucinous metaplasia is of the intestinal type.

Morphologic Differential Diagnosis. These metaplastic glands must be differentiated from the pale glands in atypical hyperplasia and in adenocarcinoma with early stromal invasion, where the nuclei are large, depolarized, and aneuploid, furthermore from secreting glands, where the nuclei are round. Distinction from mucinous adenocarcinoma is possible by the lack of stromal invasion.

Clinical Correlation and Differential Diagnosis. Endocervical metaplasia is most often found in postmenopausal women who receive hormonal replacement therapy. Thus, it is (a) usually associated with gestagenic or antiestrogenic stimulation, particularly with tamoxifen, and is frequently accompanied by abortive secretion or endometrial atrophy, or (b) results from genetic or reactive heterotopic differentiation of Müllerian epithelium.

Distinction is possible by correlation with the functional diagnosis of the endometrium and by the clinical history.

4.1.3 Papillary (Syncytial) Metaplasia

Papillary or syncytial epithelial projections with hyperchromatic nuclei may develop focally on the surface (Fig. 4.5) or in the glandular epithelium (Fig. 4.6) most often in postmenopausal women following bleeding or mechanical irritation.

Morphologic Differential Diagnosis. If such metaplastic foci arise from larger areas, they must be differentiated from early serous papillary carcinoma, which possesses polymorphic nuclei and fibrovascular cores not shown by benign metaplasia.

4.1.4 Tubal (Ciliated Cell) Metaplasia

Ciliated cell metaplasia resembles the mucosal lining of the fallopian tube. These foci consist of single-layered or pseudostratified tall, columnar ciliated cells with eosinophilic, often vacuolated cytoplasm and may form intraglandular papillae. They occur in proliferative or

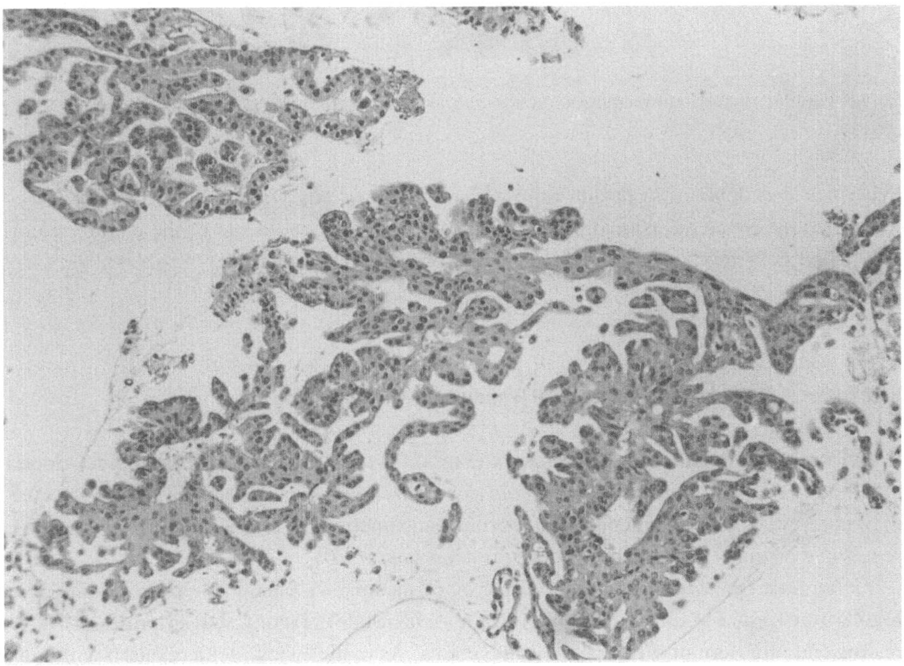

Fig. 4.5 Papillary syncytial metaplasia of the endometrial surface epithelium. H & E, ×100

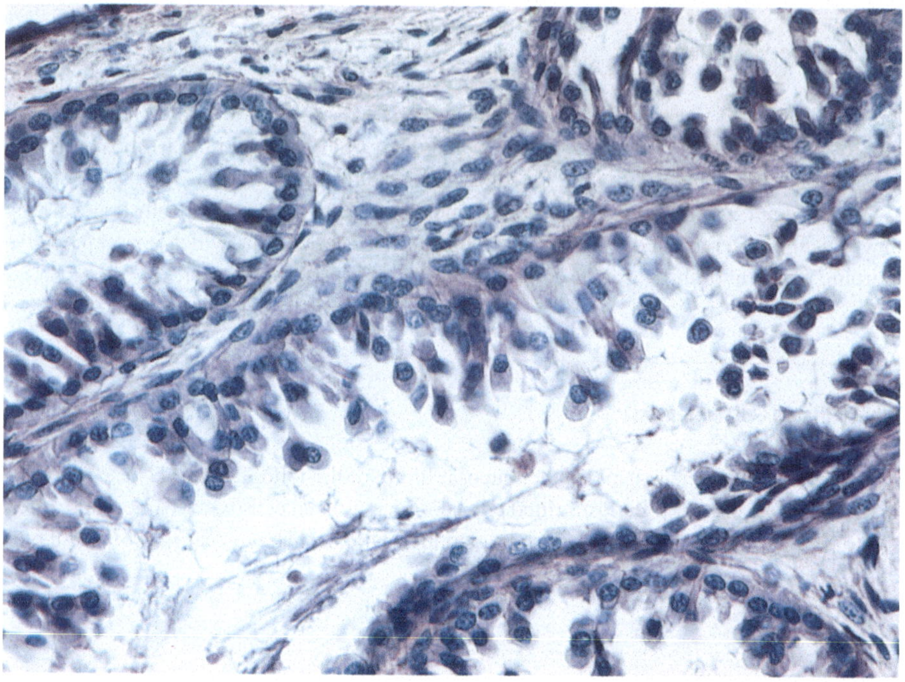

Fig. 4.6 Papillary syncytial metaplasia of endometrial glands with hobnail cell change. H & E, ×350

hyperplastic endometrium during estrogen stimulation or in women on hormone replacement therapy. Since occasional ciliated cells are normal constituents of the endometrium, only larger accumulations of these cells should be called metaplasia.

4.1.5 Rare Forms of Metaplasia of Endometrial Glandular Epithelium

Rare forms include *clear cell metaplasia* (Fig. 4.7), possibly derived from maldeveloped mucinous cells, and *eosinophilic (oncocytic) metaplasia* (Fig. 4.8). Such cells, however, may not always be truly metaplastic, but instead functional variations of glandular cells, regressive changes, or cells in disturbed mitosis (see p. 70).

Hobnail cell metaplasia, another rare type of metaplasia, contains hyperchromatic, but regular nuclei in a similar position as in the Arias-Stella reaction, but in proliferative or resting endometrium of postmenopausal patients. As in the Arias-Stella reaction with high β-human chorionic gonadotrophin (β-HCG) levels, hobnail cell metaplasia is occasionally seen in patients with elevated postmenopausal gonadotrophin levels. The Arias-Stella reaction, in contrast, is not a metaplasia and will therefore be discussed later (see p. 98).

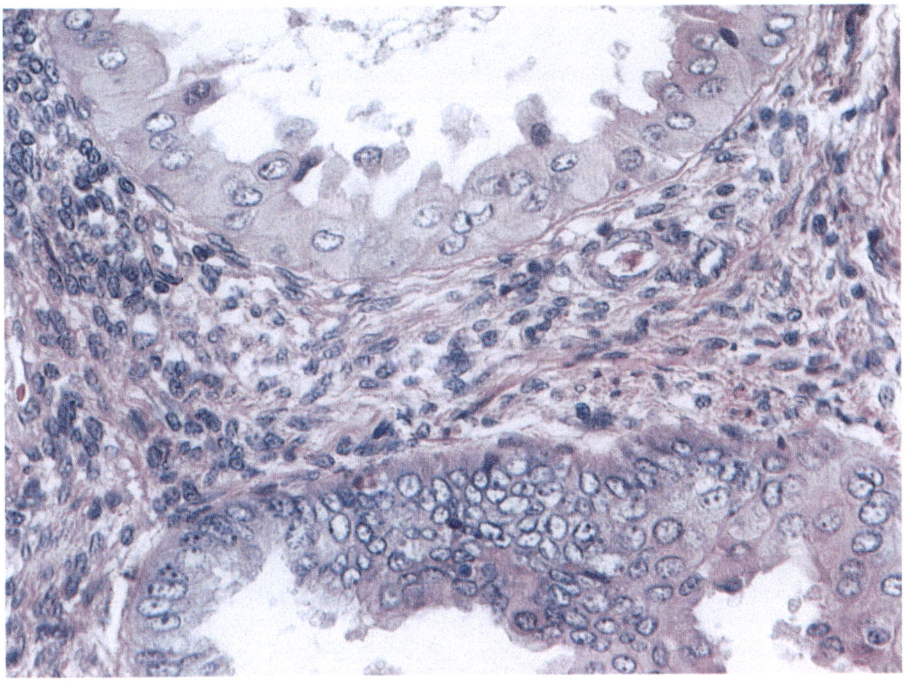

Fig. 4.7 Clear cell metaplasia with occasional hobnail cells. H & E, ×350

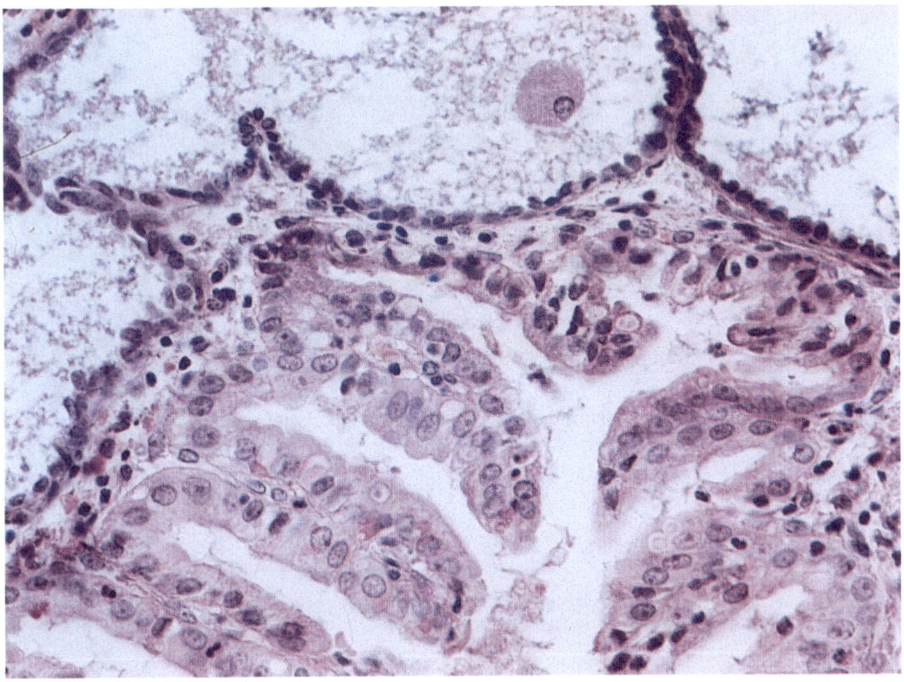

Fig. 4.8 Eosinophilic metaplasia with epithelial papillae. H & E, ×350

4.2 Stromal Metaplasia

In rare instances the endometrial stromal cells undergo metaplastic changes. Small foci of smooth muscle metaplasia may occasionally be observed (Fig. 4.9). Cartilagenous, osseous, fatty, or glial metaplasia has rarely been found.

Morphologic Differential Diagnosis. Stromal metaplasia must be distinguished from: (a) fetal remnants (the metaplastic cells merge with normal stromal cells at their periphery and do not react as foreign inclusions or growths); (b) mixed mesenchymal tumors by their minimal size and benign histologic appearance.

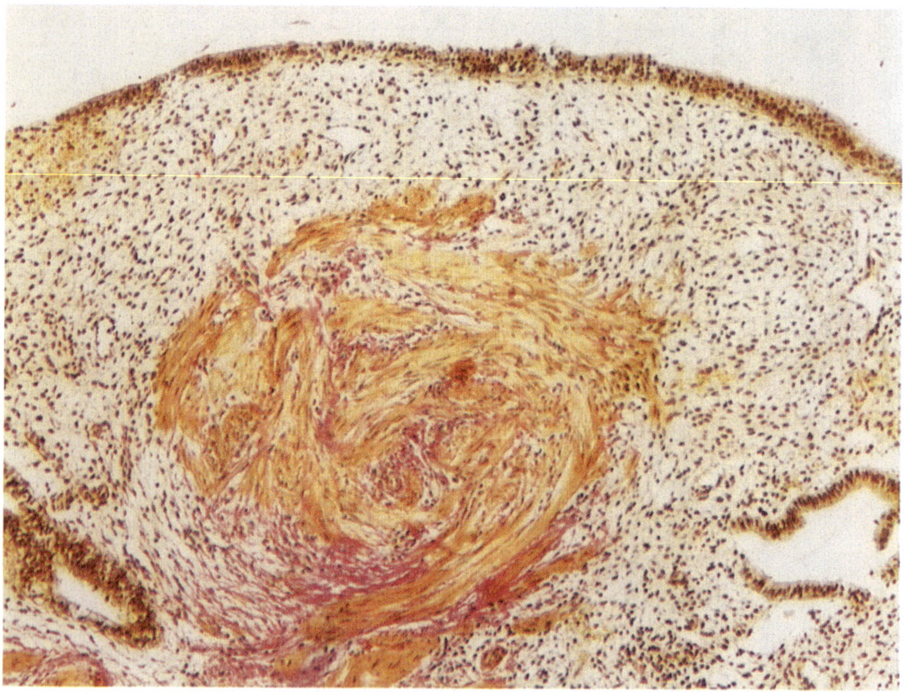

Fig. 4.9 Smooth muscle metaplasia of endometrial stromal cells. Van Gieson stain, ×100

Circulatory Disturbances 5

5.1 Pathologic Edema

In pathologic edema (Fig. 5.1) the endometrial glands are widely separated and the stromal cells pushed apart by small lakes of edema fluid or diffuse accumulation of edema between them. The reticulin fibers are extremely scanty and also pushed far apart. The small lymphatic channels in the stroma are distended. The appearance of glandular and stromal cells is otherwise within normal limits.

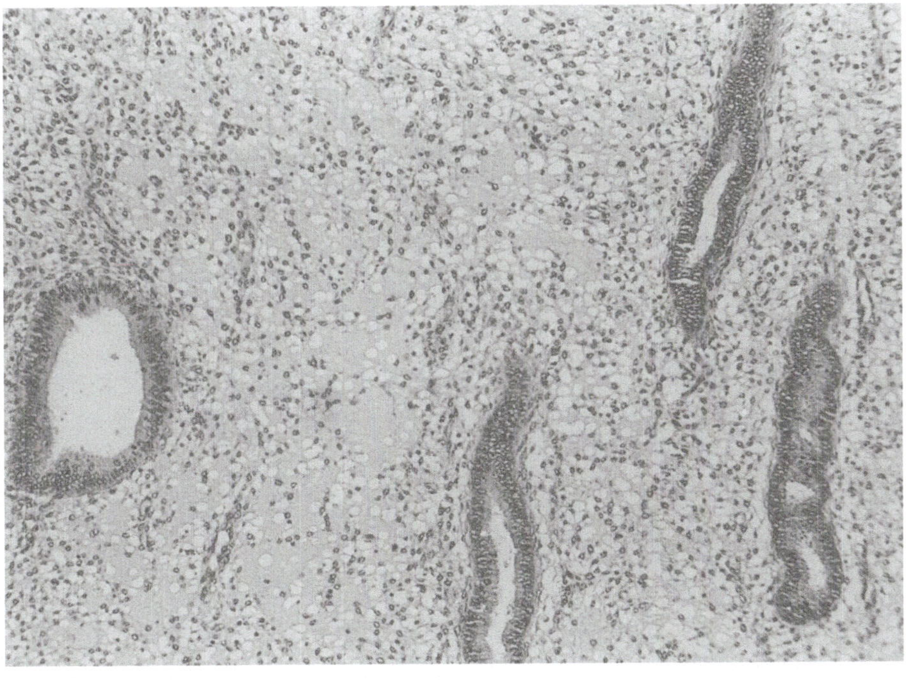

Fig. 5.1 Pathologic edema, H & E, ×100

G. Dallenbach-Hellweg et al., *Atlas of Endometrial Histopathology*,
DOI: 10.1007/978-3-642-01541-0_5,

Morphologic Differential Diagnosis. Pathologic edema must be differentiated from physiologic variations in the vascular and lymphatic circulation during the normal menstrual cycle. Stromal edema is physiologic in the midproliferative phase and on the 22nd day of the normal menstrual cycle (8th day after ovulation).

Clinical Possibilities and Differential Diagnosis. (a) Venous or lymphatic obstruction; (b) hormonal dysfunction with endogenous hyperestrogenism; (c) focal variation in hormone supply under exogenic hormones; and (d) mechanical pressure on lymphatic vessels by malposition of the uterus, submucous fibromyomas, or polyps.

Distinction is possible by correlation of edema with accompanying functional diagnosis of the endometrium and/or surrounding endomyometrium, and with the clinical history.

5.2 Lymphatic Cysts

Large lymphatic cysts (Figs. 5.2, 5.3) lined by flat endothelium can be seen in the lower parts of the functional layer, occasionally surrounded by smaller cysts and patchy, focal or diffuse stromal edema. The lymphatic cysts can be differentiated from cystically dilated glands by their very flat endothelial lining.

Clinical Possibilities. These cysts develop in the same manner as focal or diffuse stromal edema and occasionally together with it. When blood vessels are ligated during

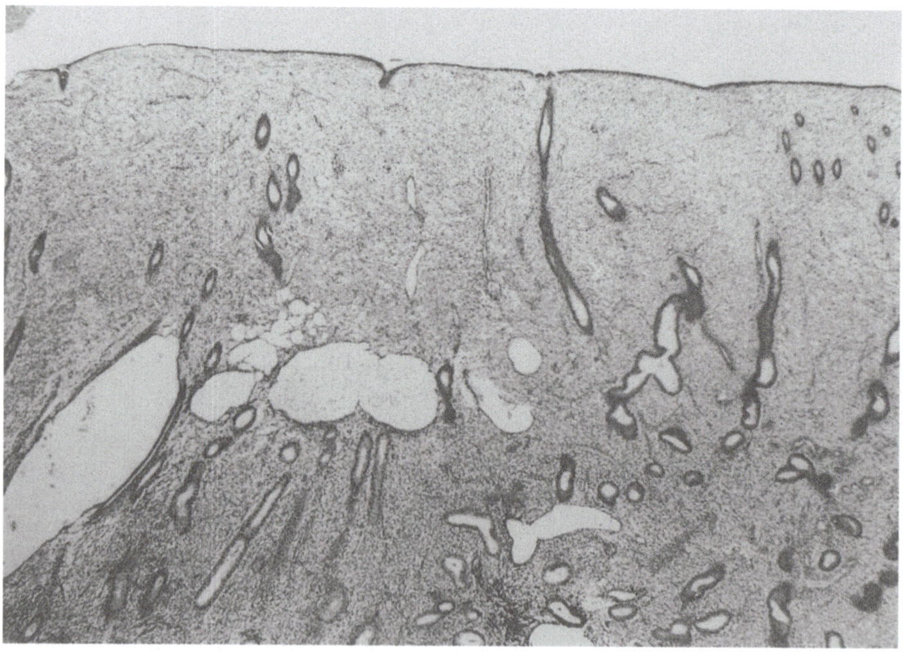

Fig. 5.2 Lymphatic cysts. H & E, ×25

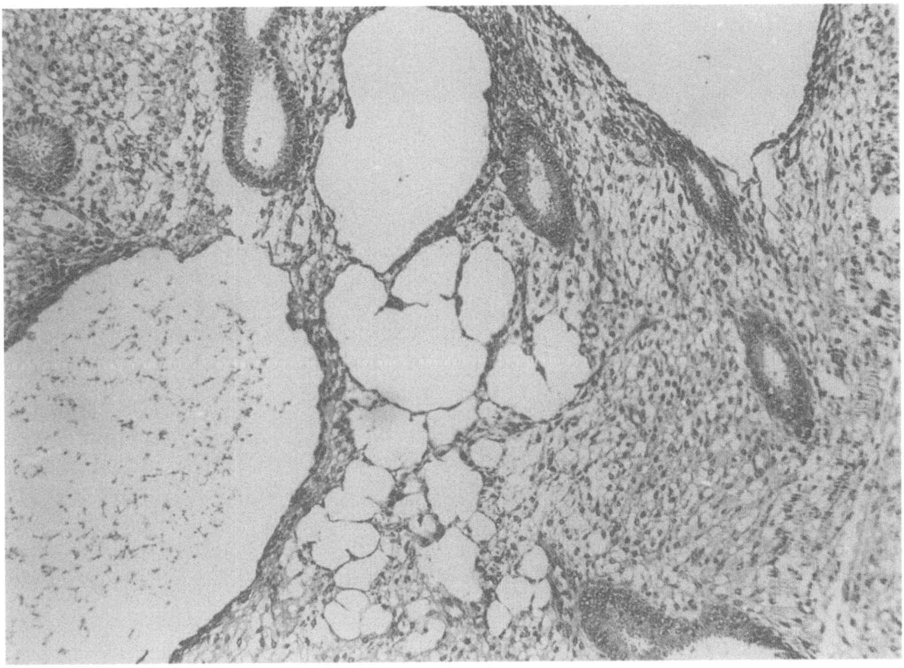

Fig. 5.3 Lymphatic cysts. H & E, ×100

hysterectomy, lymphatic channels may be blocked and become cystically dilated before the operation is finished.

Distinction from freezing artifacts (see p. 5) is possible (a) by their lack of flat endothelium around the cystic spaces (Fig. 2.1), and (b) by the technical situation: transport of endometrial specimen by mail at outside temperatures below zero.

5.3 Apoplexia Uteri

Histologically, a diffuse extravasation of blood throughout the superficial endometrial stroma is usually seen in apoplexia uteri (Figs. 5.4, 5.5). The hemorrhage is confined to the upper layer of the endometrium and ends sharply at the internal uterine os. In less recent hemorrhages, there may be necrosis of stromal cells and loss of reticulin fibers as well as degeneration of the glandular epithelium within the affected parts and, rarely, scattered aggregates of polymorphonuclear leukocytes. The endometrium is usually atrophic and reactive changes remain restricted; therefore, hemosiderin-laden macrophages are not seen.

Morphologic Differential Diagnosis. The apoplexia must be differentiated from vascular thrombosis associated with tissue necrosis, which develops in simple or complex hyperplasia or after estrogen therapy.

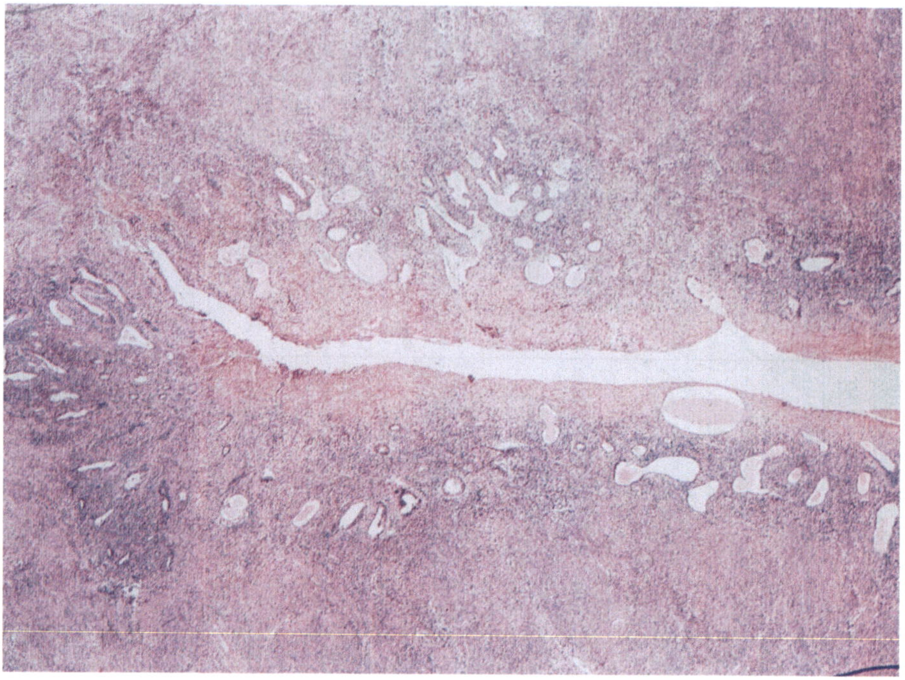

Fig. 5.4 Apoplexia uteri. H & E, ×25

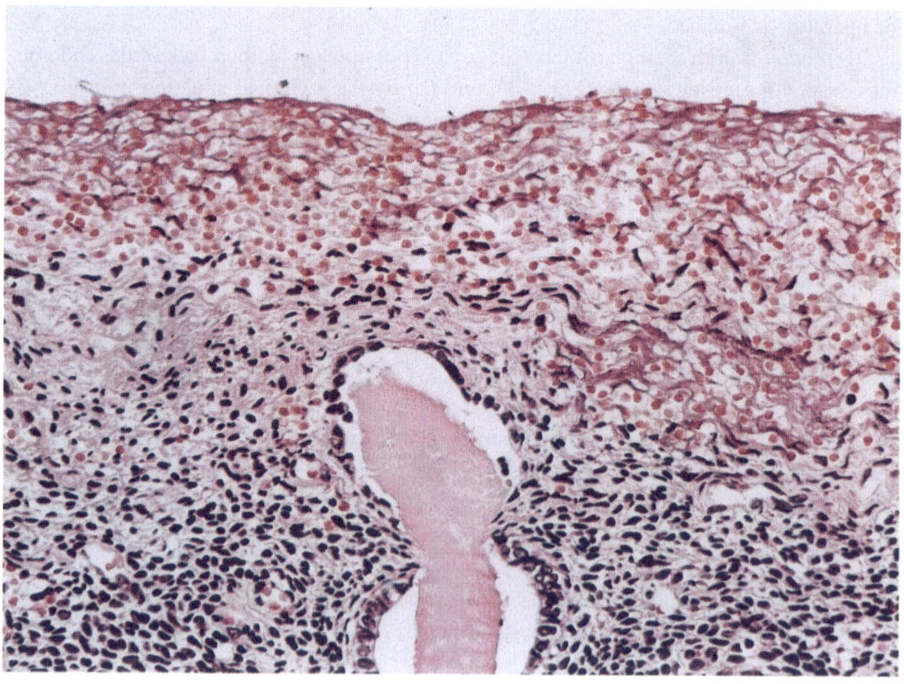

Fig. 5.5 Apoplexia uteri. H & E, ×250

Clinical Possibilities and Differential Diagnosis. (a) Chronic passive hyperemia with hemorrhages due to local mechanical obstruction of vessels by pressure from fibromyomas; (b) generalized reduced blood flow as in cardiac failure (Daly and Balogh 1968); (c) agonal or postoperative hemorrhage by impaired circulation.

Distinction is possible according to the criteria for edema, but of negligible clinical importance.

Functional Disturbances

6

If one follows the various stages of follicular maturation before and after ovulation, the arrest or persistence of this maturation can be divided into anovulatory and ovulatory disturbances. Both types of disturbance may show a spectrum of structural changes in the endometrium depending on the amount of estrogen and progesterone produced, with absolute or relative deficiency or overproduction of one or both hormones (Table 6.1).

6.1 Anovulatory Disturbances

During the reproductive period, the polycystic ovary syndrome is the most important cause of anovulation. Regardless of age, nonfunctioning ovaries or deficient or prolonged follicular stimulation by a central or ovarian defect may cause an anovulatory disturbance (see Table 6.1). Histologically, all resting or proliferative stages from atrophy to hyperplasia may be found.

6.1.1 Atrophy

Diffuse Atrophy

In diffuse atrophy (Figs. 6.1–6.3), the endometrium is very low and consists mainly of small, spindle-shaped stromal cells covered by a cuboidal surface epithelium. Only occasional basal glands are found. Most of these are narrow and lined by low cuboidal epithelial cells with small, round nuclei with dense chromatin. Mitoses are lacking. The cytoplasm is scanty. Spiral arterioles are undeveloped. In early stages, a few glands may still remain in deficient proliferation or be resting and become atrophic gradually. The extent of atrophy with total or subtotal loss of glands and more or less complete absence of enzymes and

G. Dallenbach-Hellweg et al., *Atlas of Endometrial Histopathology*,
DOI: 10.1007/978-3-642-01541-0_6, © Springer-Verlag Berlin Heidelberg 2010

Table 6.1 Functional disturbances of the endometrium in infertility

Morphology	Possible causes
Atrophy	– Nonfunctioning ovaries (central or ovarian defect) – Refractive endometrium
Deficient proliferation	– Deficient follicular stimulation (central or ovarian defect) – Anovulatory cycle
Irregular proliferation or hyperplasia	– Persistent follicle – Repeated anovulatory cycles (polycystic ovaries) – Endometrium refractive to progesterone
Deficient secretory phase with coordinated delay with dissociated delay	– Relative corpus luteum insufficiency due to high endogenous estrogen – Insufficient corpus luteum (central or ovarian defect)
Abortive secretion	– Nonovulating, insufficient follicle with sporadic luteinization
Arrested secretion	– Gestagen stimulation without ovulation, mostly exogenic
Asynchronous cycle	– Disturbance of central regulation (direct or indirect by negative feedback mechanism)

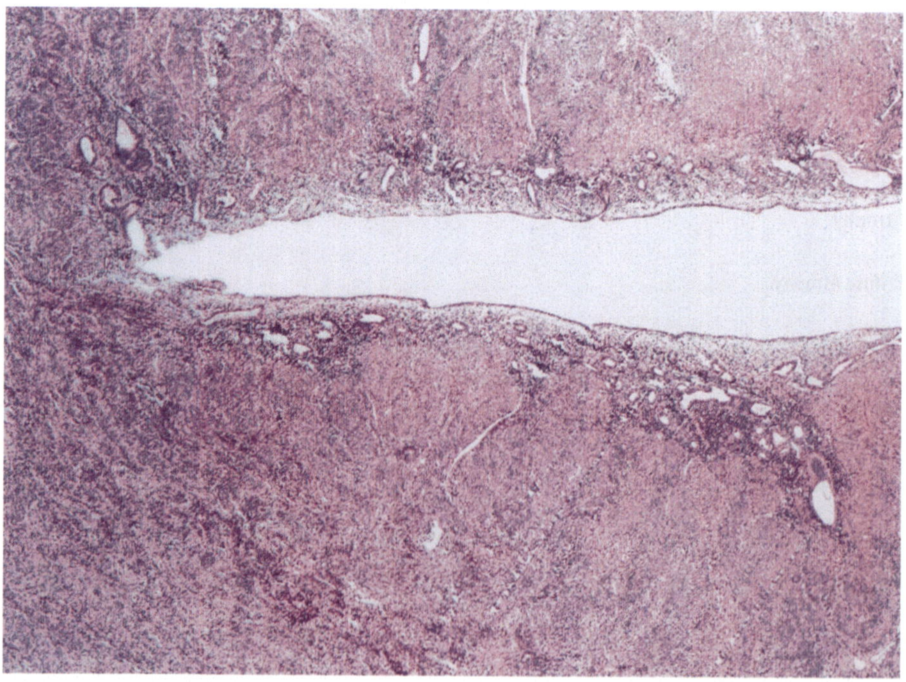

Fig. 6.1 Diffuse atrophy. H & E, ×25

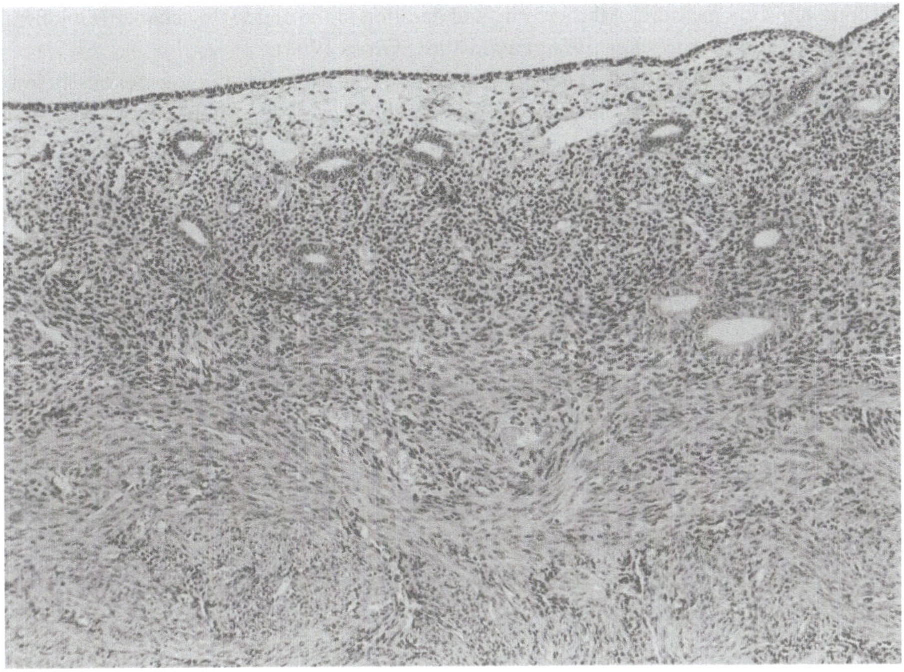

Fig. 6.2 Diffuse atrophy. H & E, ×100

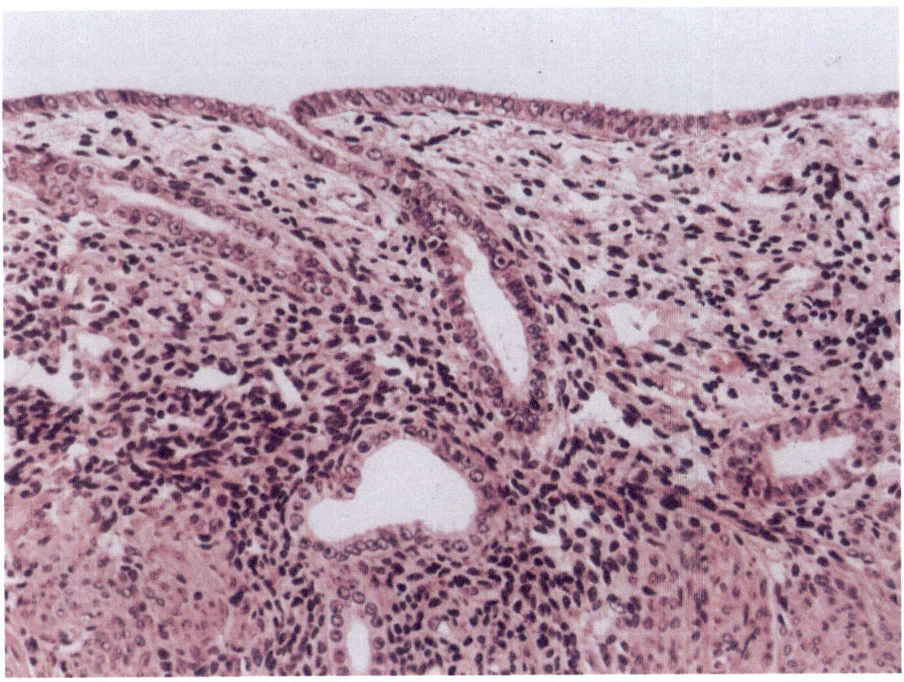

Fig. 6.3 Diffuse atrophy. H & E, ×250

glycoproteins is a measure of the severity and duration of the underlying change (Goldberg and Jones 1956; McKay et al. 1956; Lewin 1961; Gross 1964).

Clinical Possibilities and Differential Diagnosis. (a) Nonfunctioning ovaries before puberty and in the postmenopause or due to a central or ovarian defect (e.g., follicular maturation arrest); (b) refractive endometrium; and (c) iatrogenic suppression by gestagens (as with long-term use of oral contraceptives) or antiestrogens.

Distinction is possible when the histologic diagnosis is correlated with the clinical history, age of patient, hormone therapy, and basal body temperature curve.

Postmenopausal bleeding is often associated with or even caused by endometrial atrophy due to breakage of atrophic vessels.

Focal Pressure Atrophy

Focal pressure atrophy (Figs. 6.4, 6.5) shows the same features as diffuse atrophy, but is localized, either overlying or facing a submucosal leiomyoma, whereas the surrounding endometrium may be quite different. Hence, if atrophy in curettings is only focal, its cause is mechanical rather than functional.

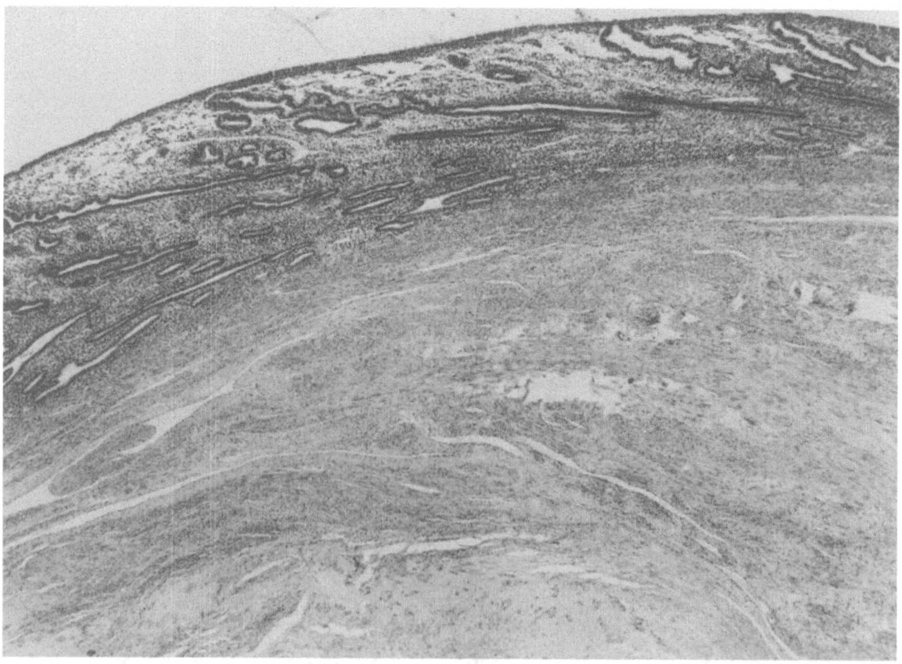

Fig. 6.4 Focal pressure atrophy. H & E, ×25

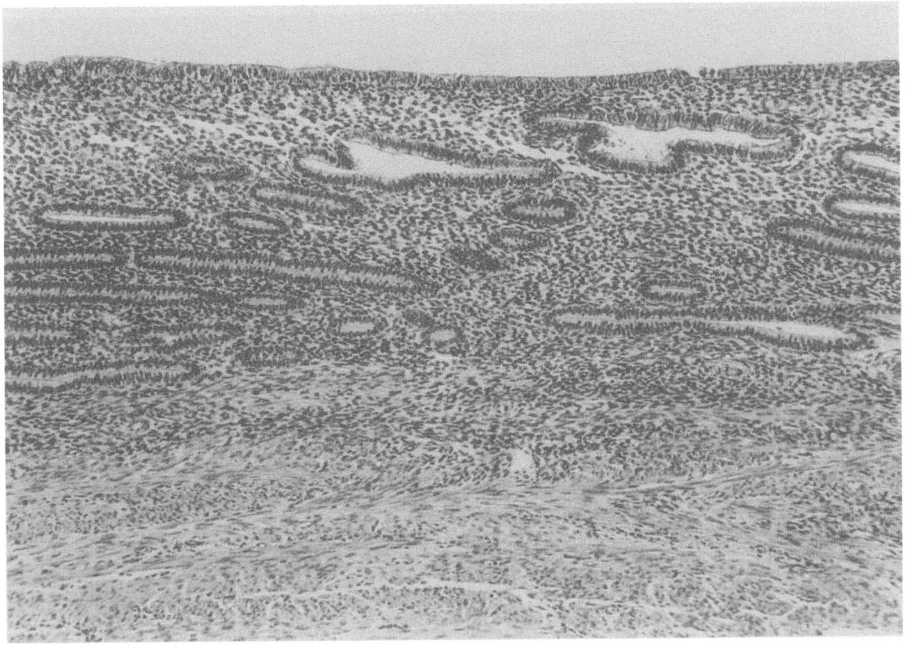

Fig. 6.5 Focal pressure atrophy with flattened glands parallel to endometrial surface. H & E, ×100

6.1.2
Resting Endometrium

Resting endometrium (Fig. 6.6) has more glands than atrophic endometrium. Most of the glands are narrow, straight, and lined by a single row of columnar epithelial cells with chromatin-rich oval nuclei lying close together. The cytoplasm is scanty. The stromal cells are spindle shaped and densely packed with very little edema focally. Mitoses are rare in glandular and stromal cells. Both cells contain only little RNA, and their enzyme activities are low. The maximum height of the resting endometrium is 3 mm.

Clinical Possibilities and Differential Diagnosis. (a) Ovarian hypofunction shortly before puberty or regression in the early postmenopausal period; (b) hypoplastic ovaries with very low estrogen production; (c) recent arrest of ovarian function (transitional stage to atrophy); and (d) iatrogenic suppression by synthetic gestagens.

Distinction as in atrophy (see above).

6.1.3
Deficient Proliferation

In deficient proliferation (Figs. 6.7, 6.8), the growth of the glands and stroma remains retarded as compared with that of the normal proliferative phase. The height of the endometrium is

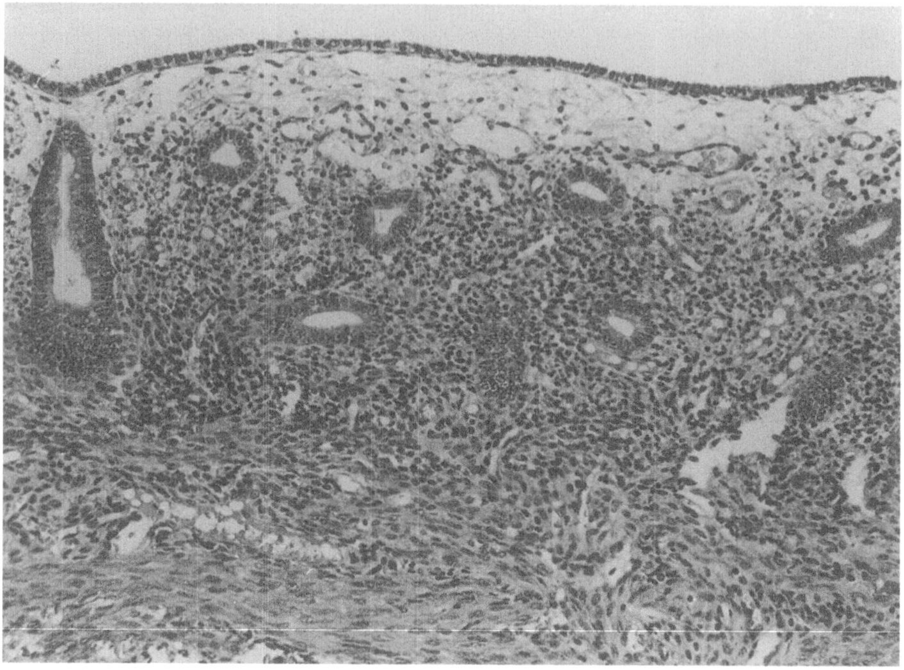

Fig. 6.6 Resting endometrium. H & E, ×100

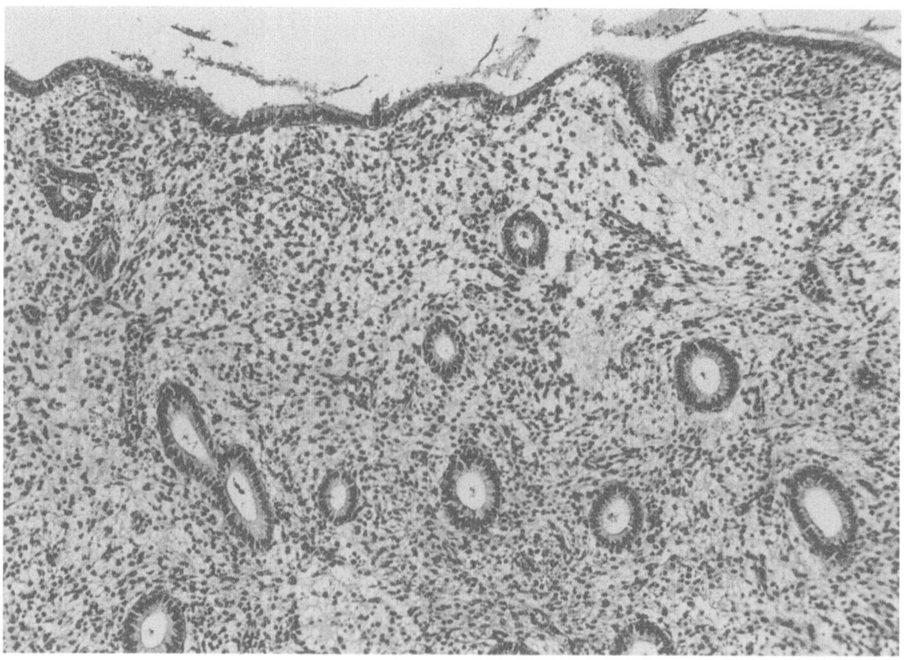

Fig. 6.7 Deficient proliferation. H & E, ×100

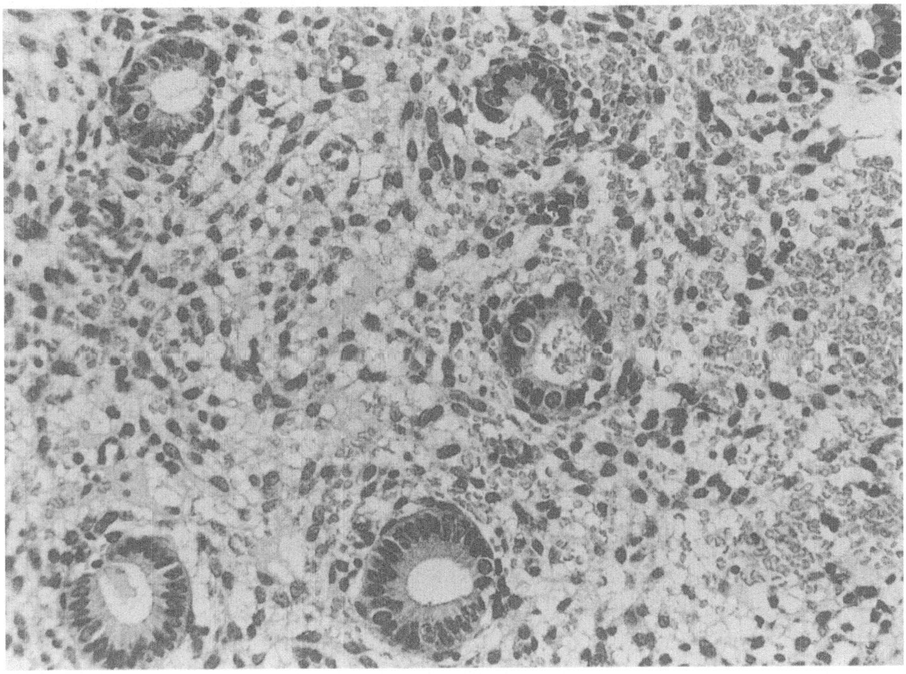

Fig. 6.8 Deficient proliferation. H & E, ×250

moderate, and the glands are slender and straight. The glandular and stromal cells are small. Proliferation, protein synthesis, and enzyme activities are reduced, but edema is usually present and more conspicuous than in the resting endometrium. There are only a few mitoses.

Clinical Possibilities and Differential Diagnosis. Premature ovarian failure by (a) gene mutations resulting in deficient follicular stimulation with early depletion of follicles as in Turner mosaicism, central or ovarian defect causing an anovulatory cycle or as a precursor stage of a deficient secretion; (b) non-genetic failure with infectious or iatrogenic suppression by hormone therapy (oral contraceptives), or following radio- or chemotherapy.

Distinction as in atrophy (see p. 55).

6.1.4 Irregular (Disordered) Proliferation

In irregular proliferation (Figs. 6.9–6.11), the growth of glands and stroma exceeds that of the normal proliferative phase. The endometrial glands are irregular in shape, width, and distribution; the lining epithelial cells are pseudostratified and form a dense row, their nuclei are large and rich in chromatin, and mitoses are frequent. The stroma is densely cellular and focally edematous. The height of the mucosa varies, but is generally considerable. The nuclear and cytoplasmic contents of DNA, RNA, estrogen receptors, and enzymes are high.

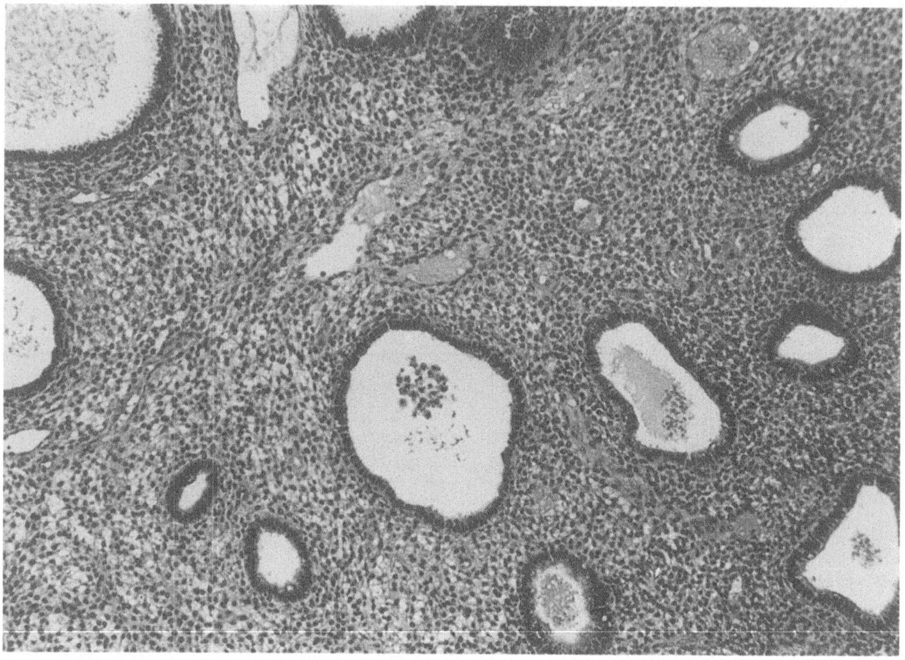

Fig. 6.9 Irregular (disordered) proliferation without signs of secretion. H & E, ×100

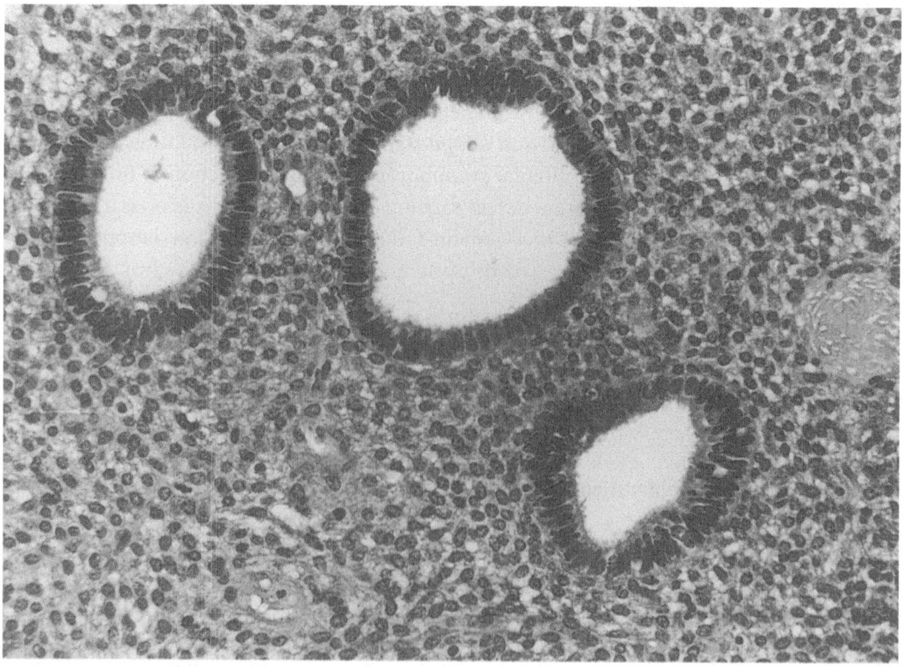

Fig. 6.10 Irregular (disordered) proliferation without sings of secretion. H & E, ×250

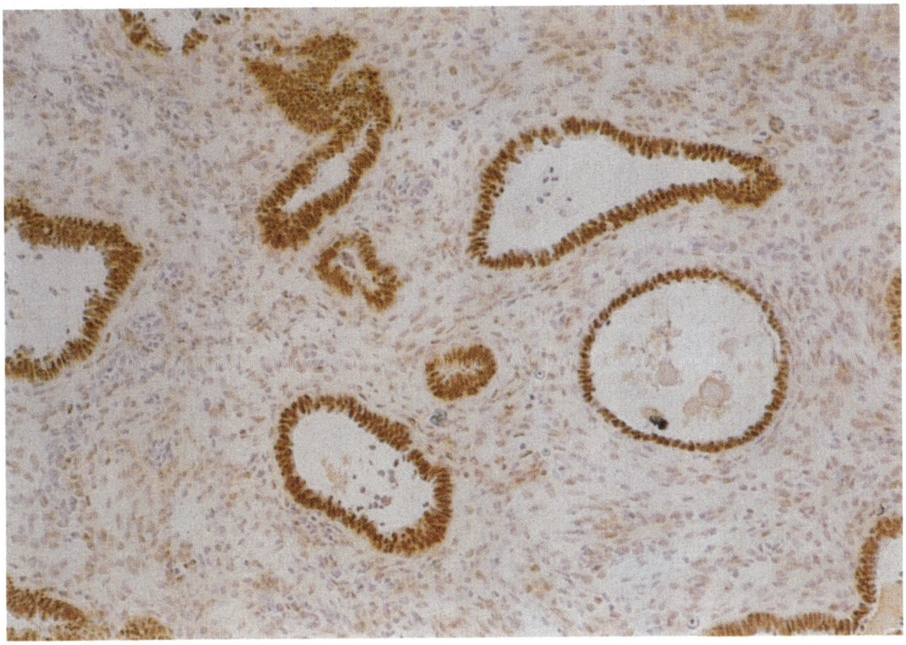

Fig. 6.11 Irregular (disordered) proliferation with high content of estrogen receptors. Immunohistochemical reaction with the ER-ICA assay, ×100

Irregular proliferation is a transitional form to simple (glandular cystic) hyperplasia.

Clinical Possibilities and Differential Diagnosis. (a) Excessive estrogen production from a persistent follicle or polycystic ovaries with repeated anovulatory cycles, ovarian stromal hyperplasia, or ovarian tumors; (b) absence of progesterone receptors in the endometrium; and (c) iatrogenic stimulation by synthetic estrogens.

Distinction as in atrophy (see p. 55).

6.1.4.1
Deficient or Irregular Proliferation with Focal Abortive Secretion

With focal abortive secretion (Fig. 6.12), the endometrial glands are either straight and narrow, as in deficient proliferation, or vary in their width and distribution, as in irregular proliferation without focal abortive secretion, but the glandular epithelium is low with small, rounded, chromatin-dense nuclei. The scanty cytoplasm contains small amounts of glycogen, often in the shape of minute, basal or apical vacuoles. The stroma corresponds to that in deficient or irregular proliferation and remains unchanged during the abortive secretion, which should not be misinterpreted as a sign that ovulation has taken place.

Morphologic Differential Diagnosis. Abortive secretion must be differentiated from late ovulation followed by absolute or relative corpus luteum insufficiency (refer to "Deficient Secretory Phase," p. 93 and Fig. 6.56).

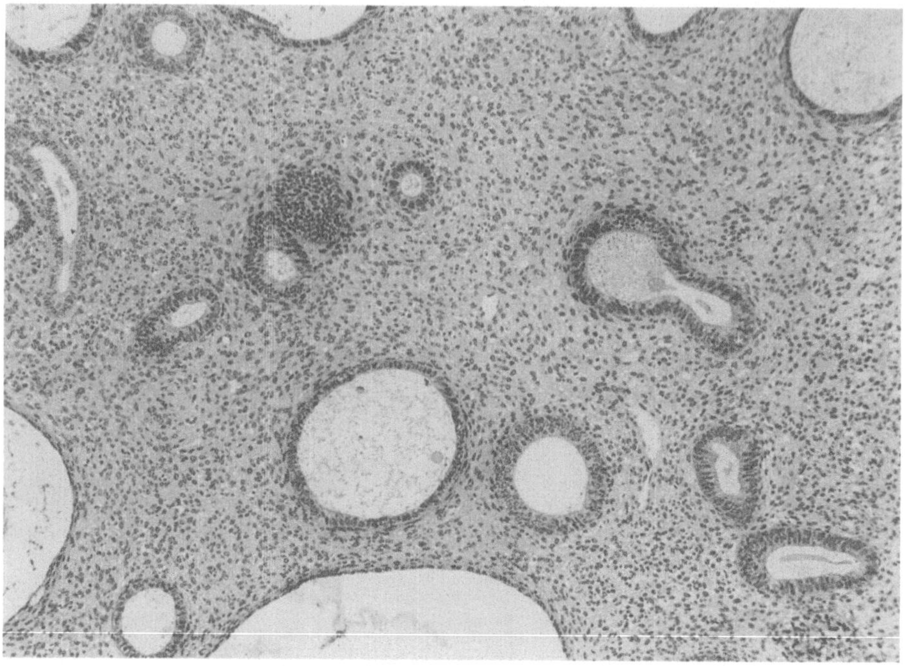

Fig. 6.12 Irregular (disordered) proliferation with focal abortive secretion H & E, ×100

Except for severe corpus luteum insufficiency, this distinction is possible by judging (or measuring) the size of glandular nuclei and vacuoles, both of which are considerably smaller in nonovulatory abortive secretion.

Clinical Possibilities and Differential Diagnosis. (a) Focal incomplete luteinization within a deficient or persistent follicle, when the luteinizing hormone (LH) does not suffice to induce ovulation; (b) use of sequential type oral contraceptives with suppression of ovulation as well as secretory transformation.

6.1.5 Anovulatory Withdrawal Bleeding

Anovulatory withdrawal bleeding (Figs. 6.13, 6.14) may follow deficient or irregular proliferation or even hyperplasia. In contrast to normal menstrual shedding, the anovulatory bleeding sets in without dissolution of reticulin fibers. In the early stages, patchy edema and vascular thrombosis can be seen, resulting in hemorrhagic infarction and necrosis. Small, necrotic foci may contain neutrophils, macrophages, and occasionally plasma cells and fibrin deposits. Fresh hemorrhages can be demonstrated around deficiently or irregularly proliferating glands. The glandular nuclei are often pyknotic due to the slow regression. In the advanced stages, fragments of tissue are shed but not dissolved properly because of the abnormal hormonal situation caused by lack of progesterone withdrawal and relaxin secretion.

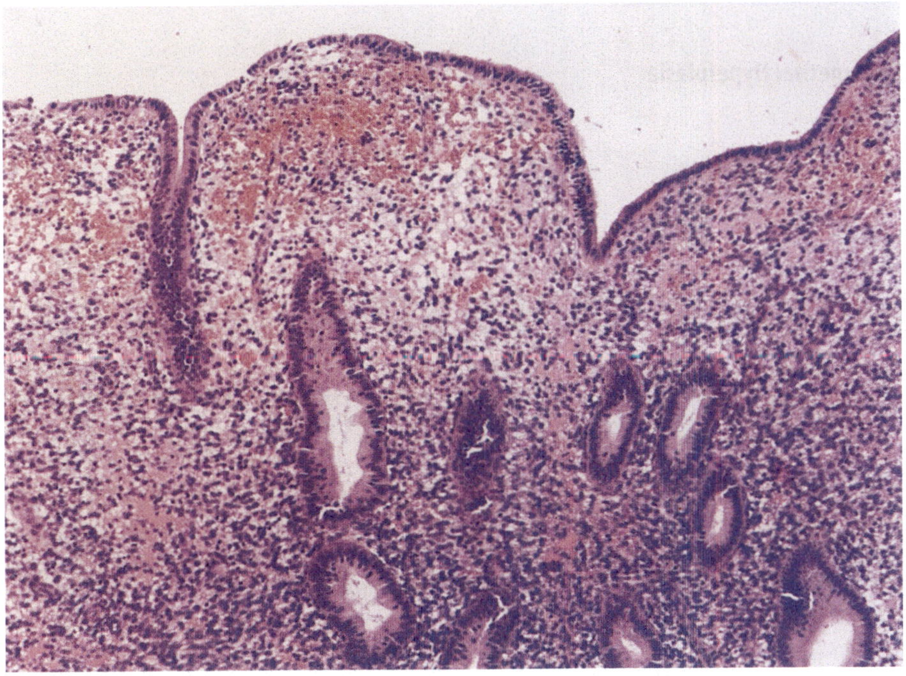

Fig. 6.13 Anovulatory withdrawal bleeding. H & E, ×100

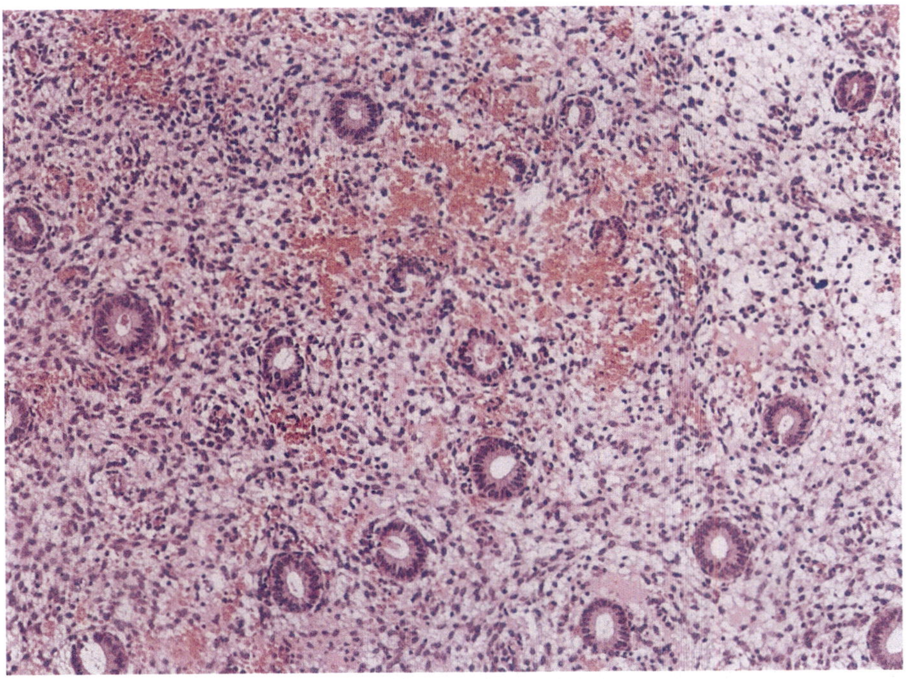

Fig. 6.14 Anovulatory withdrawal bleeding. H & E, ×100

6.2 Endometrial Hyperplasia

6.2.1 Nonatypical Hyperplasia

6.2.1.1 Simple Hyperplasia

In simple hyperplasia (Figs. 6.15–6.25), according to the extent of proliferative activity, the ratio of glands and stroma is now increased when compared with irregular proliferation. Most or all of the endometrial glands are more or less cystically dilated and lined by pseudostratified, highly proliferating epithelium with enlarged, elongated, chromatin-rich nuclei in scanty, basophilic cytoplasm rich in RNA. Mitoses are frequent and often blocked in prophase or metaphase, which may explain the occurrence of clear cells within the glandular epithelium (Fuchs 1959; see p. 50). The increase in activity of alkaline phosphatase is directly proportional to the level of estrogen (Filipe and Dawson 1968). The stromal cells are undifferentiated, densely arranged, and contain chromatin-rich nuclei in a sparse cytoplasm. Spiral arterioles are poorly developed. In contrast, the superficial capillaries and venules are numerous, dilated, and often congested or thrombosed, resulting in areas of necrosis. The ground substance is partly depolymerized, containing mucopolysaccarides and often a fibrinous exudate (Schmidt-Matthiesen 1965) or hyalin thrombi.

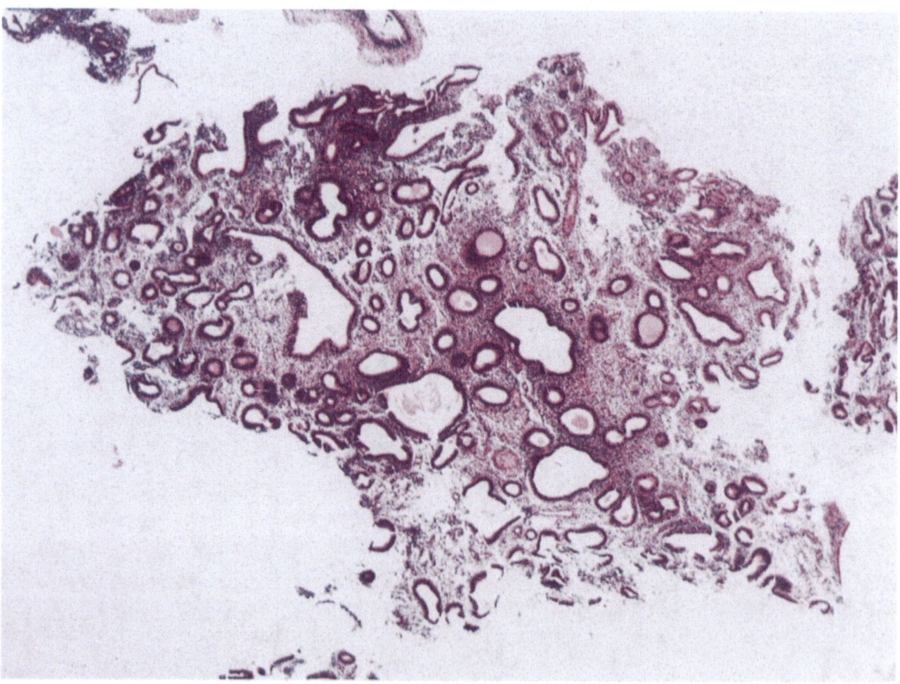

Fig. 6.15 Simple hyperplasia, early stage. H & E, ×25

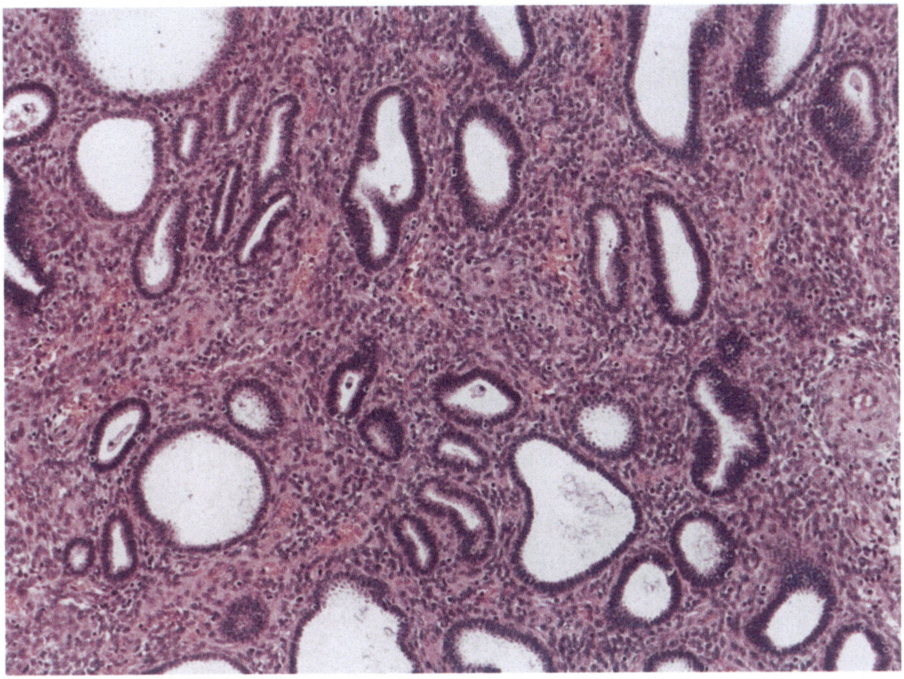

Fig. 6.16 Simple hyperplasia, early stage. H & E, ×100

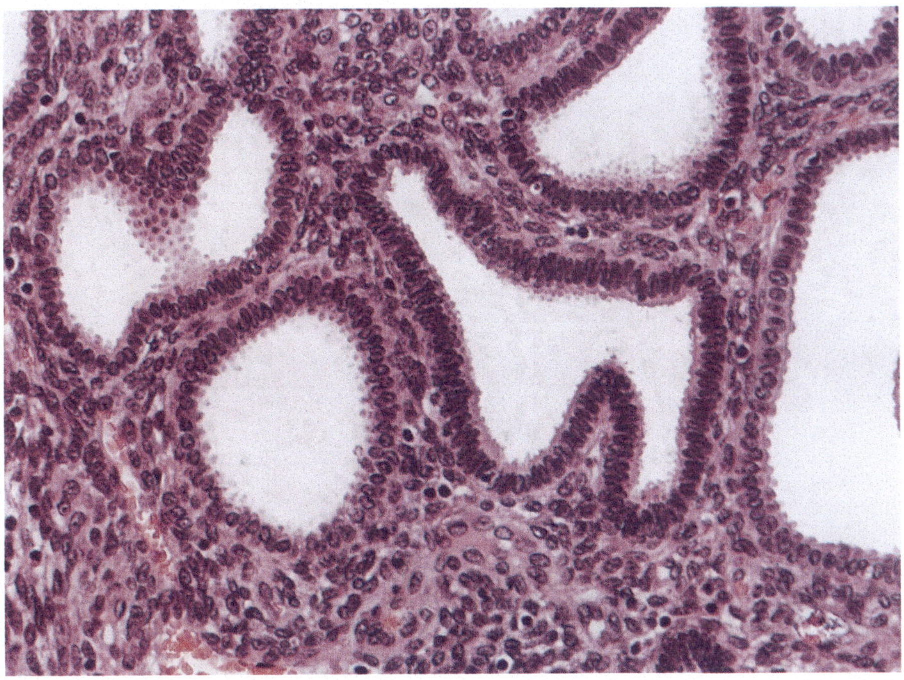

Fig. 6.17 Higher magnification of Fig. 6.16, slight. H & E, ×250

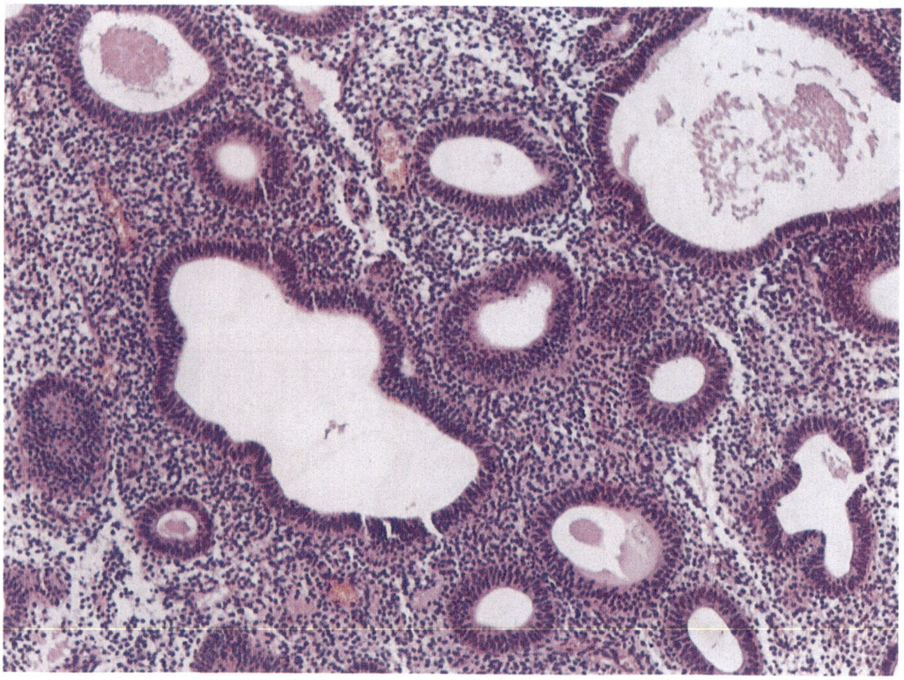

Fig. 6.18 Simple hyperplasia, advanced stage. H & E, ×100

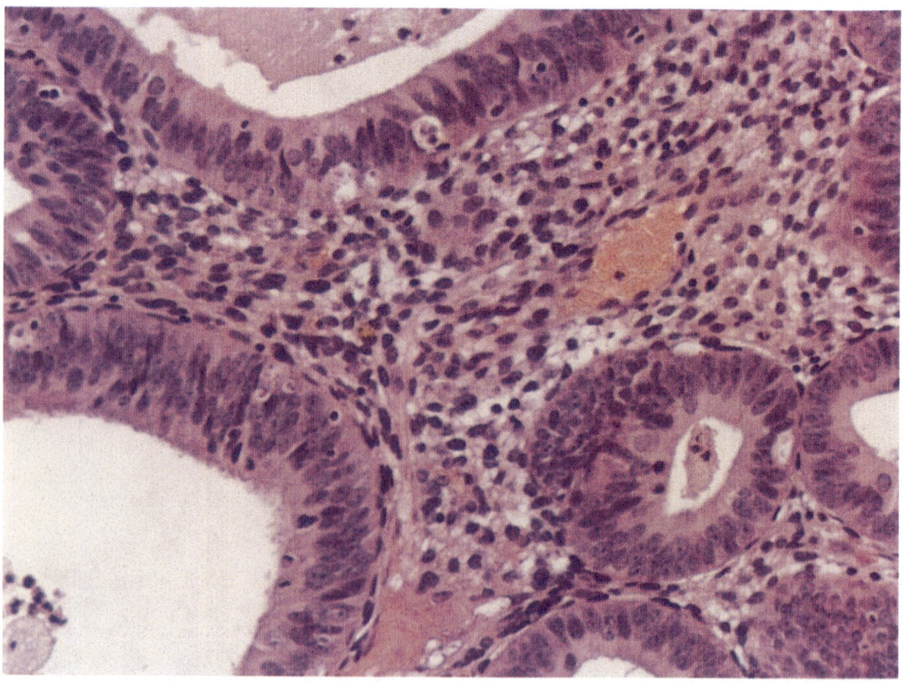

Fig. 6.19 Higher magnification of Fig. 6.18. H & E, ×250

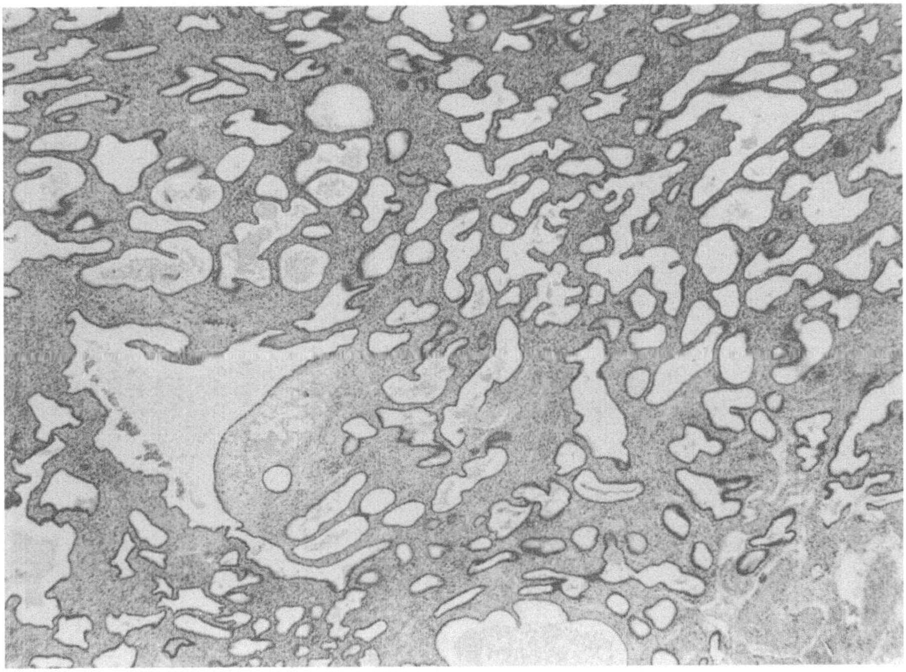

Fig. 6.20 Simple hyperplasia with secretory transformation. H & E, ×25

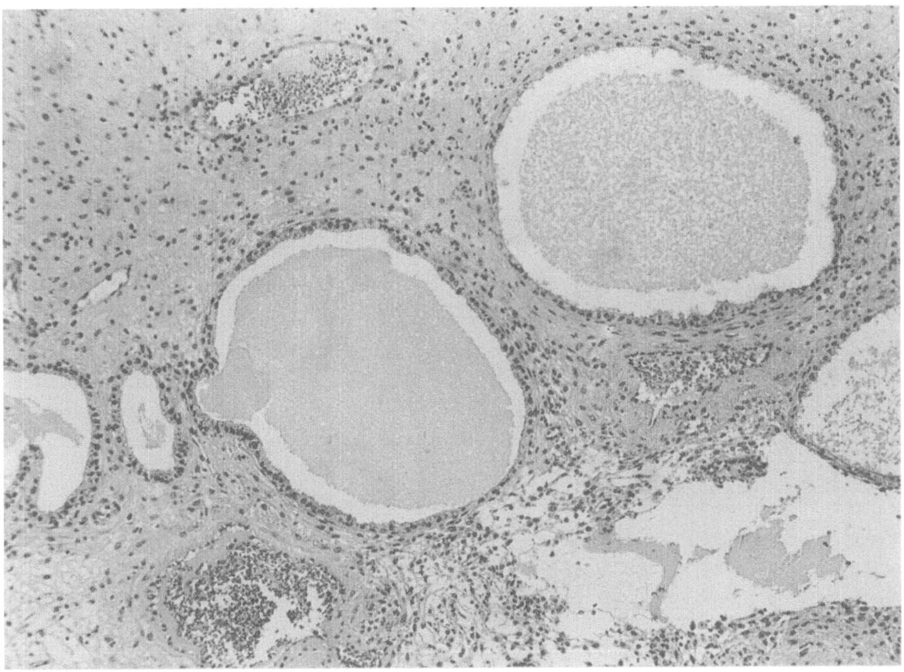

Fig. 6.21 Simple hyperplasia with secretory transformation. H & E, ×100

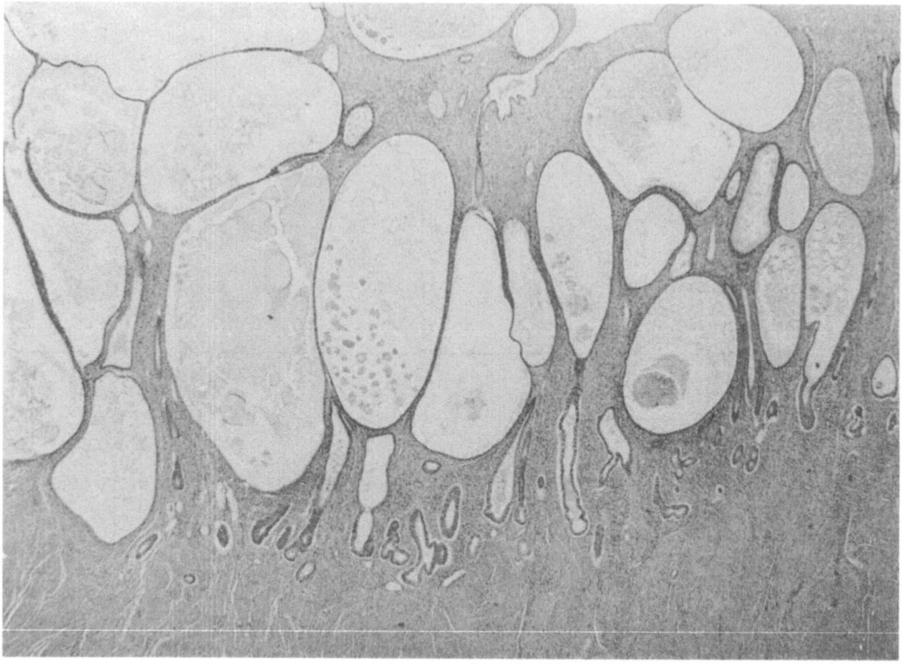

Fig. 6.22 Resting cystic hyperplasia. H & E, ×25

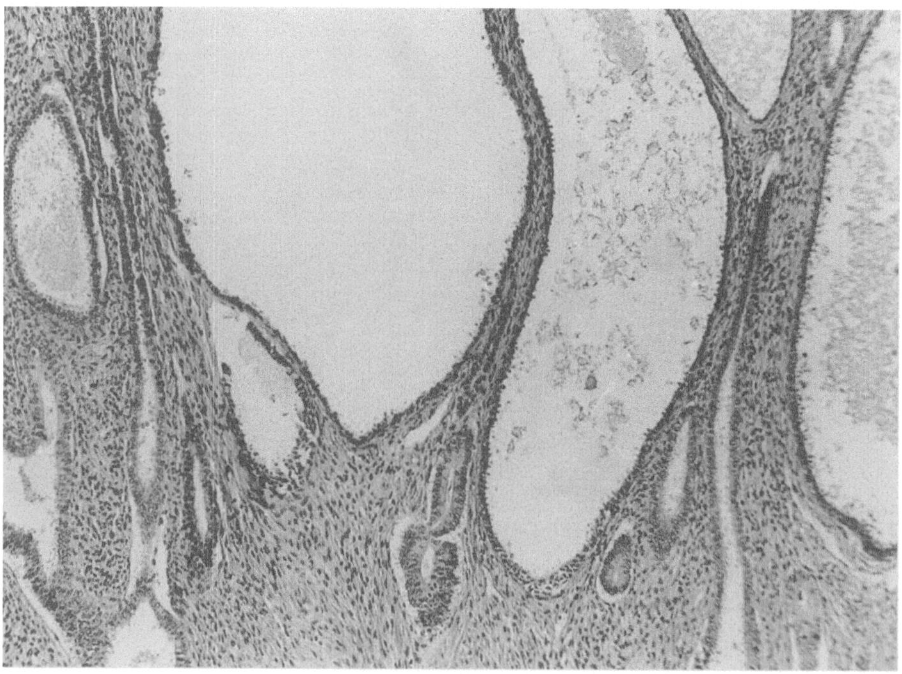

Fig. 6.23 Resting cystic hyperplasia. H & E, ×100

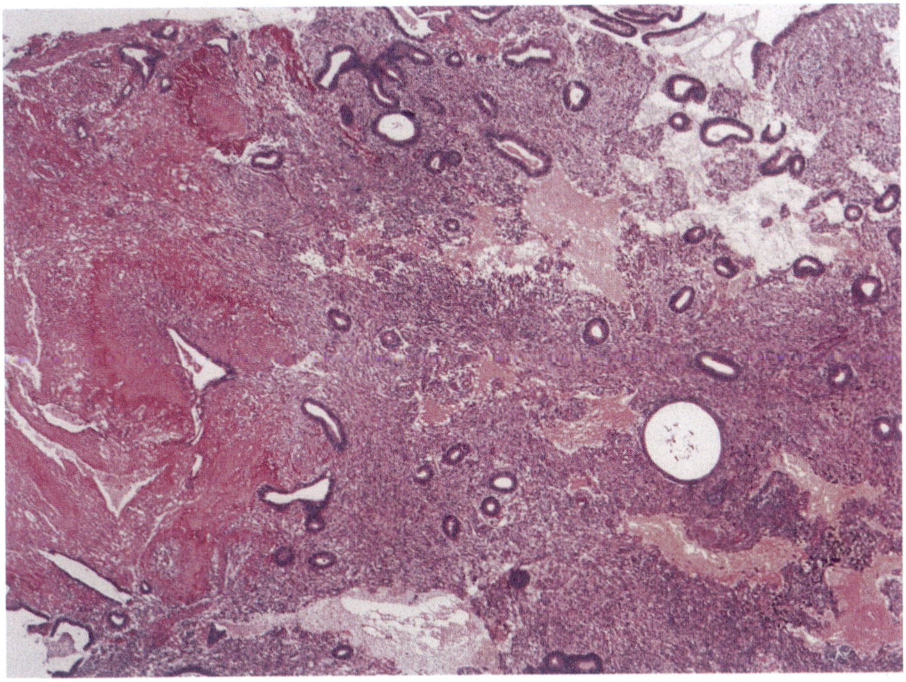

Fig. 6.24 Adaptation hyperplasia, periodic acid-Schiff (PAS) reaction, ×25

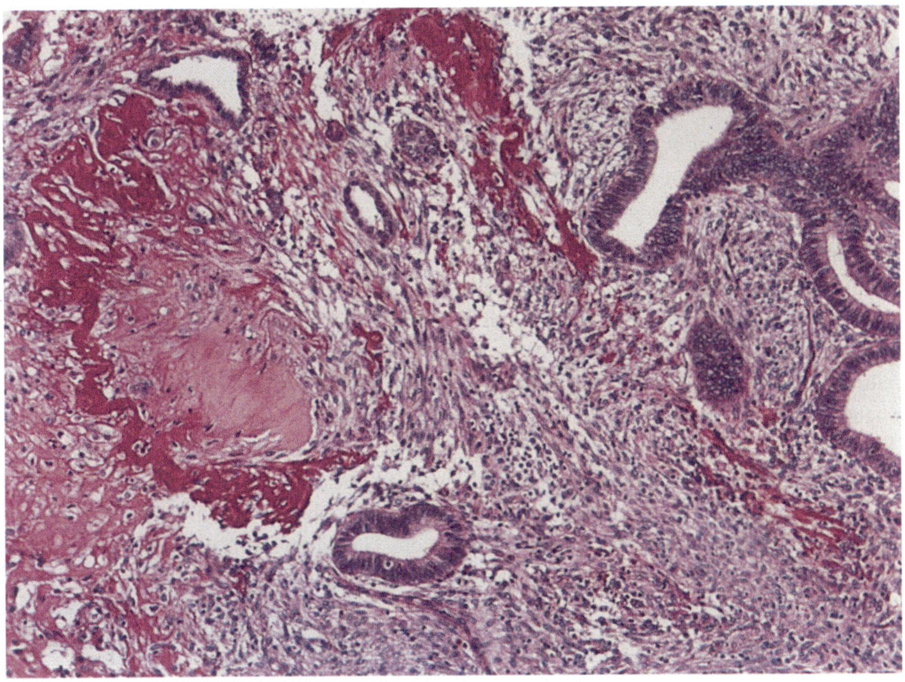

Fig. 6.25 Adaptation hyperplasia, periodic acid-Schiff (PAS) reaction, ×100

Early Stage

In the early stage (Figs. 6.15–6.17), the tall, columnar glandular epithelium may still form a single row (Fig. 6.17).

Advanced Stage

The severe form (Figs. 6.18, 6.19), however, is always accompanied by an increase in glandular crowding and pseudostratification of the glandular epithelium.

Clinical Possibilities. (a) Long-standing follicular persistence or repeated anovulatory cycles, as in polycystic ovary syndrome (hyperandrogenic ovarian insufficiency); (b) excessive endogenous estrogen production by ovarian stromal hyperplasia, by granulosa theca cell tumors or other estrogen-producing ovarian tumors, by adrenal glands, or in the fatty tissue; and (c) unopposed exogenous estrogen.

Secretory Transformation

In simple hyperplasia, secretory transformation may occur in some or most of the glands (Figs. 6.20, 6.21) and is occasionally accompanied by various degrees of stromal differentiation. The glandular epithelium becomes single layered again by intraluminal folding as in normally secreting endometrium, yet the nuclei remain small as in abortive secretion, and basal vacuoles are rarely seen. The stroma may become predecidual or even decidual and may contain abundant granular endometrial stromal cells (Fig. 6.21).

Clinical Possibilities. Secretory transformation may develop by (a) sporadic luteinization in a persistent follicle, (b) exogenous gestagen therapy, or (c) spontaneous ovulation (in the reproductive period).

Resting Cystic Hyperplasia

In the resting form (Figs. 6.22, 6.23), the glands retain their cystic appearance but their lining epithelium becomes atrophic. Since the stromal cells also undergo shrinkage and atrophy, the cystic glands lie close to each other. DNA and RNA contents of glandular and stromal cells are greatly reduced. Mitoses are rare.

Clinical Correlation. Resting cystic hyperplasia is seen following decrease of previously elevated estrogen levels and consequently almost only in the postmenopausal age group.

Adaptation Hyperplasia

Adaptation hyperplasia (Figs. 6.24, 6.25) may develop post partum or post abortum. Only some glands are cystically dilated; others are irregularly shaped and distributed. All glands are lined by highly proliferating epithelium, as in simple hyperplasia, and separated by a densely cellular stroma of large or shrunken, rounded cells. In the stroma there are characteristic patches of hyalinized decidual remnants surrounded by garland-shaped PAS-positive material (Figs. 6.24, 6.25) and by chronic inflammatory infiltrates. In contrast to simple hyperplasia, spiral arterioles are still prominent. There are also fresh focal hemorrhages (Figs. 6.24).

Clinical Possibilities. Adaptation hyperplasia is caused by post partum or post abortum persistence of follicles with prolonged anovulation. The diagnosis is aided by recognizing decidual remnants or prominent spiral arterioles.

6.2.1.2 Complex (Adenomatous) Hyperplasia

In complex (adenomatous) hyperplasia (Figs. 6.26–6.28) under the action of continuous unopposed estrogen, the glandular proliferation progresses beyond the cystic dilation by epithelial budding, branching, and formation of new glands. The tall, columnar glandular epithelium becomes pseudostratified or even stratified. In the elongated, enlarged, yet diploid nuclei DNA synthesis and mitotic activity is greatly increased (Fettig 1965; Wagner et al. 1967). The sparse, undifferentiated cytoplasm accumulates abundant RNA. The stroma becomes rarefied.

The complex proliferation of glands may be predominantly focal within a simple hyperplasia, characterized by moderate glandular convolution, crowding, and pseudostratification of proliferative glandular epithelium (Fig. 6.26).While some glands are still cystically dilated, others show beginning intraluminal infolding and budding. The spindle-celled stroma is preserved in some areas, but is focally quite sparse. The stromal cells are undifferentiated. Spiral arterioles are not prominent. There are *focal* architectural alterations of glands, but no cytologic atypia.

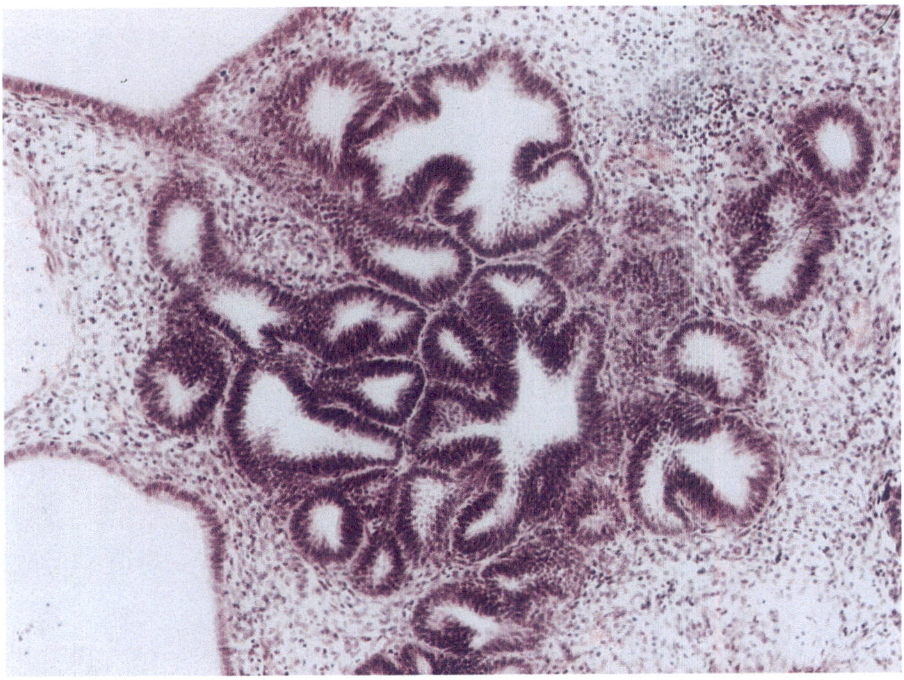

Fig. 6.26 Complex (adenomatous) hyperplasia, focal. H & E, ×75

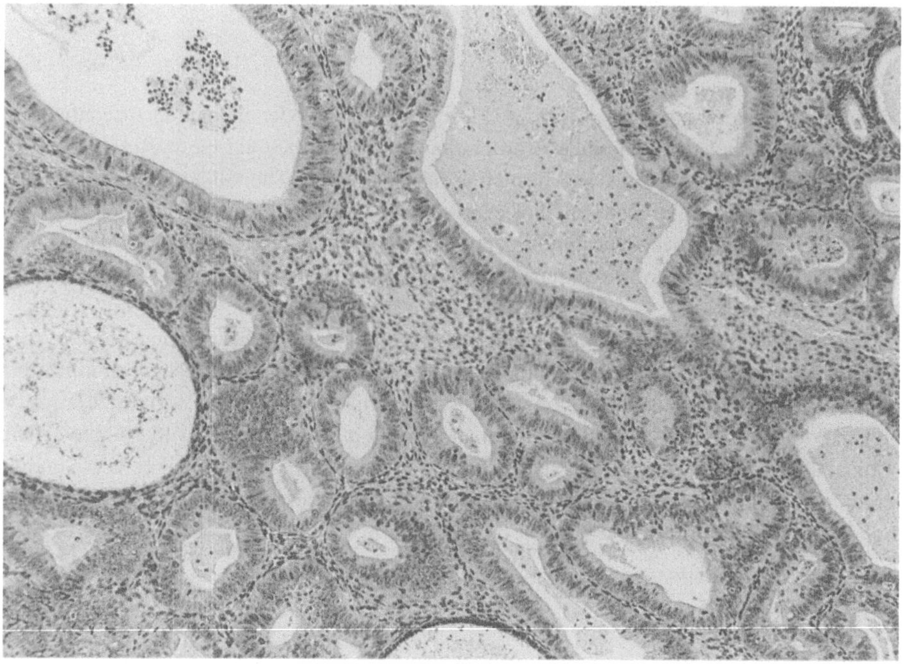

Fig. 6.27 Complex (adenomatous) hyperplasia, diffuse. H & E, ×100

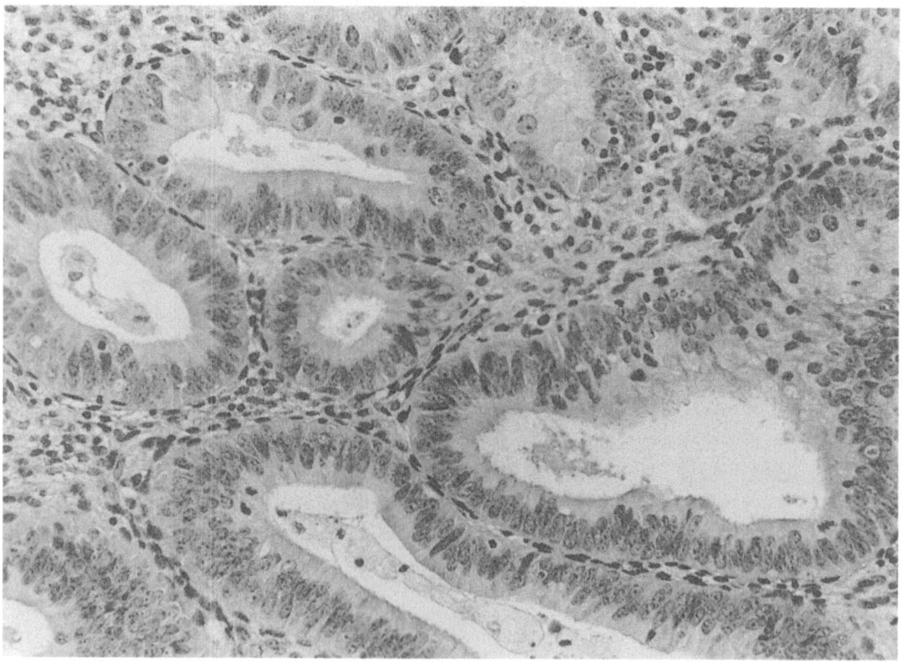

Fig. 6.28 Higher magnification of Fig. 6.27. H & E, ×250

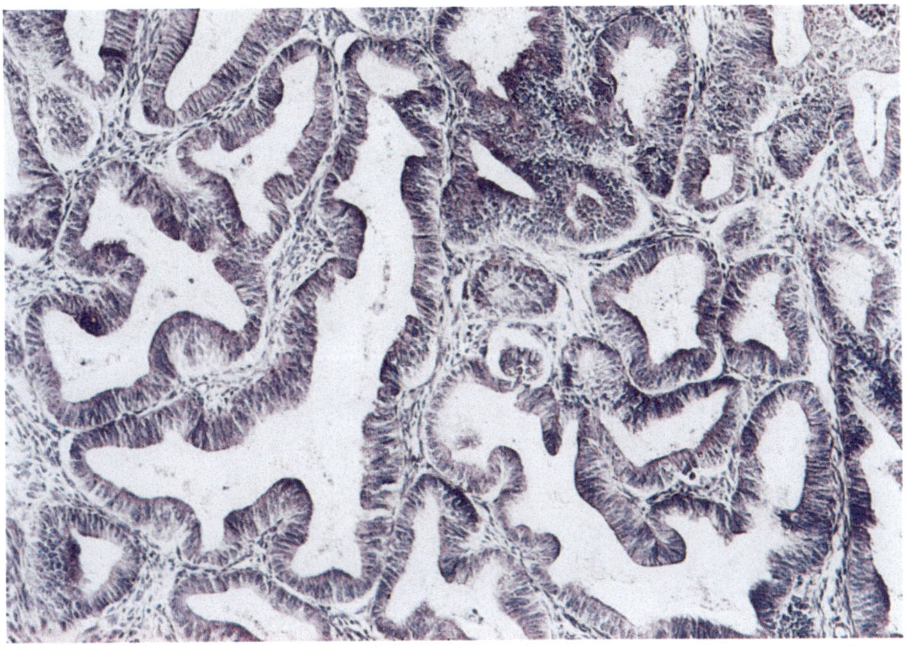

Fig. 6.29 Atypical hyperplasia, H & E, ×100

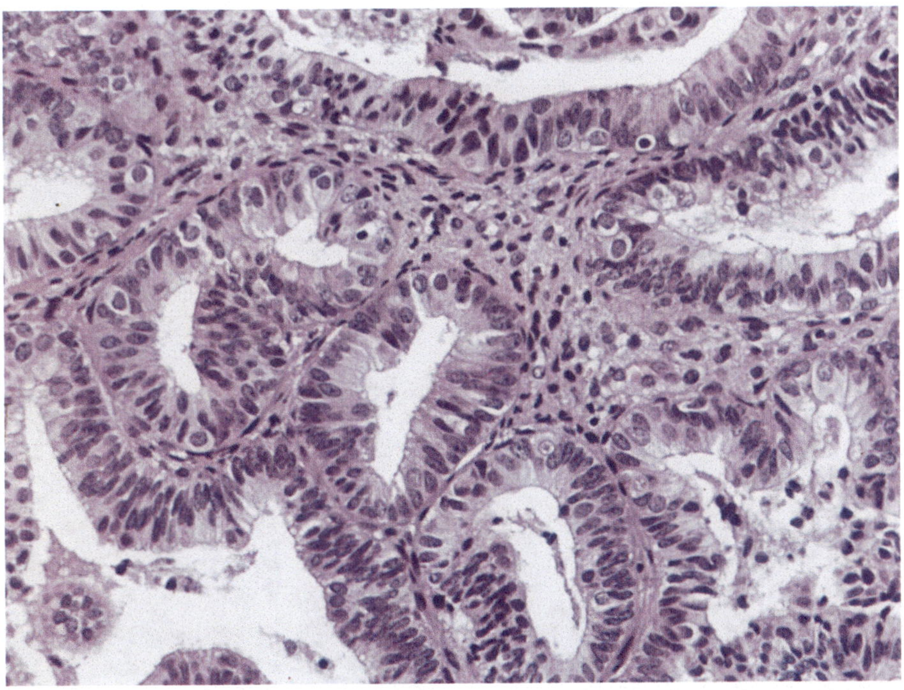

Fig. 6.30 Atypical hyperplasia, H & E, ×250

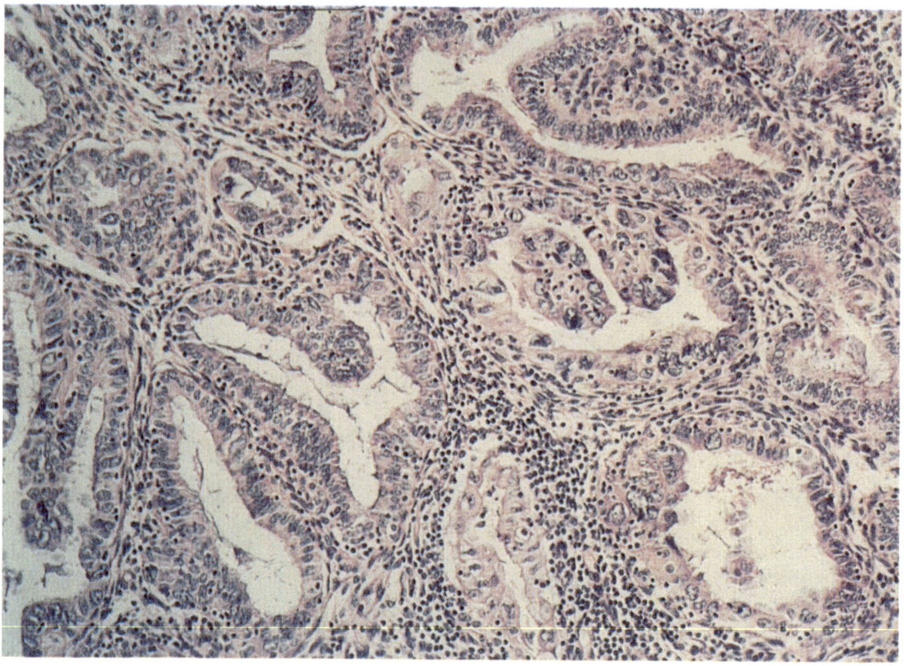

Fig. 6.31 Atypical hyperplasia with cytologic atypia. H & E, ×100

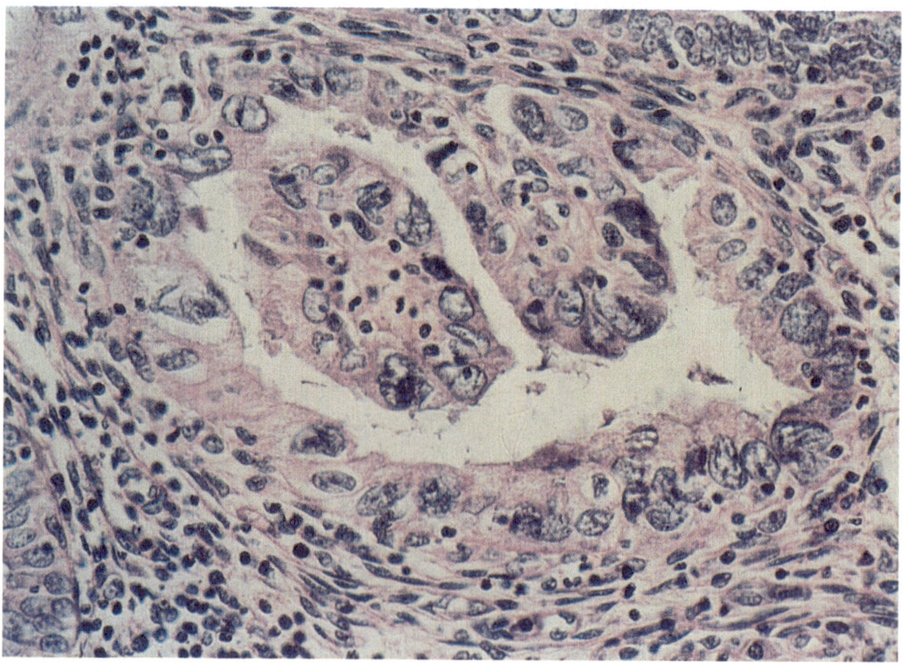

Fig. 6.32 Higher magnification of Fig. 6.31. H & E, ×350

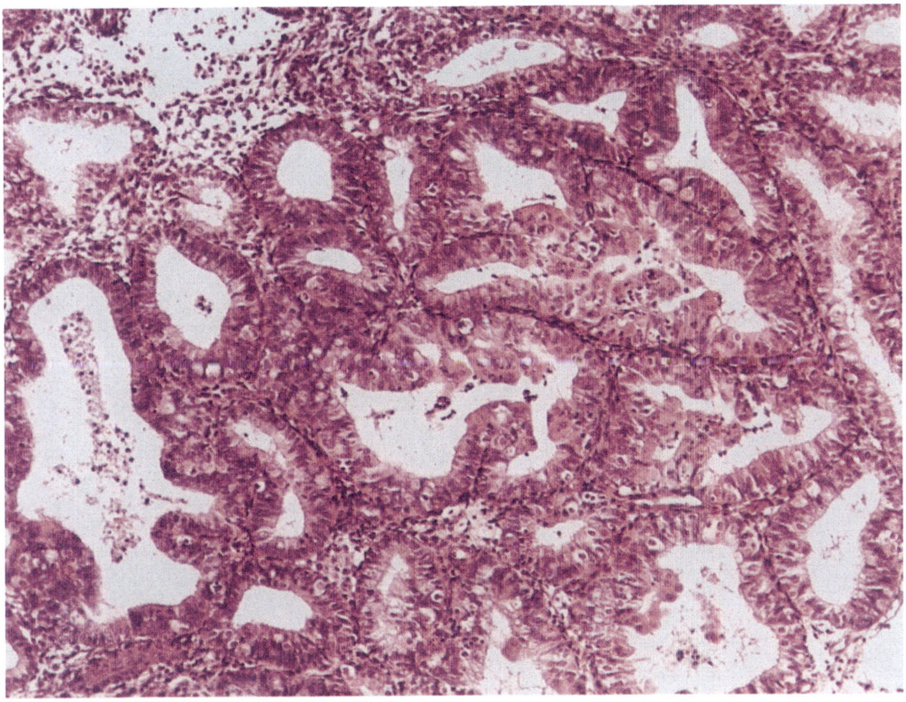

Fig. 6.33 Atypical hyperplasia. H & E, ×100

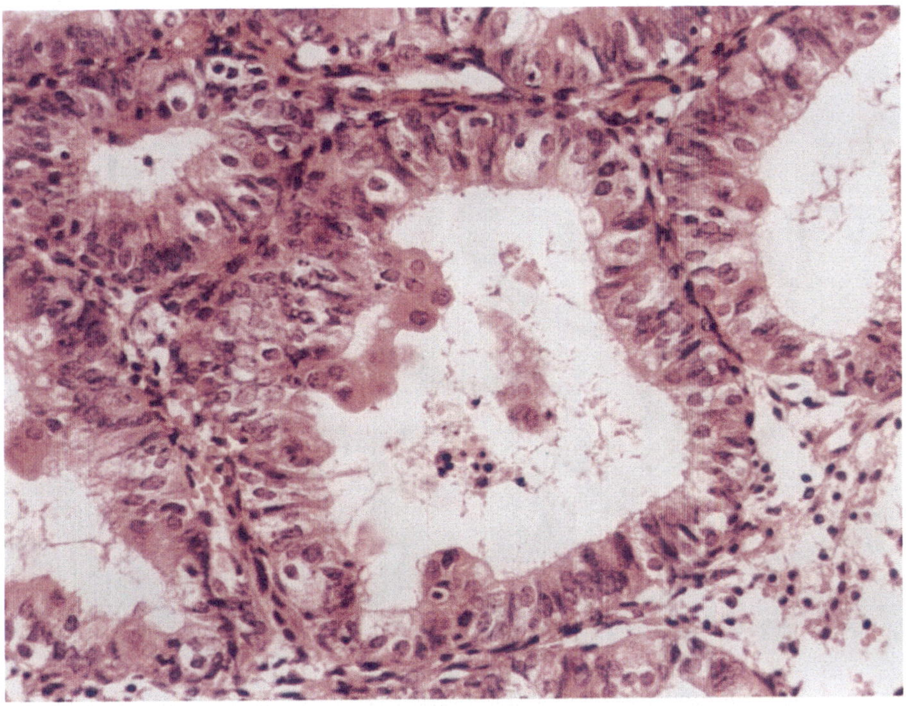

Fig. 6.34 Higher magnification of Fig. 6.33. H & E, ×250

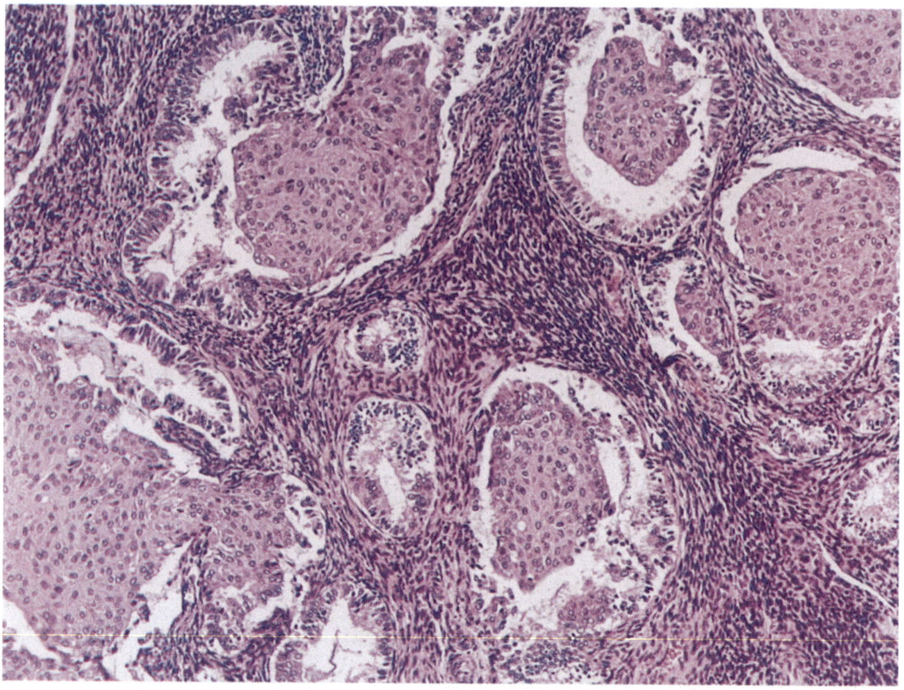

Fig. 6.35 Complex hyperplasia with squamous metaplasia (morules). H & E, ×100

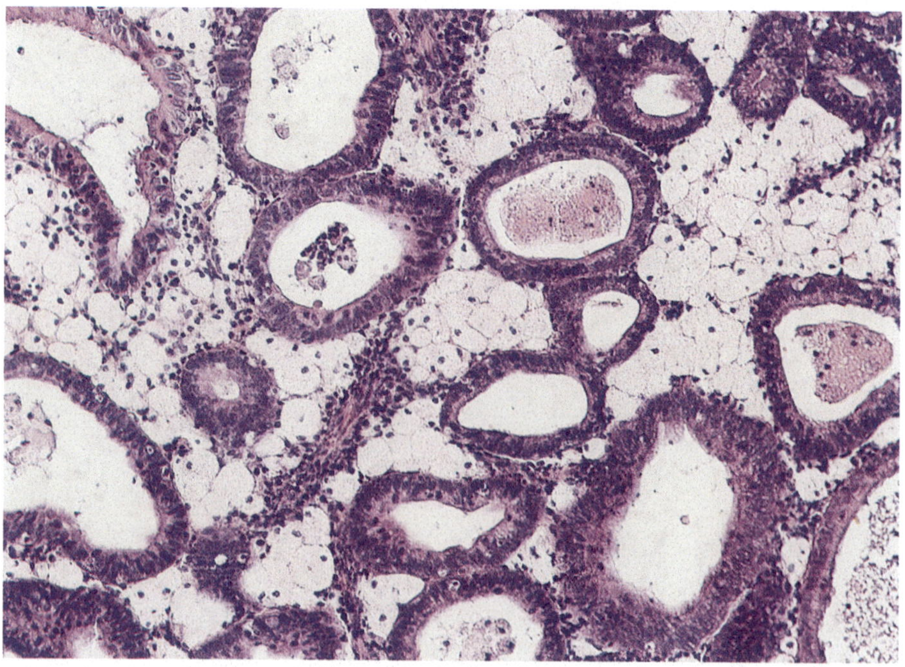

Fig. 6.36 Complex hyperplasia with stromal foam cells. H & E, ×150

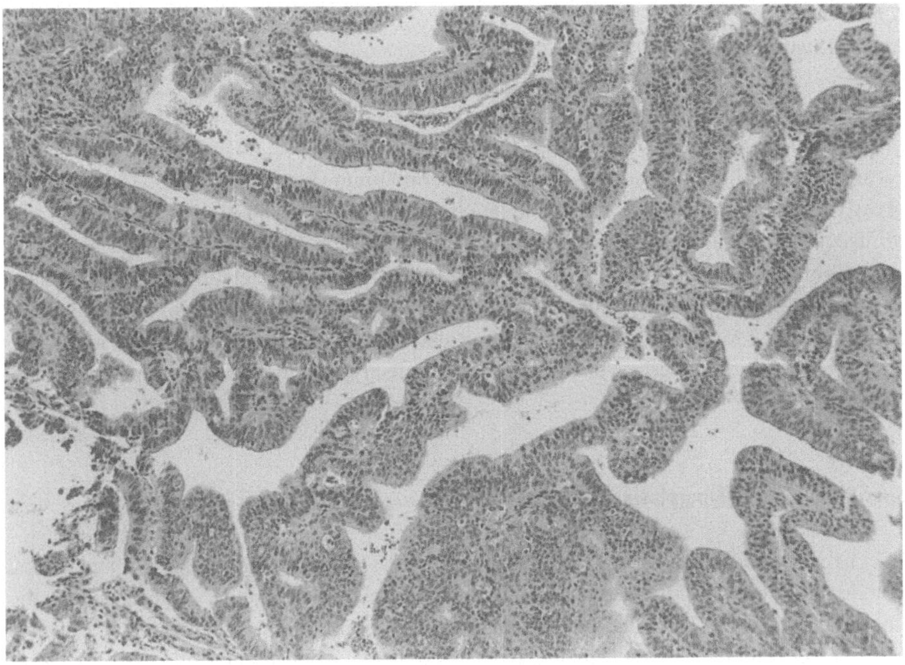

Fig. 6.37 Complex (adenomatous) hyperplasia (MSI) in a young patient with genetic instability. H & E, ×100

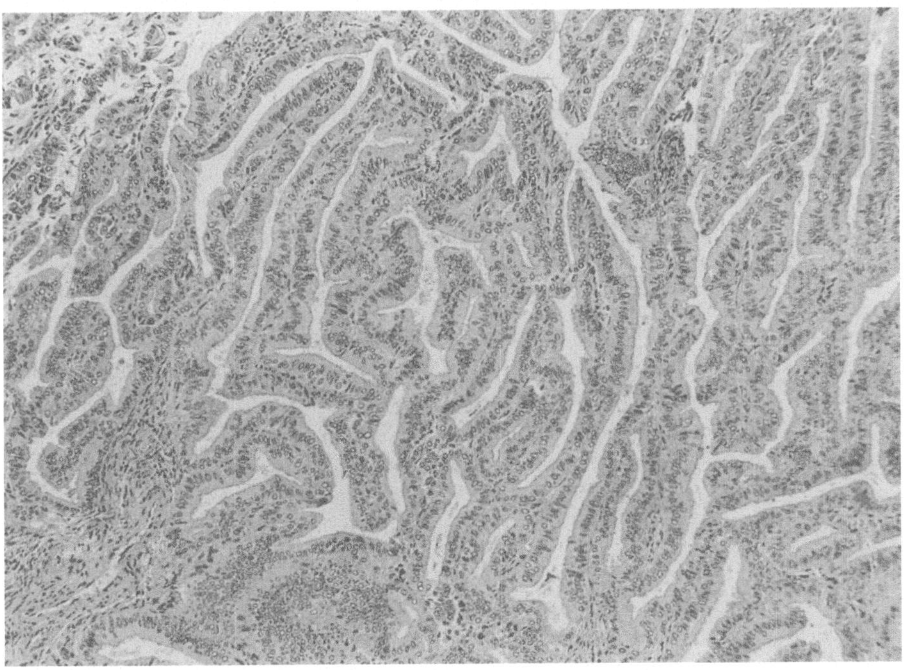

Fig. 6.38 Complex (adenomatous) hyperplasia (MSS) in a young patient with indistinct signs of luteinization. H & E, ×100

6.2.2 Atypical Hyperplasia

The atypical hyperplasia (Figs. 6.29–6.34) shows diffuse and extensive adenomatous growth with focal early microalveolar formation, increased pseudostratification or stratification, and intraluminal budding of glandular epithelium (Figs. 6.29, 6.30). The stroma is greatly reduced in most areas, resulting in a back-to-back position of the glands. There are *diffuse* architectural alterations of glands, and, in addition, areas with atypical glandular epithelium (Figs. 6.31–6.34). Large, rounded, depolarized nuclei of various chromatin density are surrounded by pale eosinophilic cytoplasm with reduced amounts of RNA (McKay et al. 1956). Consequently, there is also obvious cytologic atypia (Kurman et al. 1985). However, we have never observed a "simple atypical hyperplasia" (WHO 2003).

6.2.3 Special Findings in Hyperplasia

Foci of *squamous metaplasia* (Fig. 6.35) that replace the glandular epithelium and fill the glandular lumina develop in some endometrial hyperplasias as an individual reaction to the unopposed estrogen stimulation. The metaplastic cells contain regular nuclei in fairly abundant eosinophilic cytoplasm and are not neoplastic. They are not fully matured, however, and are devoid of intercellular bridges. Mitoses are infrequent.

Groups of *foam cells* (Fig. 6.36) may be found in the stroma of over 50% of the complex and atypical hyperplasias. They are of stromal origin and have stored lipids, which from their histochemical reactions are consistent with being cholesterol esters or estrogen derivatives (Dallenbach-Hellweg 1964; Dallenbach and Rudolph 1974). Their presence indicates high, unopposed estrogen levels. Foam cells also occur, but in a smaller percentage in simple hyperplasia, and they may persist in adenocarcinoma (Figs 9.8, 9.9).

6.2.4 Genetic Instability

In young patients below the age of 40 approximately one third of complex and atypical hyperplasias show on DNA sequencing an MMR deficiency resulting in a microsatellite instability (MSI) with a likely 100% chance of progression to invasive endometrioid carcinoma (p. 154) in contrast to microsatellite stable (MSS) hyperplasias (Figs. 6.37, 6.38) with a much lower progression rate (Sutter et al. 2003) and a high rate of regression under endogenous or exogenous progesterone stimulation in these patients, as previous studies have shown (Dallenbach-Hellweg et al. 1971; Fechner and Kaufman 1974; Moukhtar et al. 1977; Lee and Scully 1989). Microsatellite analysis therefore is a useful prognostic marker in young patients with complex and atypical hyperplasia, particularly in view of their family planning.

6.2.5
Clinical and Morphologic Distinction of Complex and Atypical Hyperplasia

Clinical Possibilities. (a) Estrogen overstimulation by long-standing unopposed endogenous estrogen production, as in persistent anovulation (polycystic ovary syndrome), ovarian tumors, ovarian stromal hyperplasia, adrenals, estrogen storage or production in fatty tissue, impaired estrogen metabolism by liver damage, long-standing estrogen therapy. Distinction is possible by evaluating the clinical history. (b) Genetic instability (MSI).

Morphologic Differential Diagnosis. Endometrial hyperplasia due to exogenous estrogen may be recognized by its focal distribution with considerable variation in morphologic appearance and by an excess of squamous metaplasia and foam cells. Atypical hyperplasia must be distinguished from early carcinoma which may already have developed focally (see p. 147). Multiple sections from the complete specimen must therefore be carefully screened for signs of early stromal invasion (Widra et al. 1995). The criteria for the distinction from early stromal invasion (see Figs. 9.1, 9.2) are listed under the discussion of early stromal invasion (see p. 147). In young patients, molecular genetic tests for MSI are advisable.

6.2.6
Hyperplasia of Glands and Stroma

In this condition (Figs. 6.39, 6.40) endometrial glands have the same appearance as in complex hyperplasia. The endometrial stroma, however, instead of being rarefied, is also hyperplastic. It consists of undifferentiated, enlarged, spindle-shaped, densely distributed cells with oval nuclei rich in DNA and sparse cytoplasm rich in RNA. Mitoses are frequent in both glandular and stromal cells. Spiral arterioles may be present (Fig. 6.40), but are not prominent (Hanson 1959).

Morphologic Differential Diagnosis. This type of hyperplasia must be differentiated from a predecidual change of the stroma, as is occasionally observed under gestagen stimulation of a complex hyperplasia, where the stromal cells are not undifferentiated but contain round nuclei and eosinophilic cytoplasm with low RNA content.

Distinction from atypical polypoid adenomyoma of the endometrium is possible by the identification of smooth muscle cells between the proliferating glands (caldesmon stain).

Clinical Possibilities. The same as in complex hyperplasia. The additional stromal hyperplasia is considered to be an individual variation due to the extensive stimulation by estrogen or its metabolic products.

6.2.7
Focal Hyperplasia

Focal hyperplasia (Figs. 6.41, 6.42) differs from the diffuse form only by its limitation to one or a few areas of the endometrium, which are usually located in the lower layers close

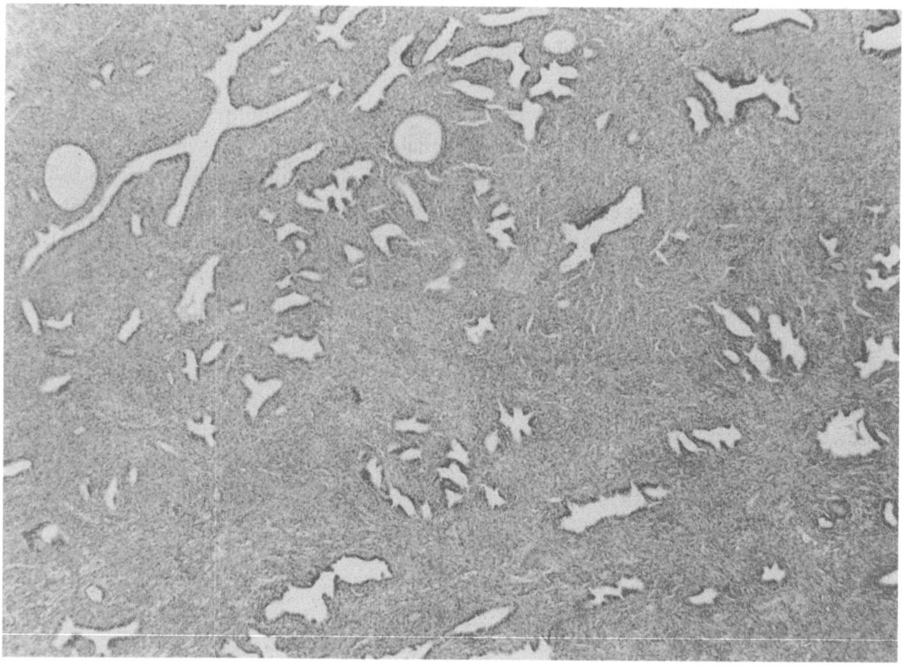

Fig. 6.39 Hyperplasia of glands and stroma. H & E, ×25

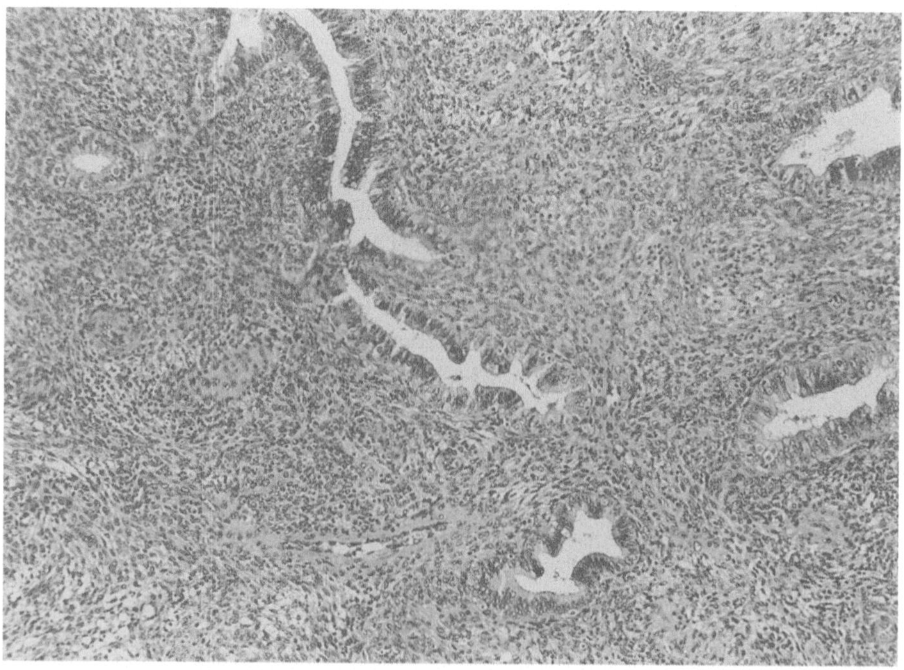

Fig. 6.40 Hyperplasia of glands and stroma. H & E, ×100

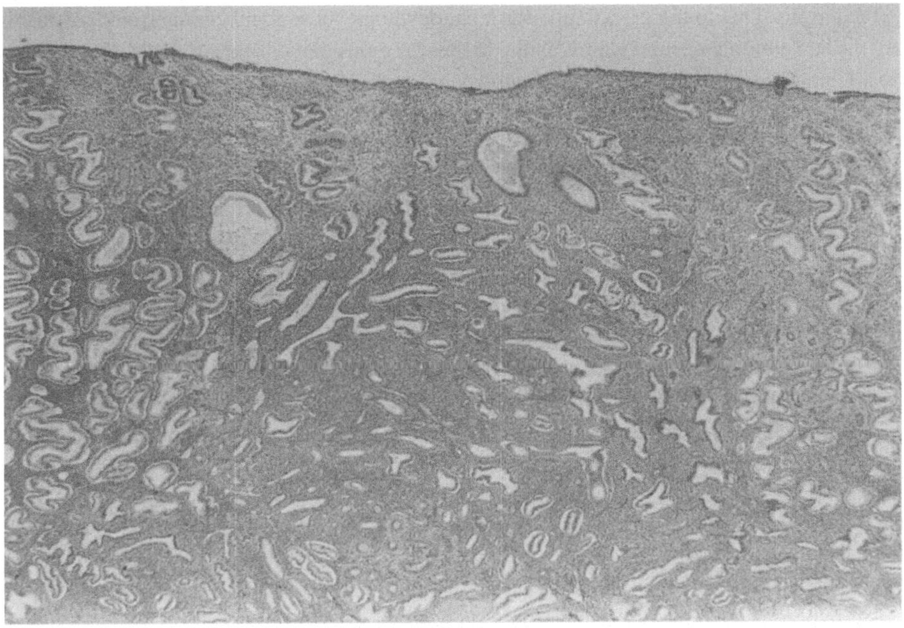

Fig. 6.41 Focal hyperplasia of glands and stroma. H & E, ×25

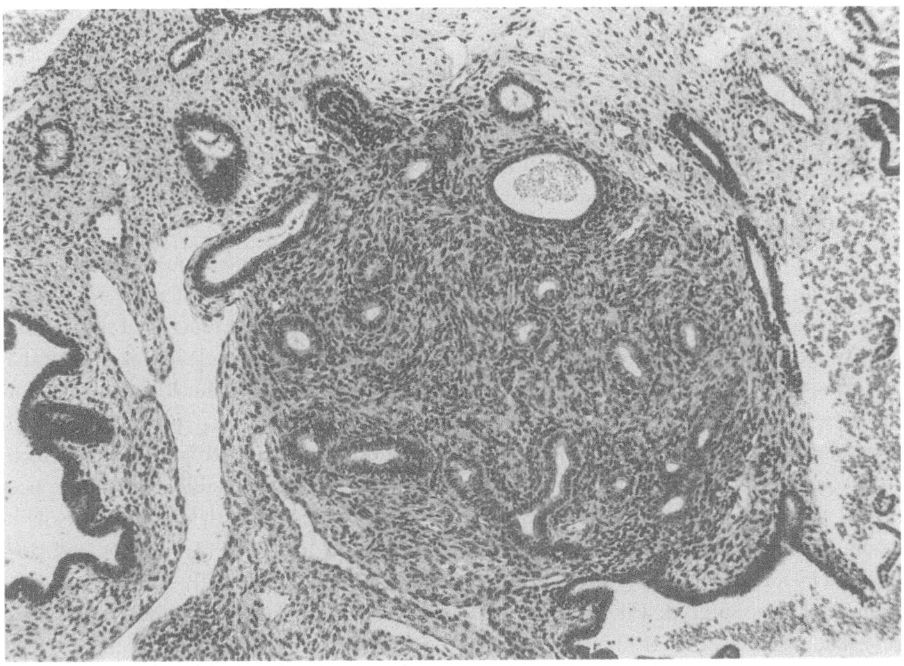

Fig. 6.42 Focal hyperplasia, mainly stromal. H & E, ×100

to the basalis. Due to the growth pressure that develops, these foci become rounded, pushing the surrounding normal glands aside. In these regions glands and stroma are hyperplastic and undifferentiated. Noteworthy is the dense packing of stromal cells within the focus of hyperplasia (Fig. 6.42). Focal hyperplasias are not shed with menstruation, but instead are pushed upwards by the regenerating endometrium of subsequent cycles to become precursors of endometrial polyps.

Morphologic Differential Diagnosis. If isolated areas of focal hyperplasia are found in curettings, they must be differentiated from polyps; these are usually covered by surface epithelium, which is not present in focal hyperplasia. In addition, polyps can be recognized with the van Gieson stain by their fibrous stroma (see Figs. 6.49, 6.50).

Clinical Possibilities and Differential Diagnosis. (a) Focal reactivity of endometrium to estrogens, while the surrounding endometrium has lost its estrogen receptor affinity; (b) focal loss of progesterone receptors with normal receptor content of surrounding endometrium.

Distinction is possible by observing the functional state of the surrounding endometrium.

6.2.8 Basal Hyperplasia

Basal hyperplasia shows the same structural features as focal hyperplasia. It may be diffuse (Fig. 6.43) or focal (Fig. 6.44) and may still be covered by the secreting endometrium which is pushed upwards. By growing up, a diffuse simple or complex hyperplasia, or, when focal, an endometrial polyp may develop.

Clinical Possibilities. The same as in focal hyperplasia (see above).

6.2.9 Endometrial Polyps

Endometrial polyps (Figs. 6.45–6.50) represent a monoclonal neoplastic proliferation of stromal cells incorporating usually a non-neoplastic glandular component. They may have a broad base (Fig. 6.45) or may be predunculated (Fig. 6.46) with a central fibrovascular core which, when visible in the plane of the section, will be a characteristic diagnostic sign. There is no universally accepted classification of endometrial polyps, but generally hyperplastic (Figs. 6.45, 6.46, 6.49, 6.50), atrophic (Figs. 6.47, 6.48) and functional polyps can be distinguished. Some polyps have a cellular fibrous stroma, most clearly seen with the van Gieson stain (Figs. 6.49, 6.50). The hyperplastic polyps may contain areas of simple or complex hyperplasias with and without atypia. They differ from the typical endometrial hyperplasia only by their polypoid shape and their fibrous stroma. Atrophic polyps which are frequently found after tamoxifen therapy have a characteristic histological appearance (Fig. 6.47): their cystic glands are lined by flat, atrophic epithelium with focal CEA-positive mucinous or serous papillary metaplasias (Schlesinger et al. 1998) (Fig. 6.48), and surrounded by a densely fibrotic stroma. The stromal cells may occasionally be focally predecidualized (Nuovo et al. 1989). These polyps are usually pedunculated and resting on a very flat atrophic endometrium (Dallenbach-Hellweg and Schmidt 1998).

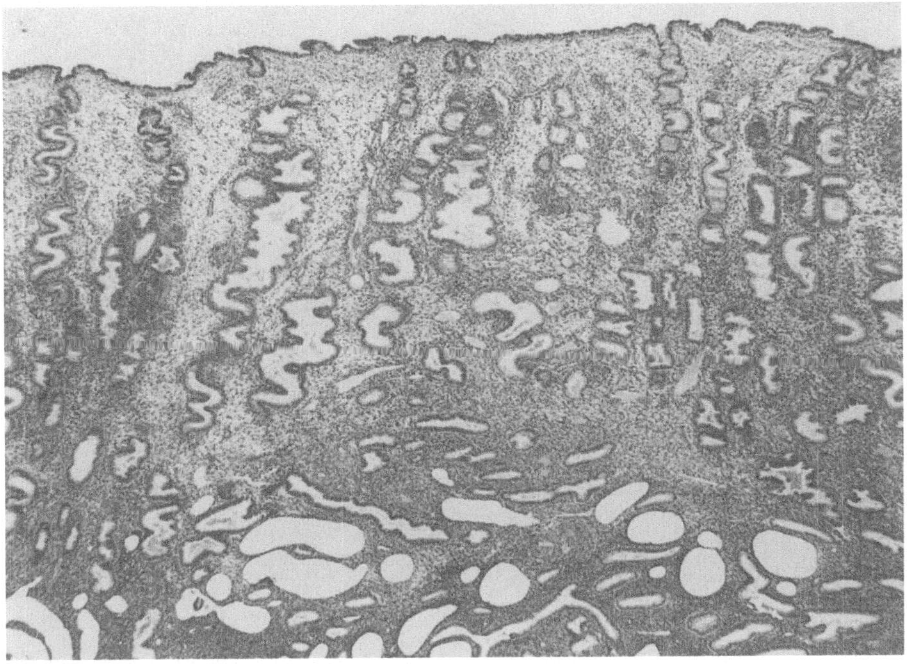

Fig. 6.43 Basal simple hyperplasia, diffuse. H & E, ×25

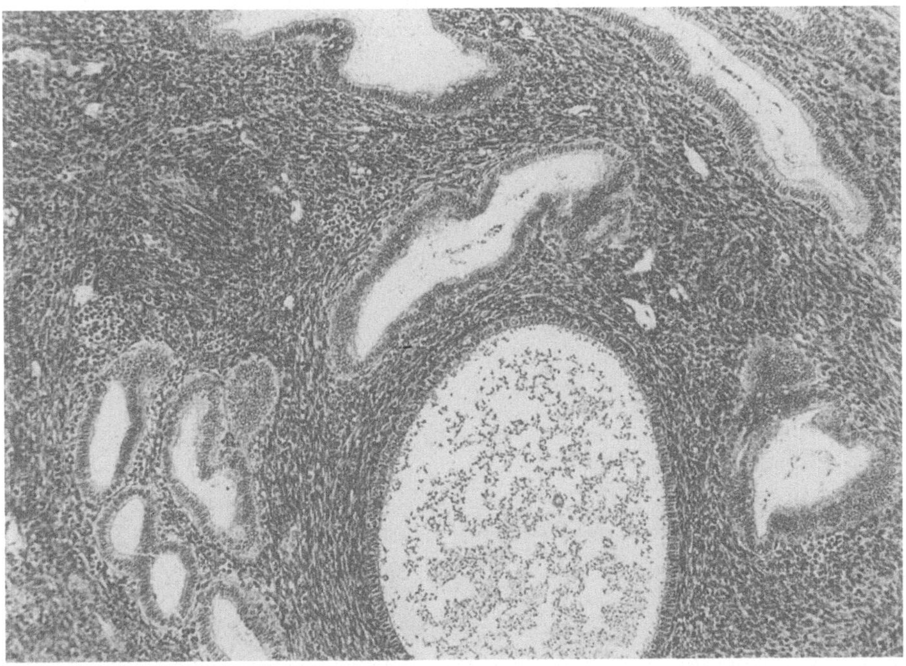

Fig. 6.44 Higher magnification of Fig. 6.43, focal. H & E, ×100

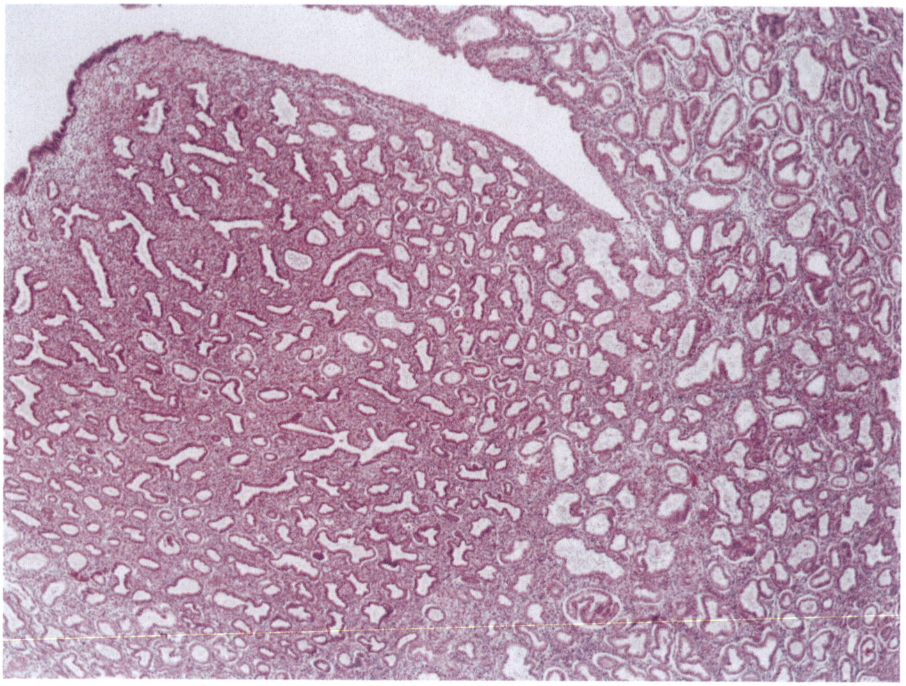

Fig. 6.45 Endometrial polyp, hyperplastic. H & E, ×25

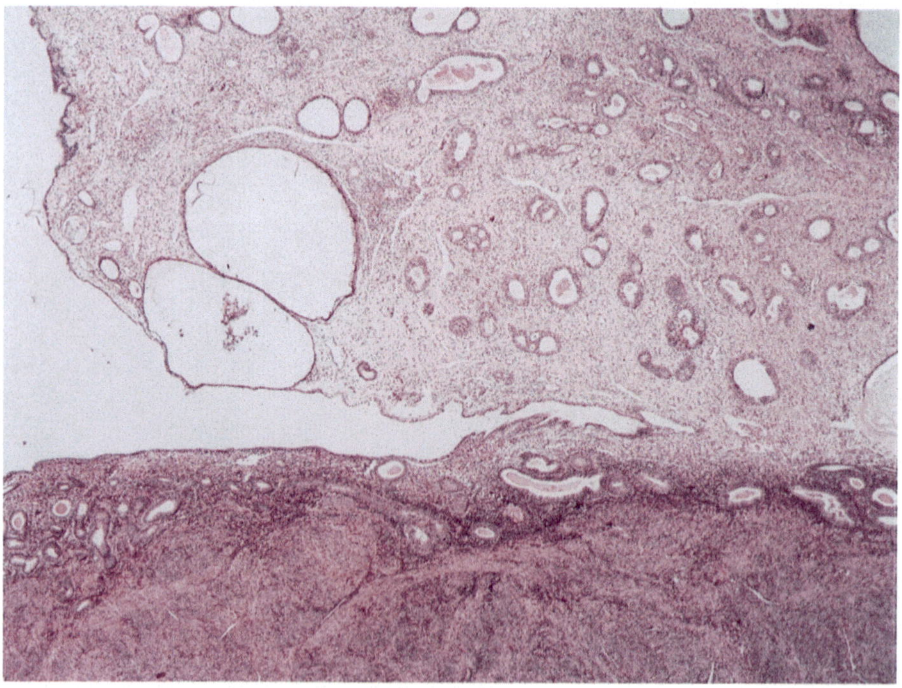

Fig. 6.46 Endometrial polyp, hyperplastic. H & E, ×25

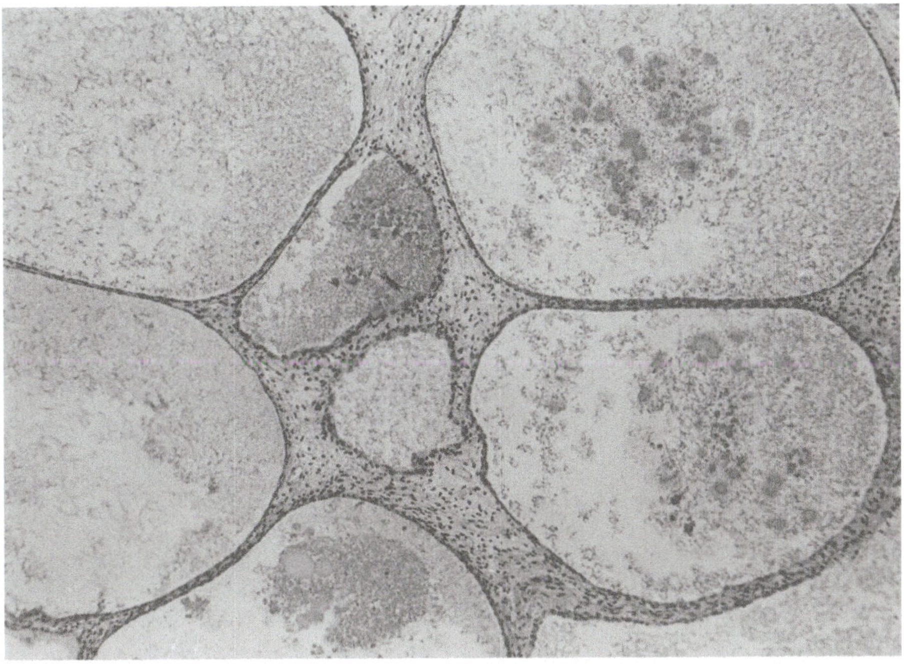

Fig. 6.47 Endometrial polyp, cystic-atrophic, after tamoxifen therapy. H & E, ×100

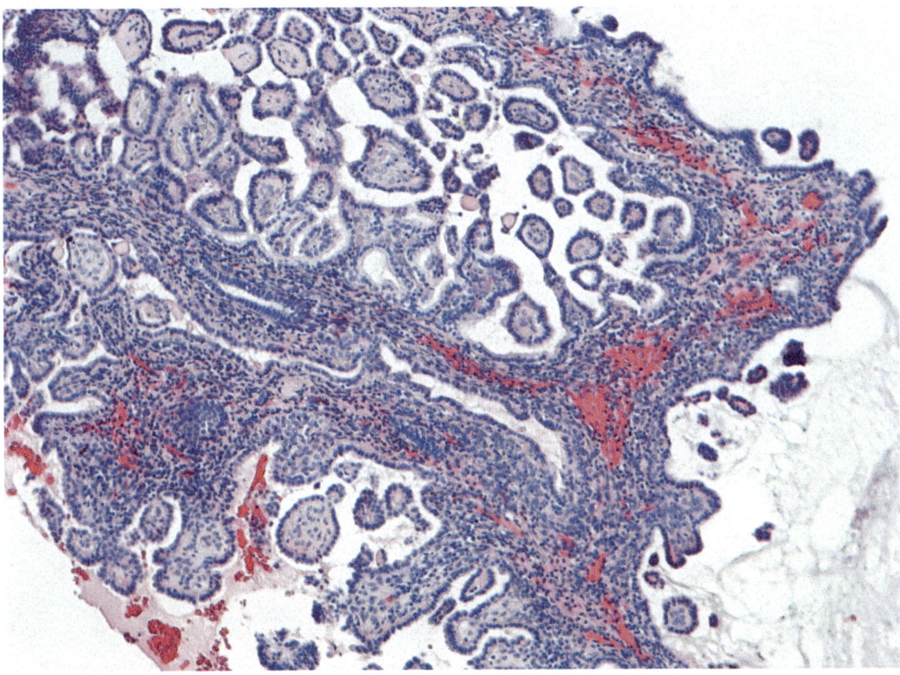

Fig. 6.48 Focal mucinous and papillary metaplasia on the surface of an atrophic endometrial polyp after tamoxifen therapy. H & E, ×75

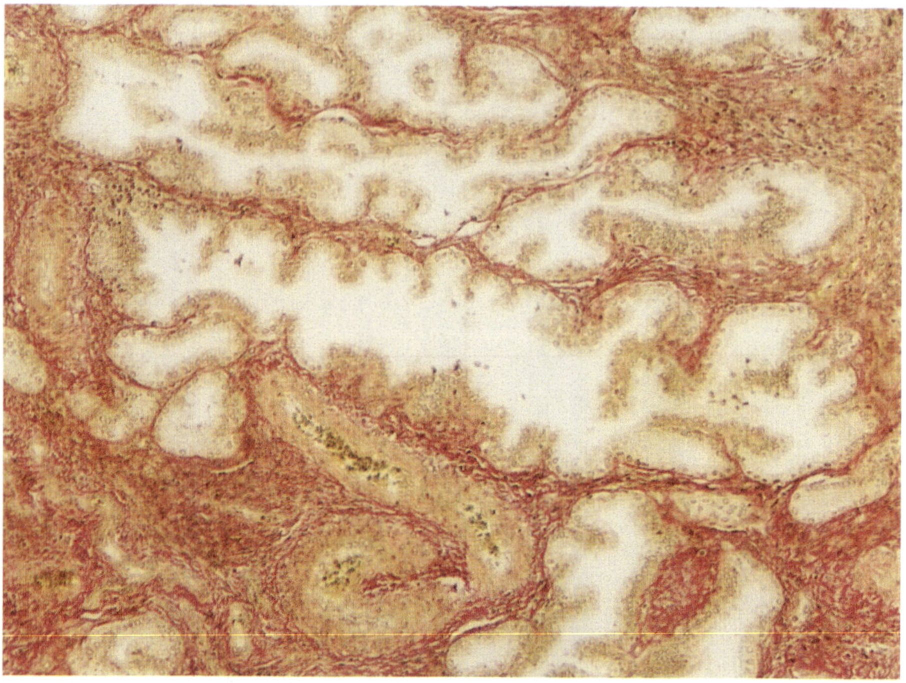

Fig. 6.49 Endometrial polyp, hyperplastic, with secreting glands, van Gieson stain, ×100

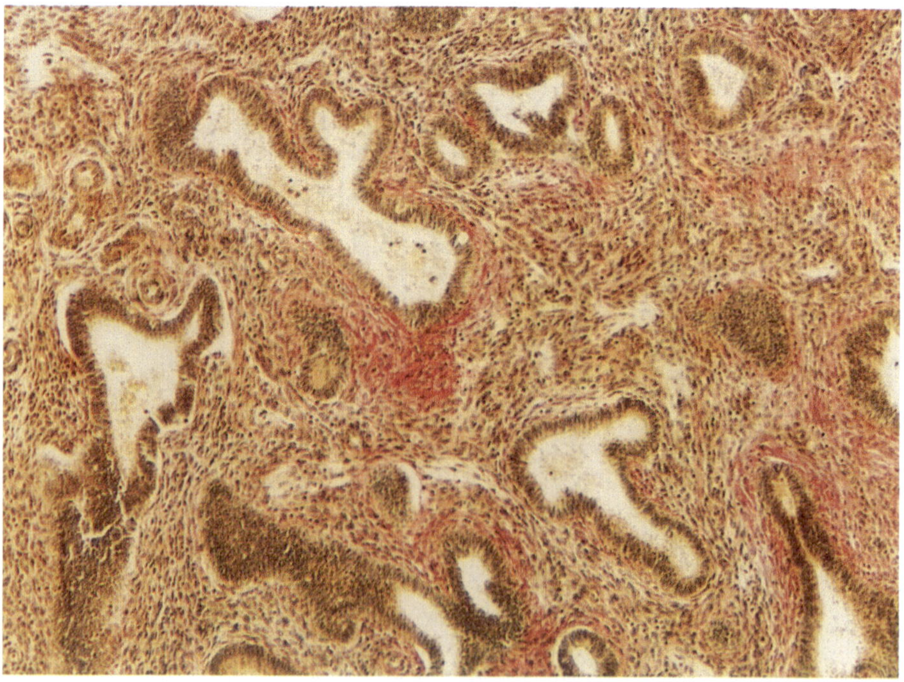

Fig. 6.50 Endometrial polyp, stroma-rich, van Gieson stain, ×100

Morphologic Differential Diagnosis. Endometrial polyps must be distinguished from adenofibroma (see p. 182). Unless a connective tissue stain is used, polyps or portions of them may not be recognized in curettings.

Clinical Possibilities. The same as in focal hyperplasia (see p. 86). Cystic atrophic polyps with dilated glands that are lined by atrophic epithelium are often seen under tamoxifen therapy (see p. 125).

6.3 Ovulatory Disturbances

All abnormalities of corpus luteum function (deficiency, persistence) induce characteristic changes in the endometrium.

6.3.1 Deficient Secretory Phase

Deficient secretory phase is a functional disturbance that causes infertility and is usually associated with an insufficient corpus luteum (Dallenbach-Hellweg 1995). The deviation from normal function varies according to the degree of insufficiency, which may have central or ovarian causes. The deficient cycle may be of normal length or shortened with early breakdown of the corpus luteum (short luteal phase). Since the result of treatment for this type of infertility depends on the accuracy of its diagnosis, a precise differentiation between the various patterns of the deficient secretory phase is of paramount importance (Gigon et al. 1970; Dallenbach-Hellweg 1984; see Table 6.1 on p. 60). Occasionally, two biopsies within the same cycle may be helpful for precise interpretation.

For a more extensive discussion of the endocrinological background of this and other ovulatory disturbances, see Runnebaum and Rabe (1994).

Deficient Secretory Phase with Dissociated Delay

In deficient secretory phase with dissociated delay (the most frequent type of deficient secretory phase; Figs. 6.51–6.54), there are unevenly spaced, poorly convoluted glands, a variation in the development of glands and stroma from region to region, and a dissociation of development between glands and their surrounding stroma. The specimen shown was taken on the 27th day of a menstrual cycle. Only very few glands even roughly correspond with the day of the cycle. Others are convoluted, lined by cells, which either still contain elongated, chromatin-rich nuclei in a sparse cytoplasm, or which have rounded nuclei with occasional basal vacuoles remaining in their cytoplasm. The secretion in the glandular lumina may have just begun or be advanced or inspissated, and the lumina may also vary in width. Some glands are straight, narrow, and lined by undifferentiated proliferative epithelium. The stromal cells are either spindle shaped and poorly differentiated or large and separated by focal edema. There are also occasional small hemorrhages. The spiral arterioles are small and underdeveloped. The general height of the endometrium varies slightly, and the surface epithelium is tall and columnar. The content of DNA, RNA, glycogen, and mucopolysaccharides in glandular and stromal cells chiefly corresponds to

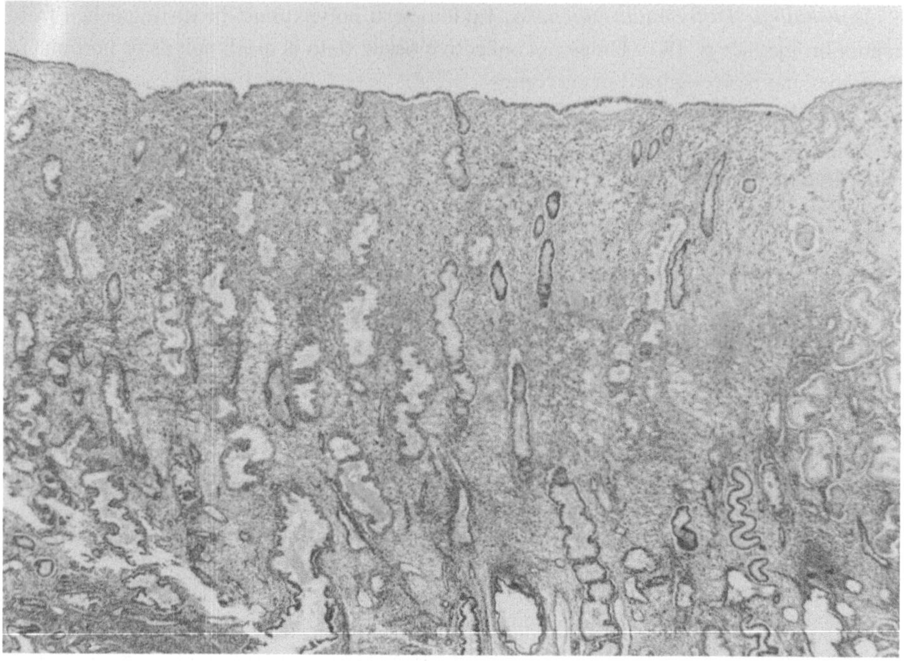

Fig. 6.51 Deficient secretory phase with dissociated delay. H & E, ×25

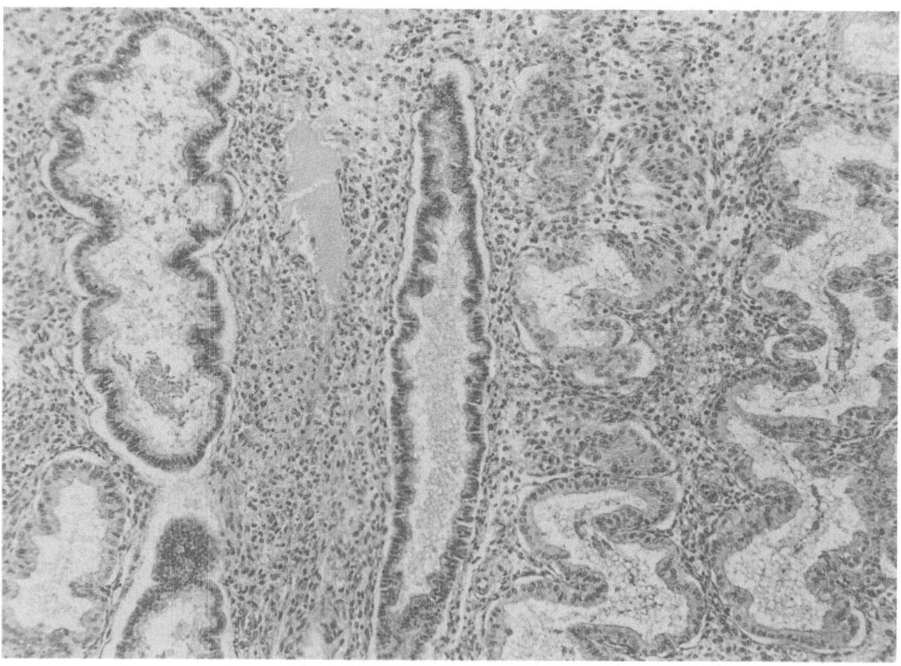

Fig. 6.52 Deficient secretory phase with dissociated delay. H & E, ×100

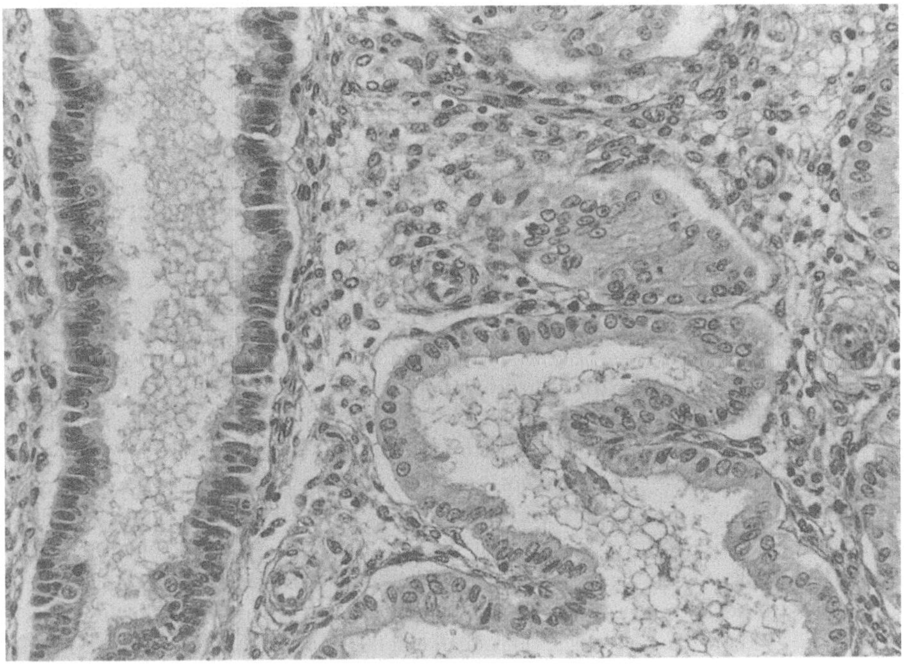

Fig. 6.53 Deficient secretory phase with dissociated delay. H & E, ×250

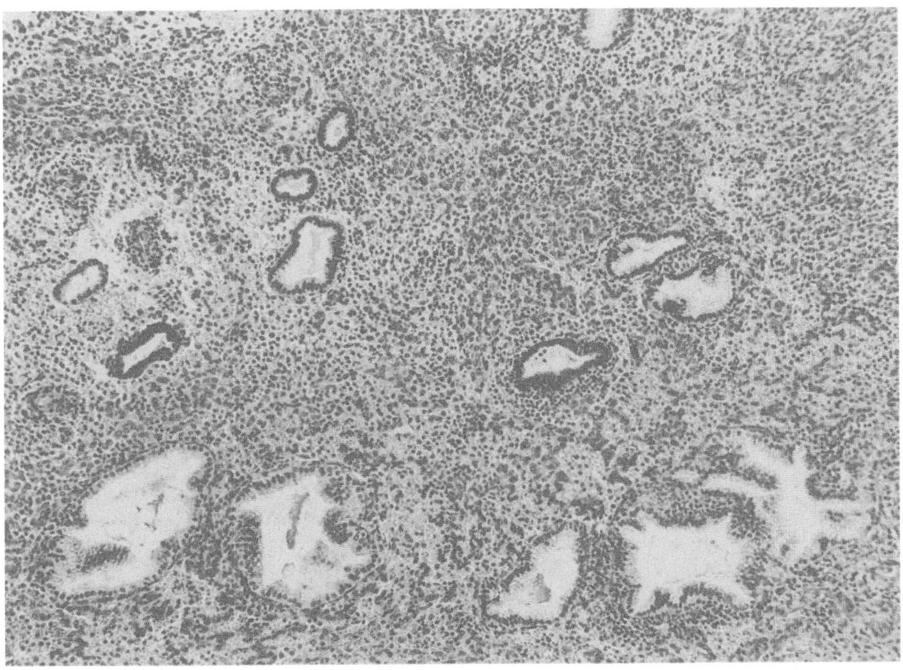

Fig. 6.54 Protracted shedding after deficient secretory phase. H & E, ×100

the degree of differentiation, as compared with the normal cycle, and therefore also varies from area to area (Hughes et al. 1964; Ancla et al. 1967; Gore and Gordon 1974).

Clinical Possibilities. (a) Deficient secretory phase due to ovarian insufficiency caused by a genetic or non-genetic ovarian or hypothalamic defect: inadequate luteinization and progesterone synthesis of granulosa cells, or suppression of progesterone release by hyperprolactinemia (this condition may be preceded by a deficient follicle with deficient endometrial proliferation); (b) deficient secretory phase caused by focal endometrial progesterone receptor defects; and (c) irregular secretion caused by a climacteric disturbance in corpus luteum function.

Distinction is possible by exact statement of the day of the menstrual cycle, by determining the plasma levels of follicle-stimulating hormone (FSH), LH, and prolactin, and by considering the general height of the endometrium (low with preceding follicular deficiency).

Deficient Secretory Phase with Coordinated True Delay

Since the morphology of the deficient secretory phase with coordinated true delay (Fig. 6.55) at the end of a menstrual cycle is virtually identical with that of a beginning normal secretory phase, the histological diagnosis can only be made by knowing the exact day of the cycle. For histologic details, we refer to Figs. 3.9 and 3.10, which could show a deficient secretory phase with coordinated true delay if taken not at the 16th but at the 26th, 27th, or 28th day of the cycle. In occasional instances when the preceding proliferation is insufficient, the glands are small and narrow, the basal glycogen vacuoles barely reach normal size, and the stromal cells remain small and undifferentiated (Fig. 6.55).

Clinical Possibilities. (a) Deficient secretory phase with coordinated true delay due to a central (hypothalamic) defect with inadequate stimulation of granulosa cells, or to an ovarian defect with impaired follicular development, or to a diffuse defect of endometrial

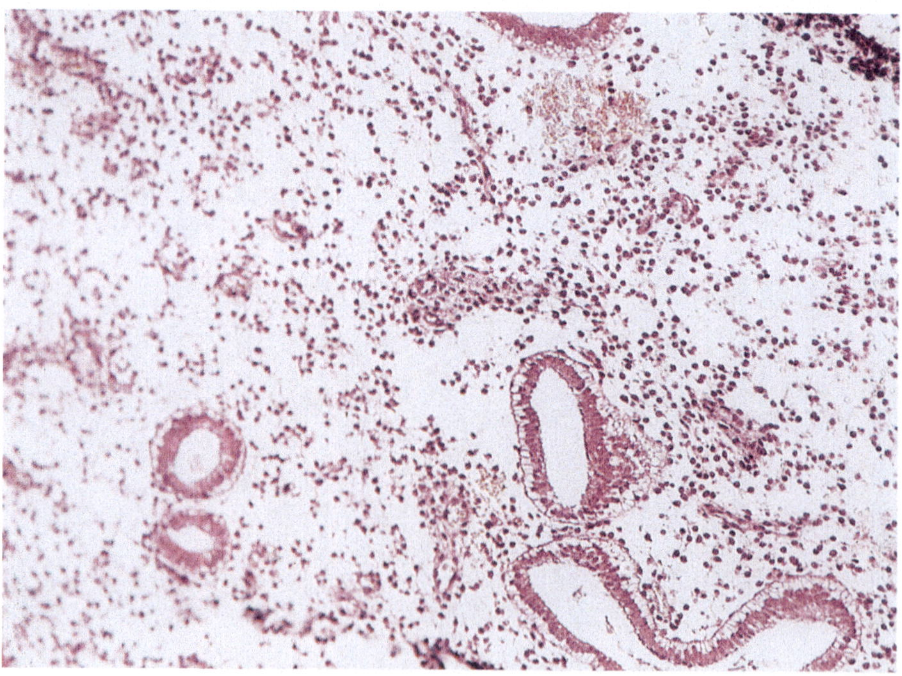

Fig. 6.55 Deficient secretory phase with coordinated true delay. H & E, ×100

progesterone receptor; (b) normal secretory phase on the 16th day of a menstrual cycle (second day after ovulation); (c) early structural changes following sequential therapy with oral contraceptives (see p. 124).

Distinction between (a) and (b) can be made by exact determination of the day of the menstrual cycle; the causes of the deficiency can be determined by measuring the plasma levels of FSH and LH.

Deficient Secretory Phase with Coordinated Apparent Delay

In deficient secretory phase with coordinated apparent delay (Figs. 6.56, 6.57), the functional disturbance is preceded by a persistent follicle with irregular proliferation and late ovulation; the secretory changes that are induced by ovulation are therefore only apparently delayed, not delayed in relation to the day of ovulation. The general height of the endometrium is considerable, but irregular. Part of the glands are cystically dilated, others narrow and only occasionally slightly convoluted. The glandular epithelium shows the beginning of secretion with basal glycogen vacuoles and slightly rounded nuclei corresponding to the second day after ovulation in a normal secretory phase. There is only slight variation in the size and extent of basal vacuoles, which are more pronounced in the glands not cystically dilated. The stromal cells are spindle shaped or large and separated by focal edema. Spiral arterioles are present and only underdeveloped focally.

Clinical Possibilities. (a) Deficient secretory phase with coordinated apparent delay due to a central defect in LH stimulation, e.g., hyperprolactinemia with a delayed LH peak following follicular persistency with overproduction of estrogen; (b) irregular proliferation in the postmenopausal age period with sporadic luteinization of a follicular cyst, or following therapy with small amounts of gestagen.

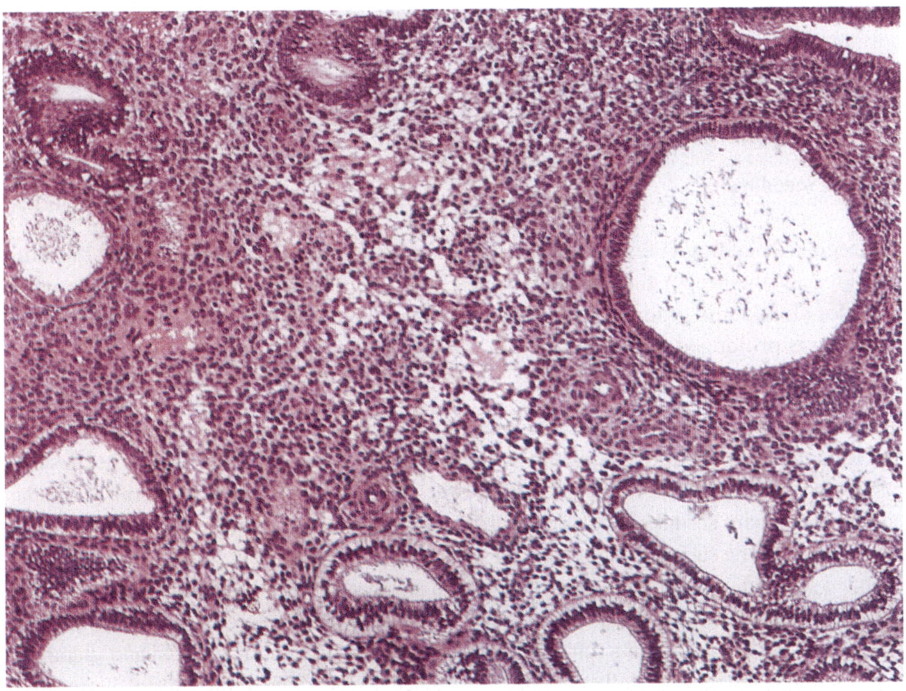

Fig. 6.56 Deficient secretory phase with coordinated apparent delay. H & E, ×100

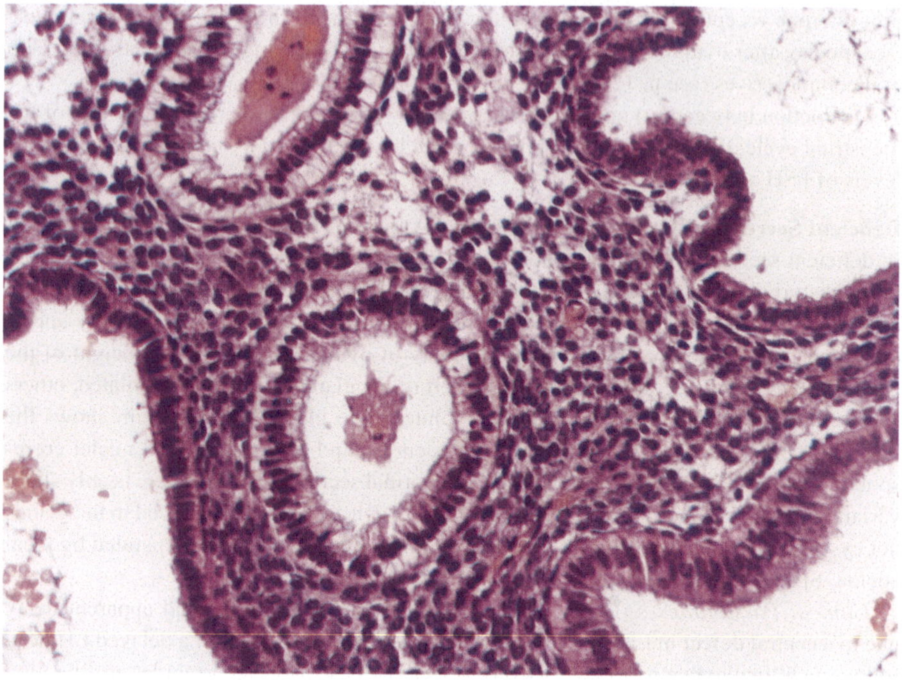

Fig. 6.57 Deficient secretory phase with coordinated apparent delay. H & E, ×250

Distinction is possible when the age of the patient, the menstrual history, and any given hormone therapy are known and, if necessary, by additional measurement of plasma levels of LH, FSH, and prolactin.

6.3.2 Irregular Shedding

In irregular shedding (Figs. 6.58–6.65), the corpus luteum develops normally but fails to regress at the proper time and continues to secrete progesterone until this secretion subsides slowly and gradually. Consequently, endometrial regression is protracted and shedding is prolonged and irregular.

Early Stages

In the early stages, there are patchy foci of hemorrhagic dissociation (Fig. 6.58) and, between these, preserved glands are seen, which have become star-shaped because of extensive shrinkage without disintegration (Figs. 6.59, 6.60). The nuclei of the glandular epithelial cells are shrunken with dense chromatin, and their cytoplasm is still fairly abundant and pale. The surrounding preserved stroma consists of densely packed, shrunken, yet rounded stromal cells and granular endometrial stromal cells still retaining their granules, thereby possibly indicating a disturbed function of relaxin (compare p. 33). Consequently, the network of reticulin fibers remains intact (Fig. 6.61), preventing stromal and glandular dissociation (Dallenbach-Hellweg and Bornebusch 1970). The spiral arterioles are often thrombosed, in part because of the prolonged bleeding.

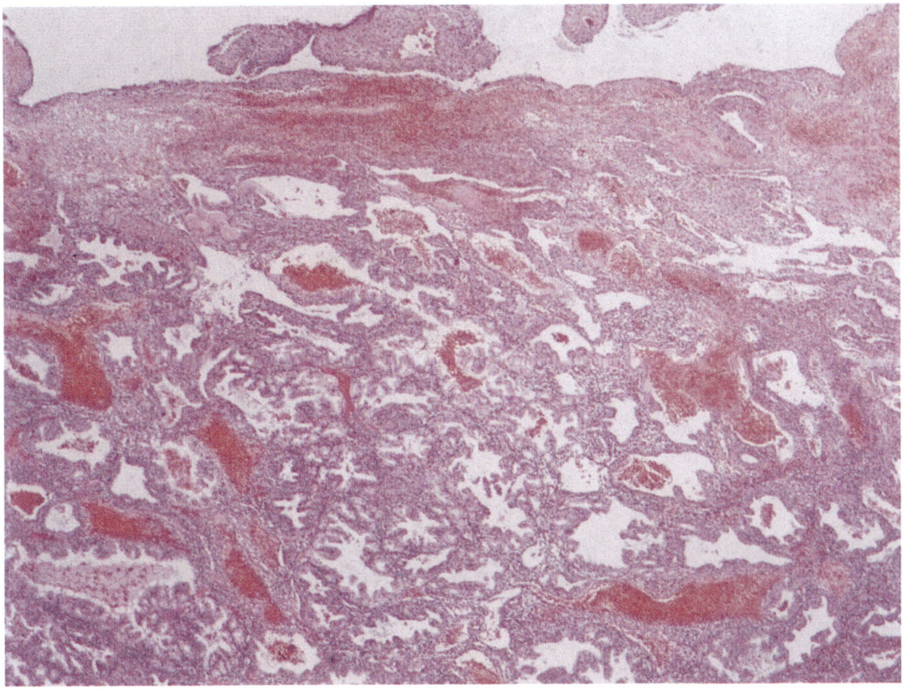

Fig. 6.58 Irregular shedding, early stage. H & E, ×25

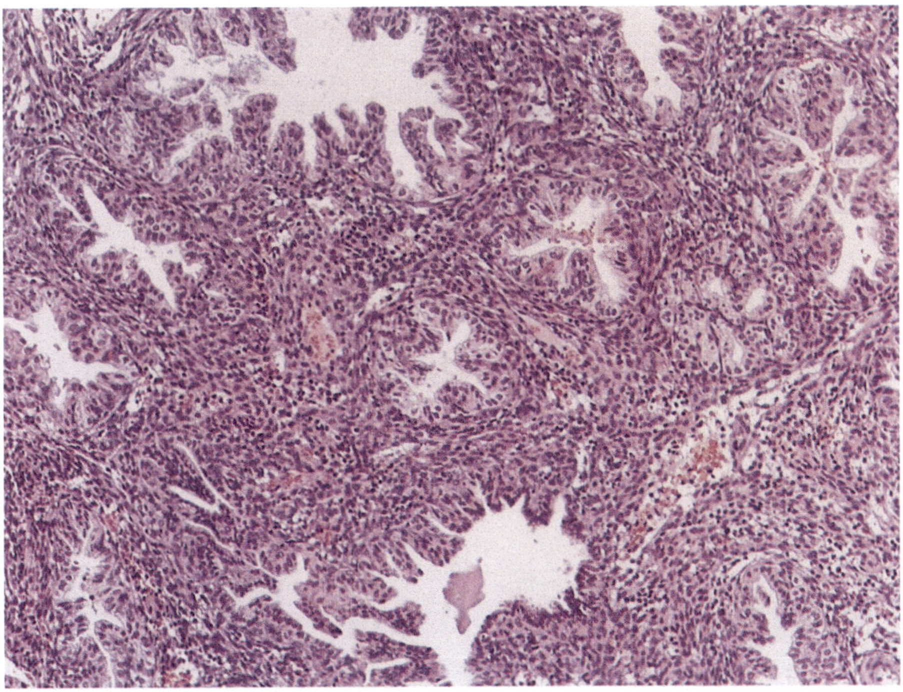

Fig. 6.59 Irregular shedding, early stage. H & E, ×100

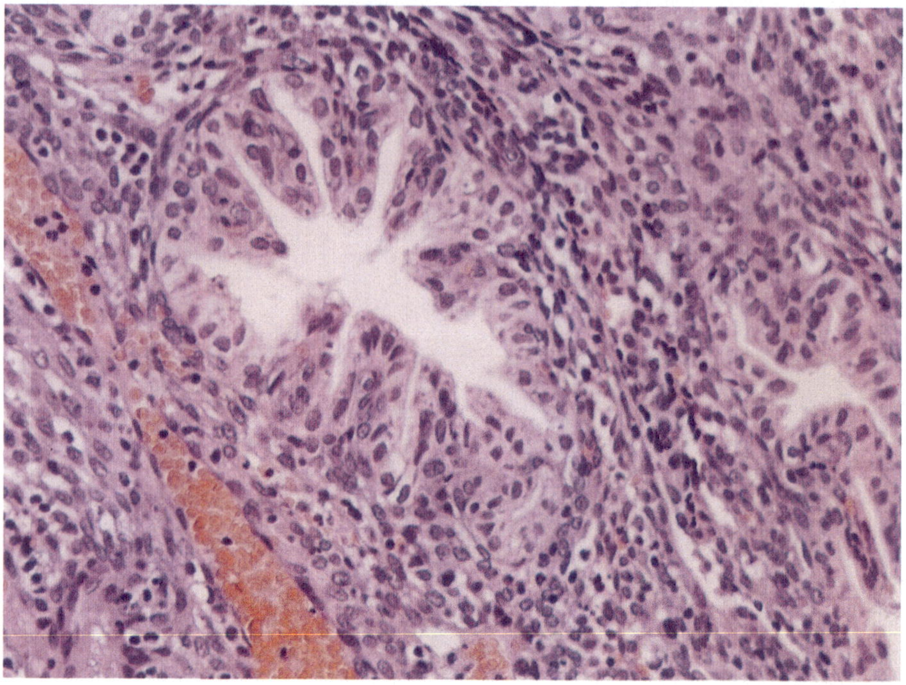

Fig. 6.60 Irregular shedding, early stage. H & E, ×250

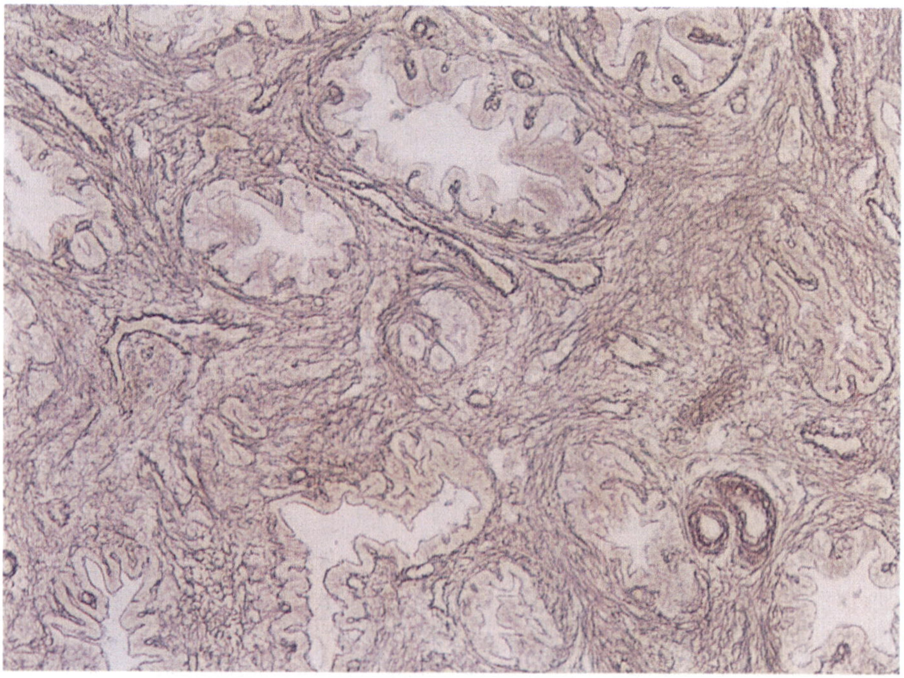

Fig. 6.61 Irregular shedding, early stage, Reticulum stain, ×100

Late Stages

In the late stages, larger regions of the endometrium undergo disintegration and hemorrhagic necrosis. The intervening regions, however, are still intact. Their glands are further regressed, and their original star shape is less pronounced but still apparent.

The nuclei of the lining epithelial cells are greatly shrunken and chromatin dense, and the cytoplasm is usually sparse, but more abundant and clearer focally. Occasionally deeper glands may already show regenerative or early proliferative changes, since they will become incorporated into the next cycle. The densely cellular stroma consists of small, spindle-shaped cells (Figs. 6.62, 6.63). Since regeneration of the endometrium takes place only after complete detachment of the shedding portions, the regenerative phase after irregular shedding is greatly prolonged and usually deficient (Philippe and Ritter 1987).

Arias-Stella Reaction

In some instances the glandular epithelial cells are greatly enlarged, yet with chromatin-dense and pleomorphic nuclei abnormally located in a clear cytoplasm. This peculiar change known as the Arias-Stella reaction (Arias-Stella 1954; Figs. 6.64, 6.65) is associated with high levels of gonadotropin produced by viable trophoblast. There may be leukocytic infiltration of the stroma, which is not different from that of irregular shedding without the Arias-Stella phenomenon.

Histologic recognition and differential diagnosis of irregular shedding is not easy for the inexperienced pathologist. The characteristic finding is the diverse admixture of endometrial fragments in various stages of regression and dissociation. The condition must be distinguished morphologically from regressing simple hyperplasia with hemorrhage following secretory transformation; here, part of the glands are still cystically dilated, and star-shaped glands are less conspicuous.

Clinical Possibilities and Differential Diagnosis. (a) Persistence of the corpus luteum by hyperstimulation from placental gonadotropin (in intra- or extrauterine pregnancy when the fetus has died or with hydatidiform mole causing multiple corpus luteum cysts), or from pituitary gonadotropin (during the first post partum or post abortum menstruation or in climacterium); (b) spontaneous polyovulation (Pepler and Fouche 1968); (c) preceding deficient corpus luteum with gradual drop in progesterone secretion (Fig. 6.54); and (d) gestagen therapy before the onset of or during menses (Holmstrom and McLennan 1947).

Distinction is possible and of clinical importance particularly between irregular shedding due to hyperstimulation by placental remnants and that not associated with previous pregnancy; in premenopausal women a positive Arias-Stella reaction is always indicative of a recent intra- or extrauterine abortion, even when placental remnants cannot be found in the curettings. The presence of endometritis or hyalinized arterioles may help differentiate intra- from extrauterine pregnancy, whereas remnants of necrotic decidua may be found in both conditions. In the absence of previous pregnancy, precise clinical data are exceedingly valuable in the accurate interpretation of the underlying cause of irregular shedding.

A positive Arias-Stella reaction with or without irregular shedding may, though rarely, be seen in postmenopausal patients under hormone replacement therapy with gestagen predominance or with tamoxifen (Huettner and Gersell 1994a, b). In such instances, the Arias-Stella reaction must be distinguished (a) from clear cell metaplasia (Fig. 4.7) (lack of nuclear atypia in metaplastic cells) and (b) from clear cell adenocarcinoma (Fig. 9.28) (lack of stromal invasion).

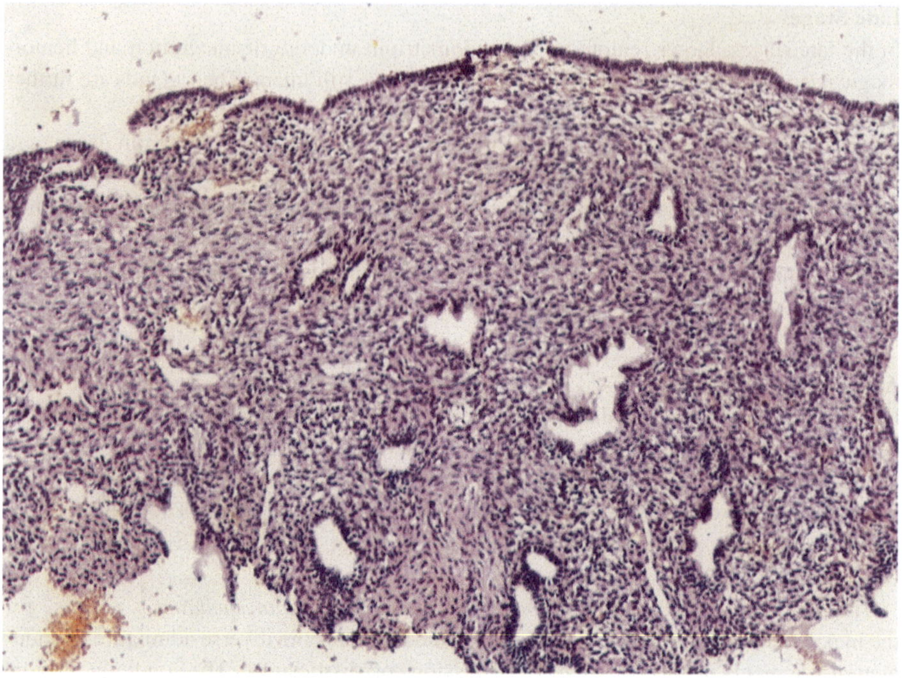

Fig. 6.62 Irregular shedding, late stage. H & E, ×100

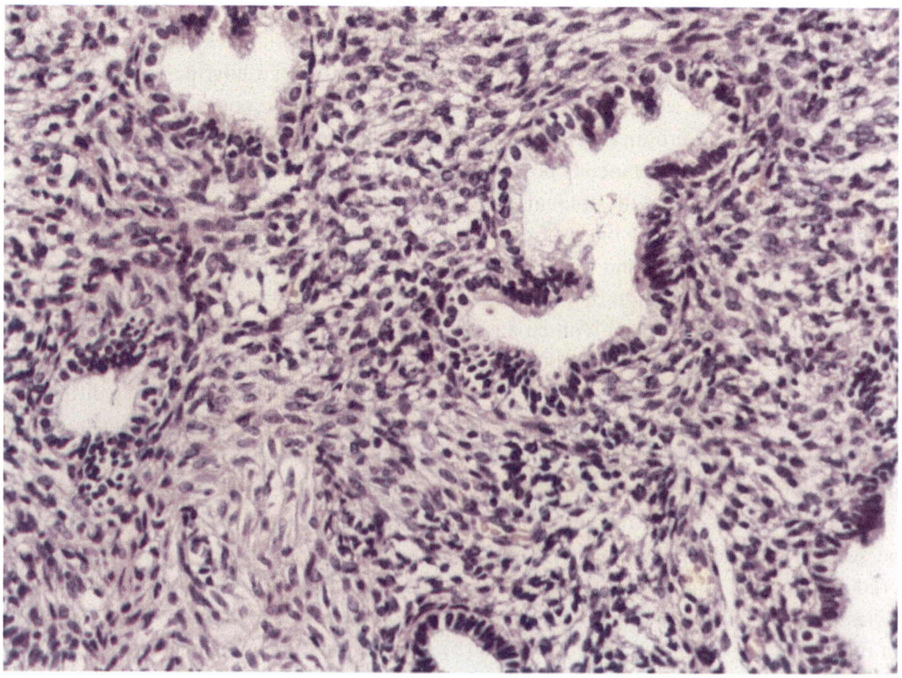

Fig. 6.63 Irregular shedding, late stage. H & E, ×250

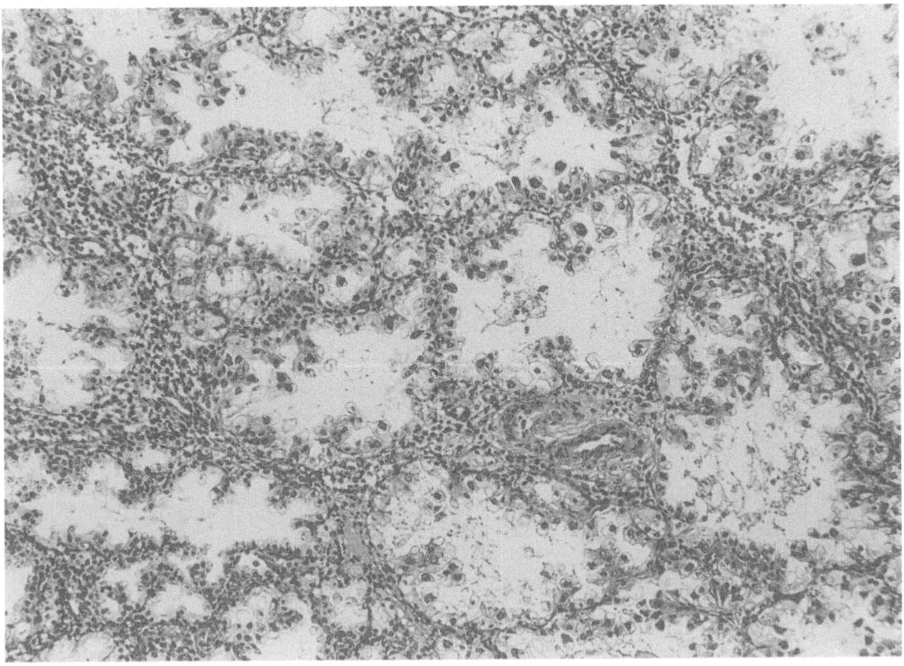

Fig. 6.64 Irregular shedding with Arias-Stella reaction. H & E, ×100

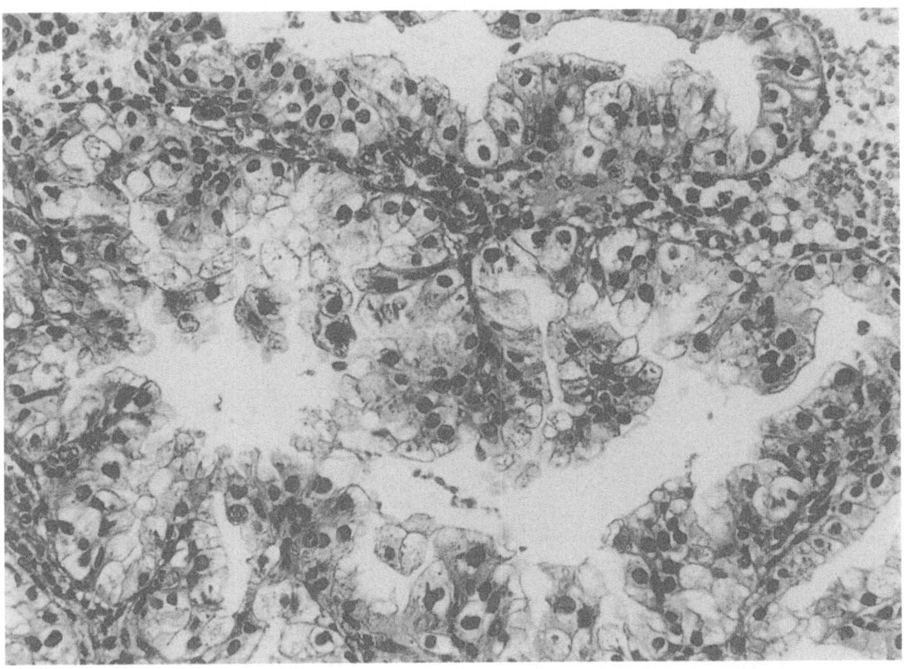

Fig. 6.65 Irregular shedding with Arias-Stella reaction. H & E, ×250

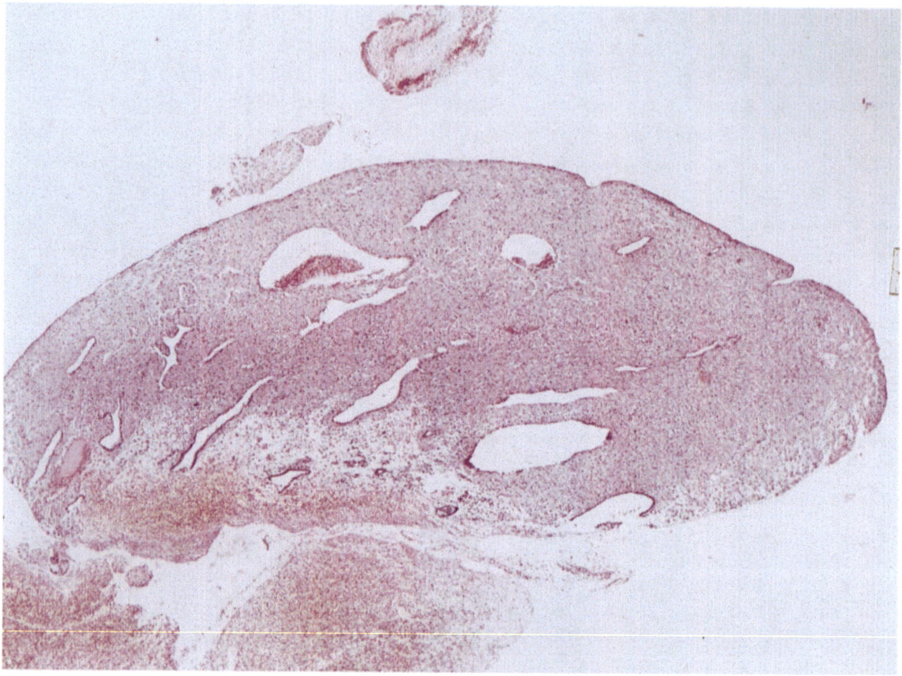

Fig. 6.66 Decidual cast shed from dysmenorrhea membranacea. H & E, ×25

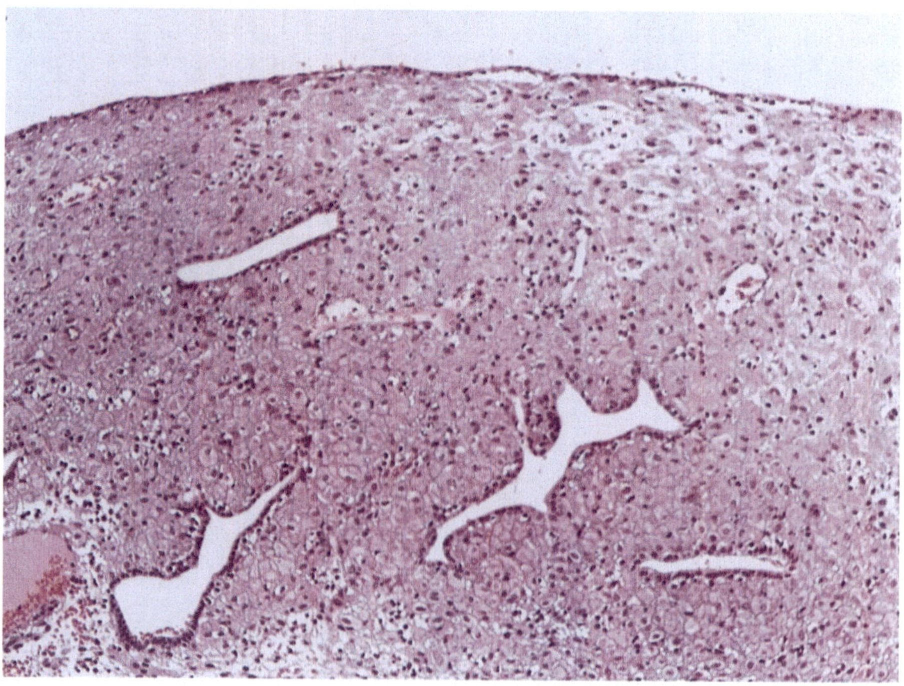

Fig. 6.67 Higher magnification of Fig. 134. H & E, ×100

6.3.3
Abnormal Decidual Shedding

A special type of abnormal endometrial shedding corresponds with the clinical diagnosis of **dysmenorrhoea membranacea**. Its morphologic substrate (Figs. 6.66, 6.67) is the finding of large, sheet-like pieces of more or less well preserved predecidual or decidual endometrium which have been shed undissociated from the uterine cavity. The plane of separation is clearly recognized by the zone of hemorrhagic necrosis (Fig. 6.66). The endometrial glands are more or less convoluted and are lined by low cuboidal cells with round nuclei in a sparse cytoplasm. The glandular lumina may be narrow or wide, but are usually devoid of secretion. The abundant endometrial stroma consists of predecidual or decidual cells. Occasionally, inflammatory infiltrates extend beyond the line of demarcation.

Morphologic Differential Diagnosis. It may be difficult to distinguish between the dysmenorrhea membranacea that follows intra- or extrauterine abortion and that induced by a persistent corpus luteum not associated with pregnancy when placental remnants or characteristics of an Arias-Stella reaction are lacking, since persistent progesterone stimulation may also transform the endometrial cells into decidual cells indistinguishable from those of a pregnancy (Spechter 1953).

Distinction is possible, however, when the endometrial glands are nonconvoluted, narrow, and lined by atrophic epithelium; such an "arrested secretion," which can also be shed in the shape of a decidual cast, is seen only after gestagen therapy (see Fig. 7.6).

Clinical Interpretation and Differential Diagnosis. The same as for irregular shedding (p. 103). A decidual cast may be expelled in one piece when disintegration of reticulin fibers fails to occur in the absence of relaxin release. Relaxin is retained with persistent progesterone secretion or during gestagen therapy. Decidual casts may then be discharged when gestagen therapy is discontinued ("hormonal curettage").

6.4
Functional Endogenous Changes During the Perimenopausal Period

At the end of the reproductive period, functional disturbances of the endometrium increase in frequency. The spectrum of changes regarded as still being physiologic, however, is much broader than that for the reproductive years. Only persistent changes that can be correlated with a well-recognized histopathologic entity should be regarded as abnormal: Long-standing hormonal imbalance (absolute or relative) due to excess estrogen leads to endometrial hyperplasia (see p. 70); secretory hypertrophy results from progesterone overstimulation; and with focal receptor defects polyps form (see p. 88).

6.4.1
Secretory Hypertrophy

Secretory hypertrophy (Figs. 6.68–6.72) is observed only in the preclimacteric period. The hypersecreting endometrium may measure 1 cm in height. Two types may be distinguished, but combinations of the two are also seen.

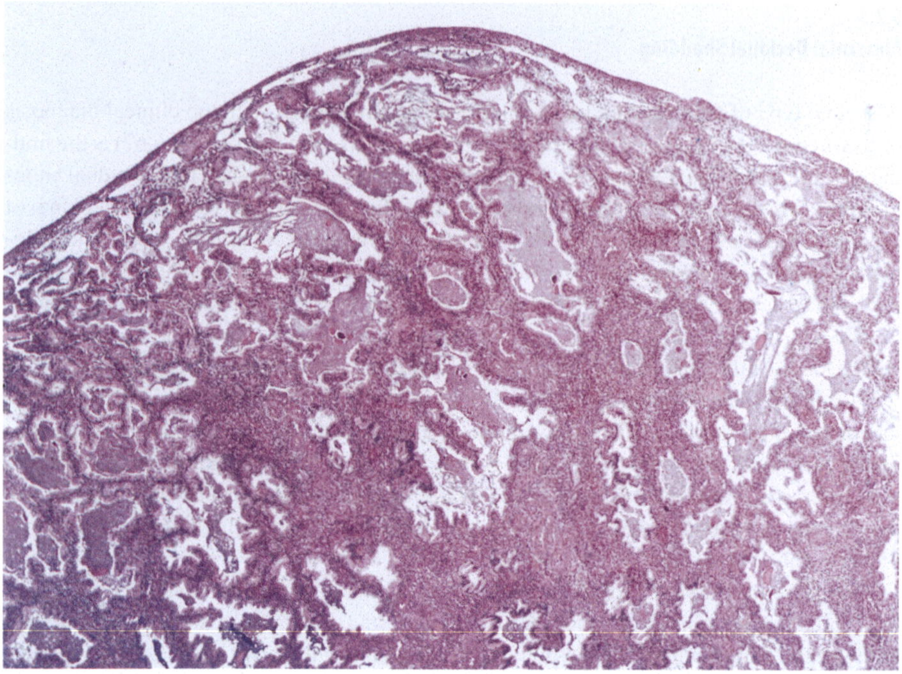

Fig. 6.68 Secretory hypertrophy, glandular type. H & E, ×25

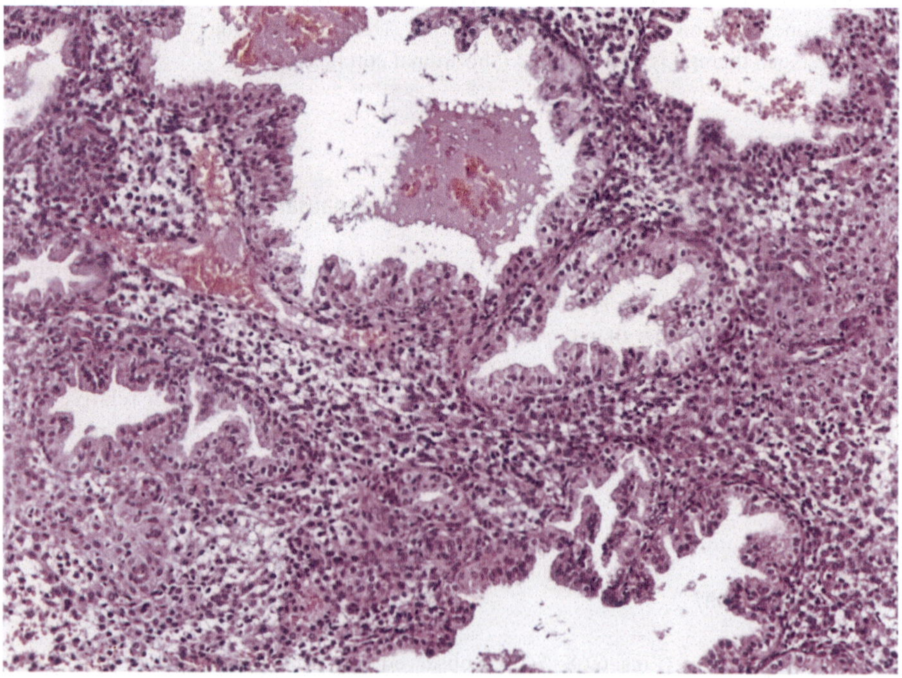

Fig. 6.69 Secretory hypertrophy, glandular type. H & E, ×100

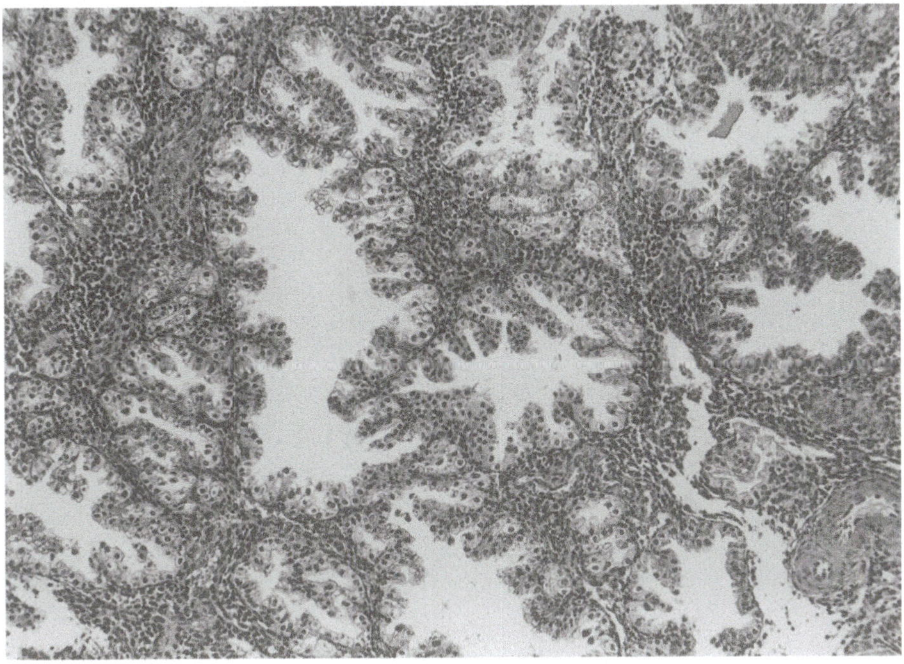

Fig. 6.70 Secretory hypertrophy, glandular type. H & E, ×100

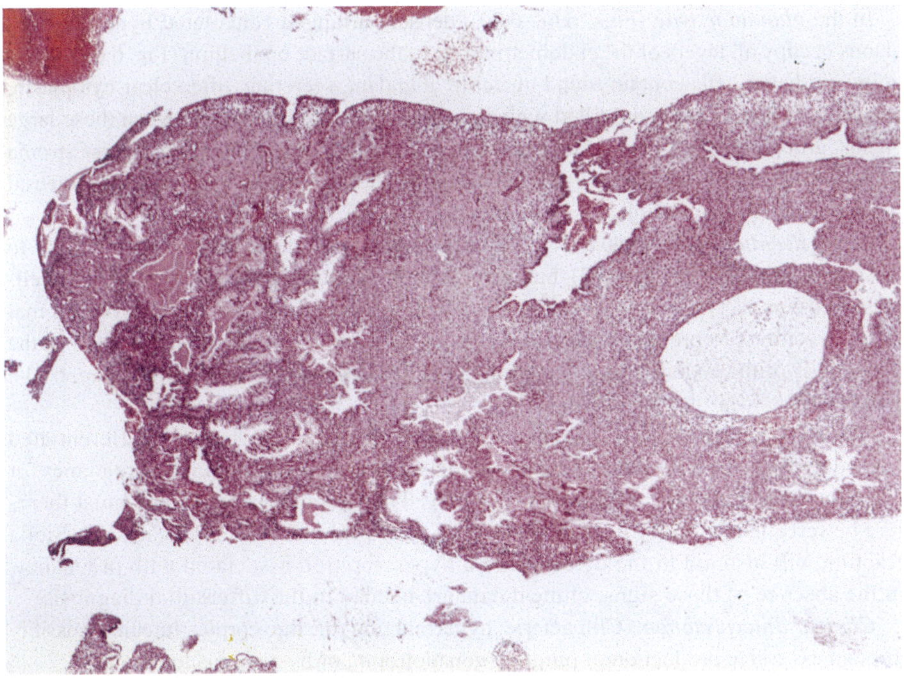

Fig. 6.71 Secretory hypertrophy, decidual type. H & E, ×25

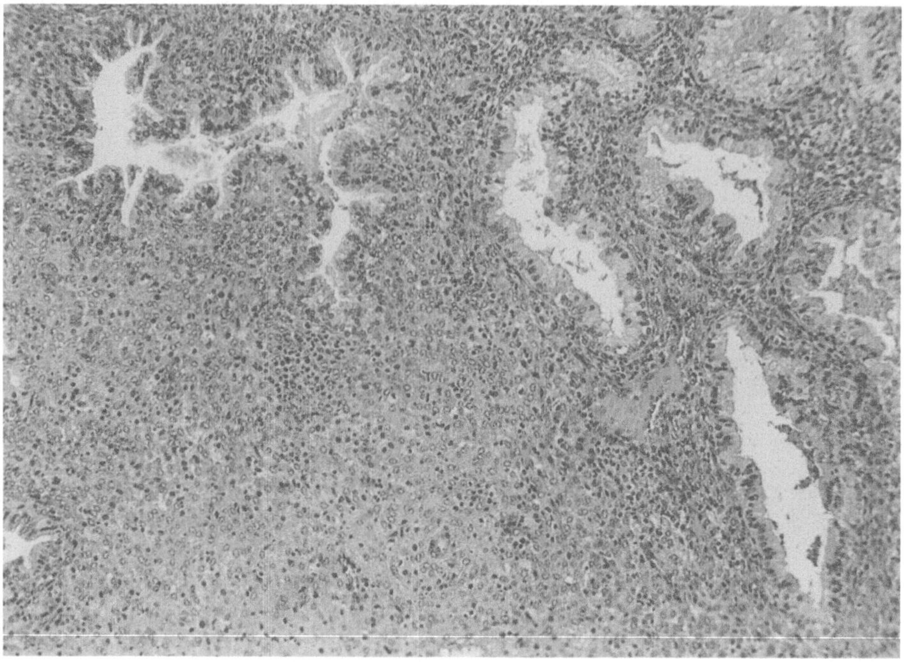

Fig. 6.72 Secretory hypertrophy, decidual type. H & E, ×100

In the *glandular type* (Figs. 6.68–6.70), densely arranged convoluted hypersecreting glands occupy all layers of the endometrium up to the surface epithelium (Fig. 6.68). Their lining epithelial cells contain round nuclei in abundant, secreting, often clear cytoplasm, and their serrated lumina are filled with secretion (Figs. 6.68, 6.69). Between these large glands, groups of slightly underdeveloped glands can be distinguished. The sparse stroma consists of densely arranged, large, rounded predecidual cells and granular endometrial stromal cells. Spiral arterioles are prominent (Fig. 6.70).

In the *decidual type* (Figs. 6.71, 6.72) the endometrial glands appear very similar to those described above (Fig. 6.72), but are in scattered groups, widely separated by a well-preserved compact stroma consisting of predecidual cells and granular endometrial stromal cells. In contrast to premenstrual endometrium, the compact stroma is not limited to the upper layer of the endometrium, but arranged in patches throughout all layers (Fig. 6.71). There may be focal stromal edema.

Morphologic Differential Diagnosis. Secretory hypertrophy must be differentiated from decidual transformation in early implantation of an intrauterine pregnancy or that accompanying an extrauterine pregnancy. The endometrial specimen must therefore be screened carefully for trophoblasts or early placental villi. A focal Arias-Stella reaction will also aid in the detection of a hypersecretion associated with pregnancy. In the absence of these signs, clinical data are needed in the differential diagnosis.

Clinical Interpretation. Climacteric hyperfunction of the corpus luteum, possibly through excessive production of pituitary gonadotropin, or by a corpus luteum cyst.

Iatrogenic Changes 7

7.1 After Hormone Therapy

Besides oral contraception in young women, hormone replacement therapy (HRT) in the peri- and postmenopausal period has become important. HRT has changed from estrogen therapy alone to combined estrogen-gestagen preparations to avoid estrogen-induced carcinogenesis.

To prevent irregular functional bleeding, intermittent spottings, or neoplastic changes a precise functional histologic diagnosis of the endometrial biopsy before and possibly during hormone therapy is essential to prevent over- or understimulation of the sensitive endometrial target cells.

Since the endometrium reacts precisely and predictively to any hormonal stimulus, the optimal dose to achieve such equilibrium and to prevent adverse reactions can be accurately estimated. The physiologic variations of the peri- and postmenopausal endometrium (see p. 41) as well as its functional endogenous changes (see p. 59) have already been discussed. They should be considered as the basis for any hormonal substitution.

Most synthetic hormones are extremely potent, since the target cells they stimulate, provided they contain receptors, are highly responsive even to low concentrations and react promptly with characteristic changes, which may differ from those induced by natural hormones. Whereas the changes caused by exogenous estrogens are very similar to those caused by endogenous estrogenic hyperstimulation, this does not hold true for the gestagens administered; most of the synthetic gestagens are much more potent than natural progesterone and overstimulate the more sensitive glandular epithelia, causing early atrophy, whereas the less sensitive stromal cells become prematurely decidualized (see p. 113).

Estrogens and antiestrogens apparently differ less in their mode of action than in their site of action: whereas estrogens stimulate endometrial glandular growth as potential precursors of endometrial carcinomas, antiestrogens like synthetic gestagens and tamoxifen induce endometrial atrophy. They stimulate, however, proliferation of endocervical glands and reserve cells and may induce endocervical-type metaplasias in the resting or atrophic endometrium as potential precursors of endocervical-type atypical hyperplasias and non-endometrioid carcinomas (see Table 7.1; Dallenbach-Hellweg et al. 2000).

G. Dallenbach-Hellweg et al., *Atlas of Endometrial Histopathology*,
DOI: 10.1007/978-3-642-01541-0_7, © Springer-Verlag Berlin Heidelberg 2010

Table 7.1 Antagonistic effects of exogenous hormones on endocervix and endometrium

	Endocervix	Endometrium
Estrogen (endog. or exog.)	Differentiation with mucus production → Cystic hyperplasia	Hyperproliferation → Simple, complex, atypical hyperplasia
Gestagen (synthetic)	Hyperproliferation → Microglandular and reserve cell hyperplasia	Arrested secretion → Atrophy → Endocervical-type (muc., clear cell, ser.) metaplasia

7.1.1 Estrogen-Induced Hyperplasia

In the reaction to synthetic estrogens, individual variations and the age of the patient must be taken into account (Hempel et al. 1977). With prolonged administration of small doses of estradiol (20–100 μg daily), various stages of endometrial hyperplasia (Figs. 7.1–7.5) develop from simple to complex and atypical hyperplasia or even carcinoma. Estrogen therapy alone therefore has become obsolete in patients with an intact uterus.

In *young women* below 40 years of age, the hyperplasia is often focal (Fig. 7.1), but within each focus the hyperplastic glands are evenly distributed and show an adenomatous growth with pseudostratification of the epithelial cells (Fig. 7.2). Their nuclei are elongated and chromatin rich, occasionally slightly rounded when tiny vacuoles become

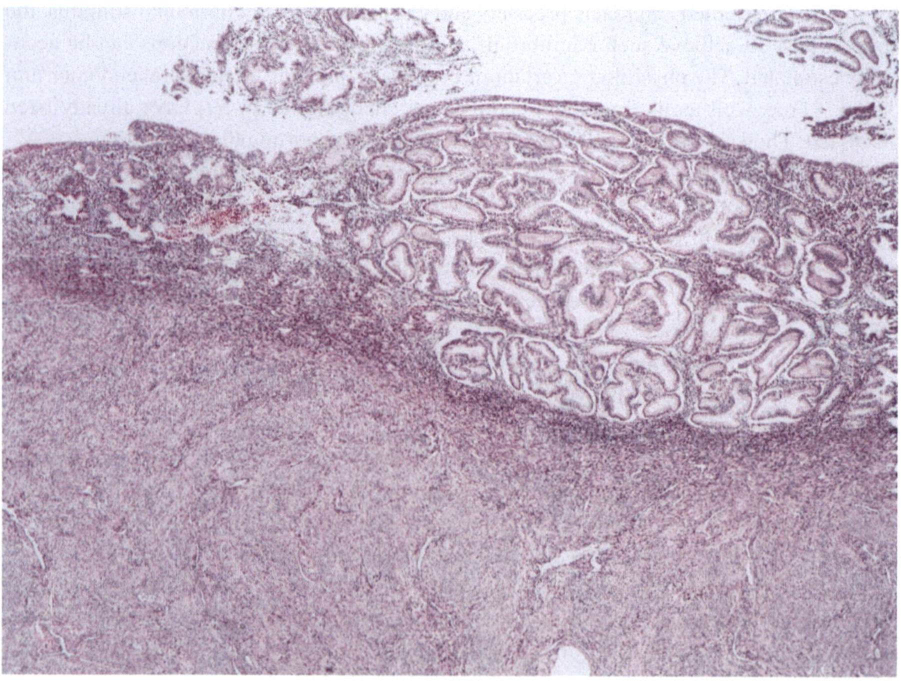

Fig. 7.1 Estrogen-induced hyperplasia in a young woman, corresponding to focal complex hyperplasia developing in deficient secretory endometrium (left). H & E, ×25

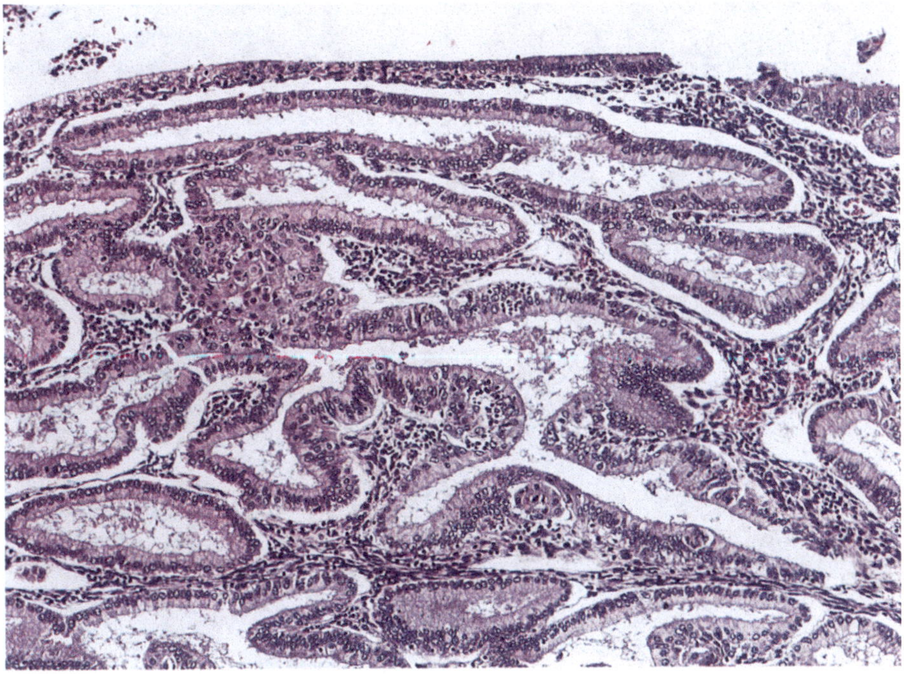

Fig. 7.2 Estrogen-induced hyperplasia in a young woman. H & E, ×100

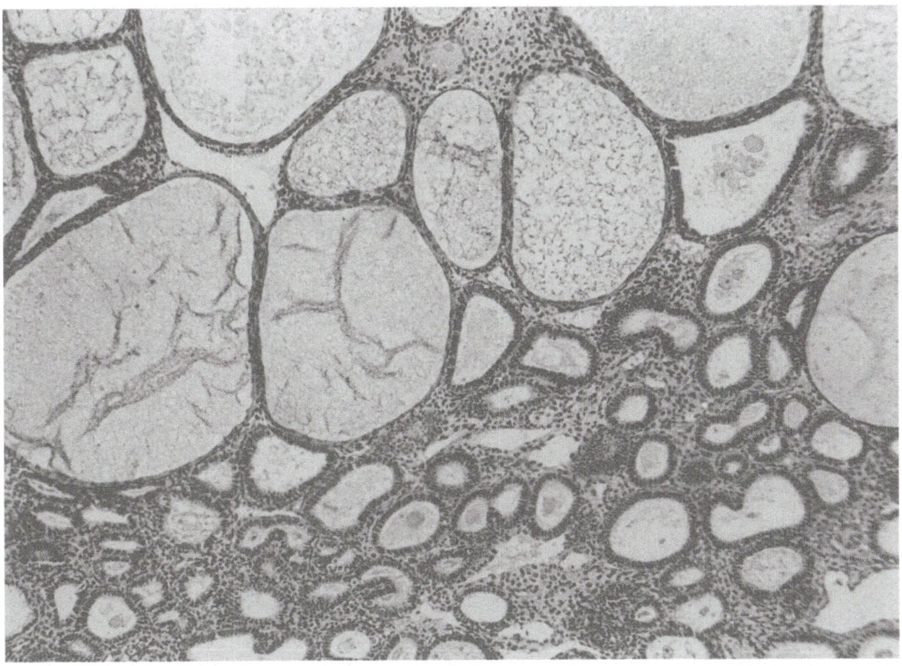

Fig. 7.3 Estrogen-induced hyperplasia in old age (see also Figs. 6.18 and 6.19, endogenous hyperplasia). H & E, ×100

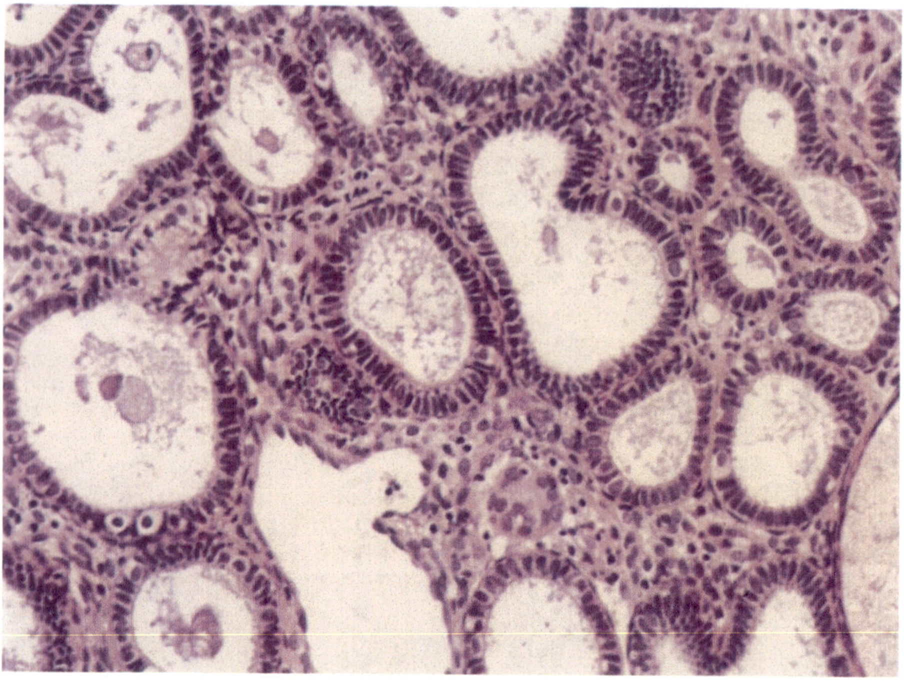

Fig. 7.4 Estrogen-induced hyperplasia in old age. H & E, ×250

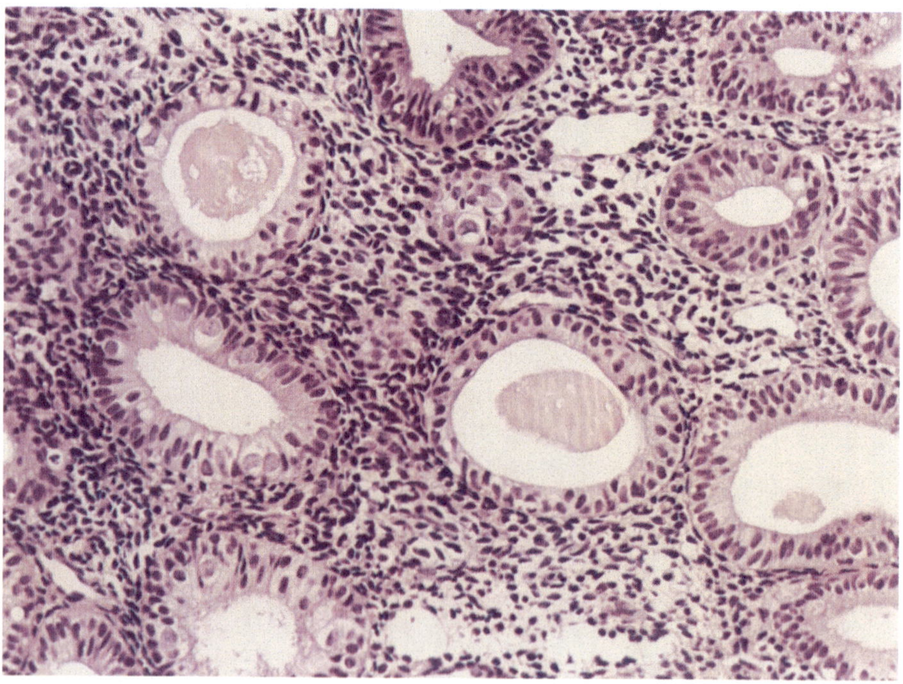

Fig. 7.5 Estrogen-induced hyperplasia in old age. H & E, ×250

visible in the cytoplasm, which is otherwise slightly eosinophilic. Nodules of squamous metaplasia may be numerous. The stroma is sparse and in some regions absent. Mitoses are frequent in the glandular epithelium, whereas the stromal cells are inactive.

In *old age* (Figs. 7.3–7.5), many endometrial glands are cystically dilated (Fig. 7.3). Their lining epithelium varies from gland to gland (Fig. 7.5); it may be pseudostratified or stratified. The nuclei are large, round, or elongated, pale or chromatin rich, and depolarized. Mitoses are frequent. The glandular cytoplasm may be sparse and basophilic, eosinophilic, or clear when the whole cell appears swollen. The remaining stroma between the abundant glands is undifferentiated, dense, or focally edematous and may contain groups of endometrial foam cells, which store estrogen metabolites. Spiral arterioles are very scanty or absent.

Morphologic Differential Diagnosis. In contrast to the hyperplasias caused by endogenous estrogen, those developing after estrogen therapy are often multicentric or polypoid, show great variation in structure from gland to gland, and may contain numerous foci of squamous metaplasia. Diffuse hyperplasia as caused by endogenous estrogen may, however, be seen, although much less frequently.

Clinical Possibilities and Differential Diagnosis. (a) Long-term estrogen therapy; (b) endogenous hyperestrogenism.

7.1.2 Gestagen Therapy

The synthetic gestagens used for contraception or in hormone replacement therapy (Figs. 7.6–7.10) differ both chemically and metabolically from natural progesterone. Because of their great potency, their action on the target cells is exaggerated. The intensity of the morphologic changes depends not only on the potency of the gestagen used but also on the dosis, length of administration and hormonal status of the patient.

7.1.2.1 Arrested Secretion

Arrested secretion (Figs. 7.6, 7.7) generally develops after 3 months of gestagen therapy when a feedback mechanism has inhibited the secretion of FSH and thereby prevented proliferation of endometrial glands. Consequently, the glands are sparse, narrow, and lined by atrophic epithelium, whereas the stroma is decidualized and rich in granular endometrial stromal cells. The arrest in secretion is the result of the preceding suppression of proliferation, whereas the stroma still shows a very distinct gestagen effect.

Clinical Possibilities. Therapy with synthetic gestagens only (gestagen preparation alone or combined with low-dose estrogen as oral contraceptives). There is no known endogenous disturbance which results in arrested secretion.

7.1.2.2 Fibrous Atrophy

Fibrous atrophy (Fig. 7.8) develops from arrested secretion when the gestagen therapy is continued for 6 months or longer (Charles 1964); here the glands have almost completely

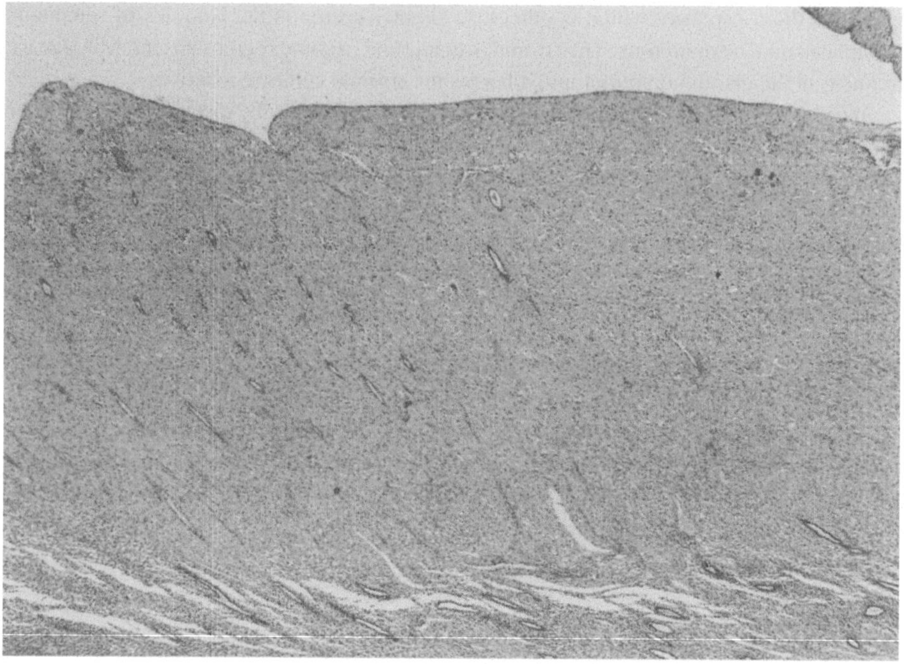

Fig. 7.6 Arrested secretion after gestagen therapy. H & E, ×25

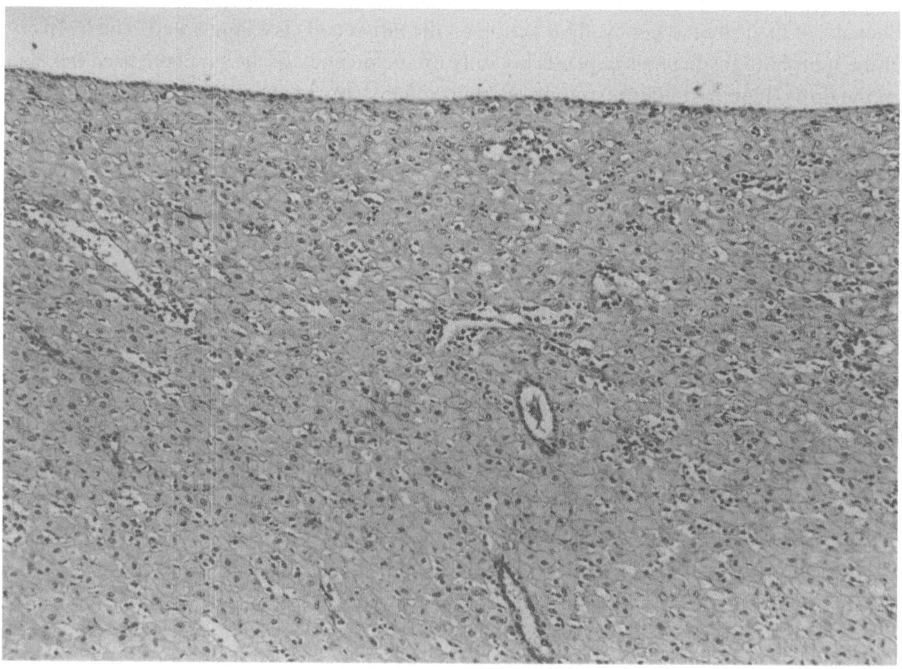

Fig. 7.7 Arrested secretion after gestagen therapy. H & E, ×100

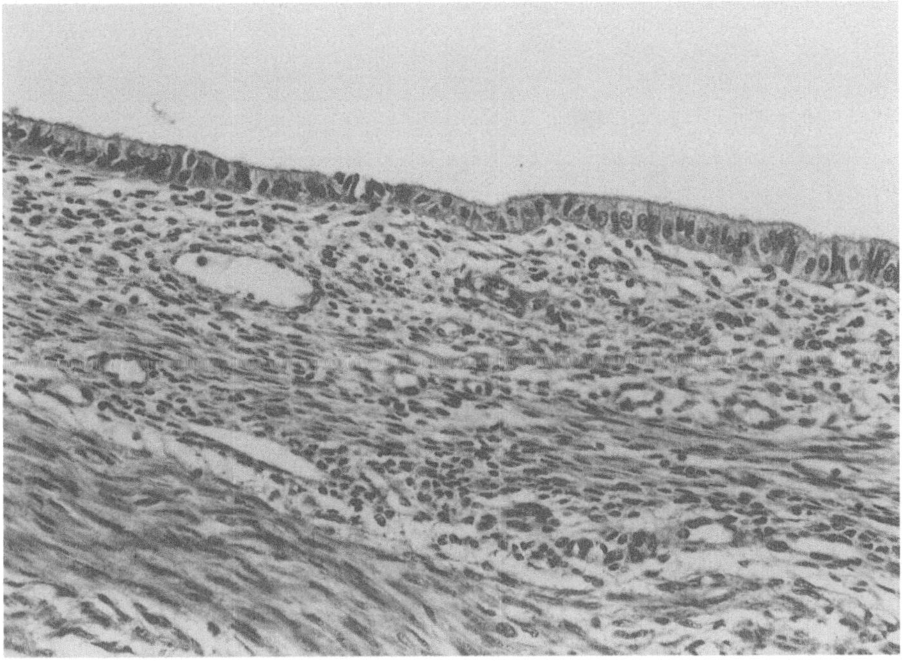

Fig. 7.8 Fibrous atrophy after gestagen therapy. H & E, ×250

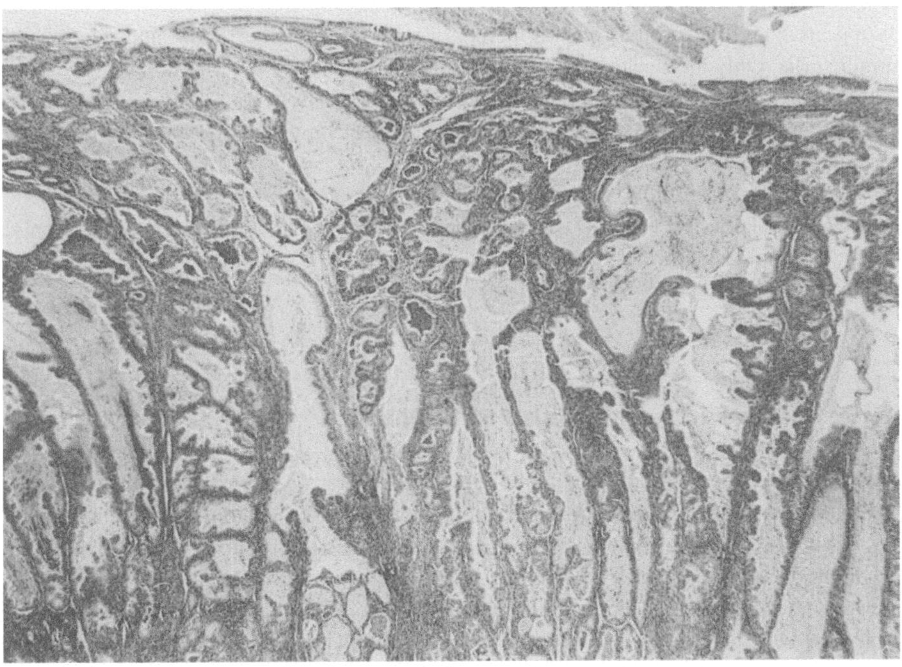

Fig. 7.9 Incomplete secretory transformation after gestagen therapy of atypical hyperplasia. H & E, ×25

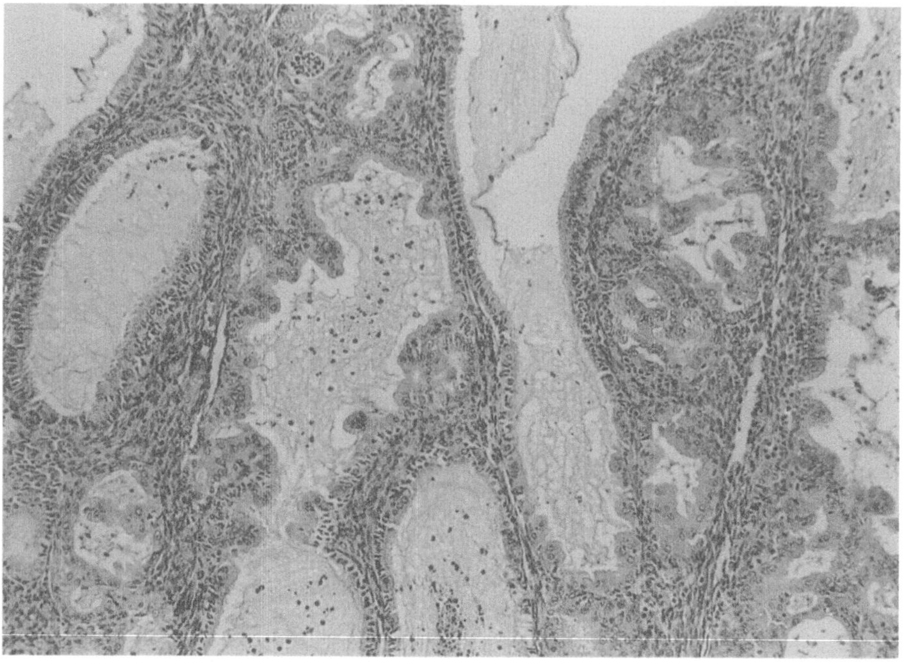

Fig. 7.10 Higher magnification of Fig. 7.9. H & E, ×100

disappeared, and the stroma consists merely of very few layers of small, undifferentiated spindle cells. Only the surface epithelium is still distinctly proliferating.

Morphologic Differential Diagnosis. Atrophy from endogenous causes is seldom as complete as that seen following long-term gestagen therapy; pressure atrophy is always focal (see Fig. 6.4).

Clinical Possibilities and Differential Diagnosis. (a) Long-term therapy with synthetic gestagens; (b) complete arrest of ovarian function in old age or after bilateral ovarectomy; (c) endometrial refractoriness to hormones; and (d) pressure atrophy.

Distinction is possible by evaluating the clinical history.

7.1.3
Gestagen Therapy of Atypical Hyperplasia or Adenocarcinoma

In atypical hyperplasia or adenocarcinoma, gestagen therapy results in more or less incomplete secretory transformation of the previously proliferating glandular epithelium (Figs. 7.9, 7.10). The nuclei become round, mitoses are inhibited (Nordqvist 1964), and the cytoplasm may show signs of early, advanced, or abortive secretion (John et al. 1974), whereas the sparse stroma remains almost unchanged. Since considerably more endogenous estrogen has to be counteracted than in a normal cycle, the stage of arrested secretion will only be reached after gestagen therapy in very high doses (150–250 mg daily) for 6–12 months or even longer (Kistner 1959; Kistner et al. 1965; Eichner and Abellera 1971). Whereas atypical hyperplasia may disappear completely after high doses of gestagen over a long period of time, only a growth arrest can usually be achieved in invasive carcinoma, whereby the interval between gestagen therapy and tumor recurrence may depend on many diverse factors involved (cf. to pertinent literature).

Clinical Possibilities and Differential Diagnosis. (a) Gestagen therapy of atypical hyperplasia or adenocarcinoma; (b) endogenous production of progesterone, e.g., spontaneous ovulation in a young woman with complex or atypical hyperplasia; and (c) secretory type of adenocarcinoma.

Distinction between (a) and (b) is possible only by evaluation of the clinical history.

7.1.4 Combination Therapy

In combination therapy (Figs. 7.11–7.21), the combined action of the two hormones is the precise result of dose and potency of each hormone given and the level of endogenous hormones available for reaction. Oral contraceptives and peri- and postmenopausal replacement hormones (HRT), as the most frequently used combined preparations, usually have a predominant gestagen effect, resulting in abortive secretion.

7.1.4.1 Abortive Secretion

In patients with abortive secretion (Figs. 7.11–7.14), the endometrial glands are diminished in number, narrow, straight, and lined by flat epithelium with small, round, chromatin-

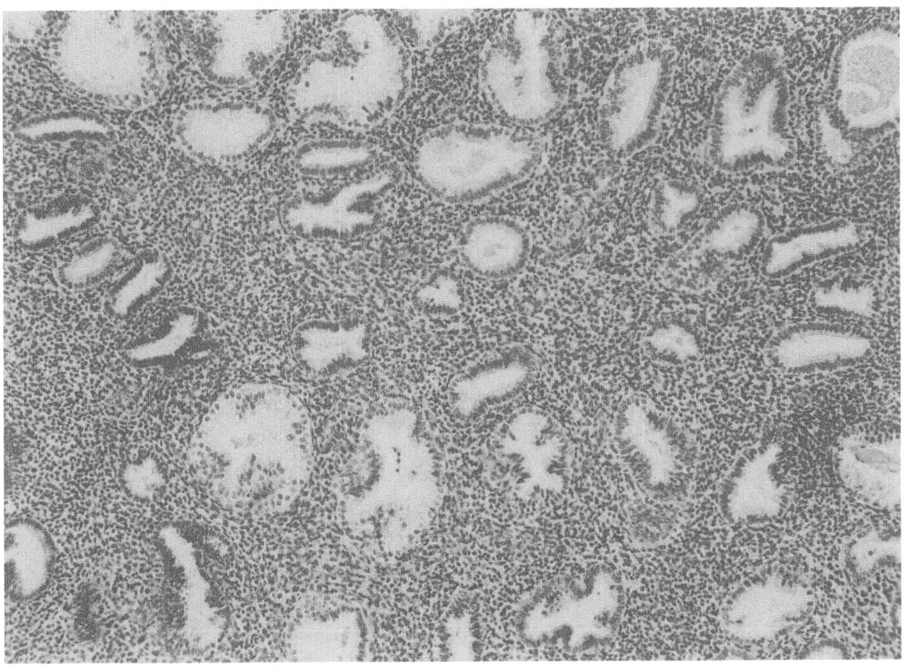

Fig. 7.11 Abortive secretion after combined hormonal treatment, early stage. H & E, ×100

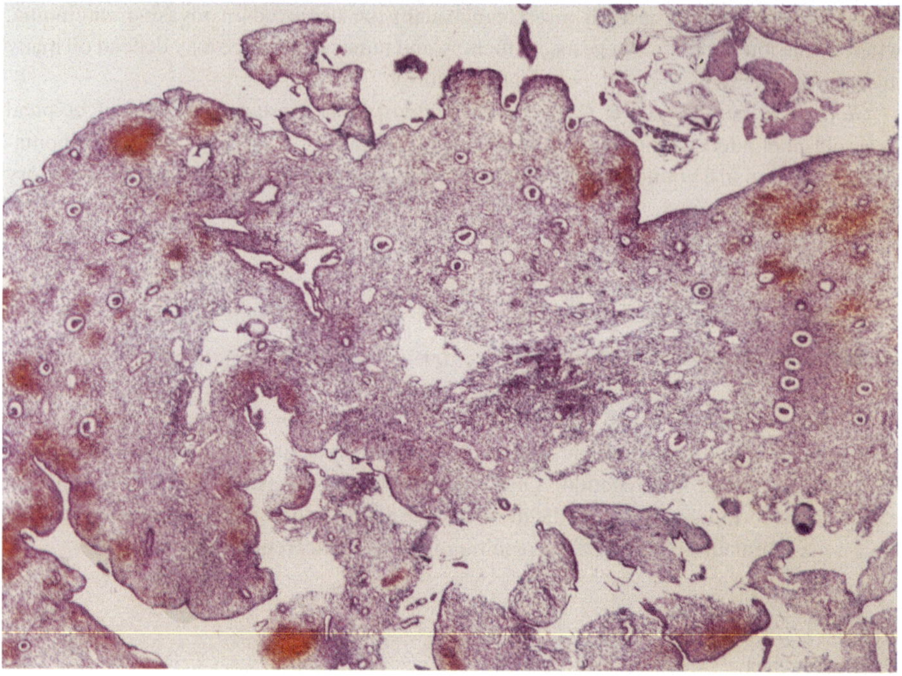

Fig. 7.12 Abortive secretion after combined hormonal therapy, late stage. H & E, ×25

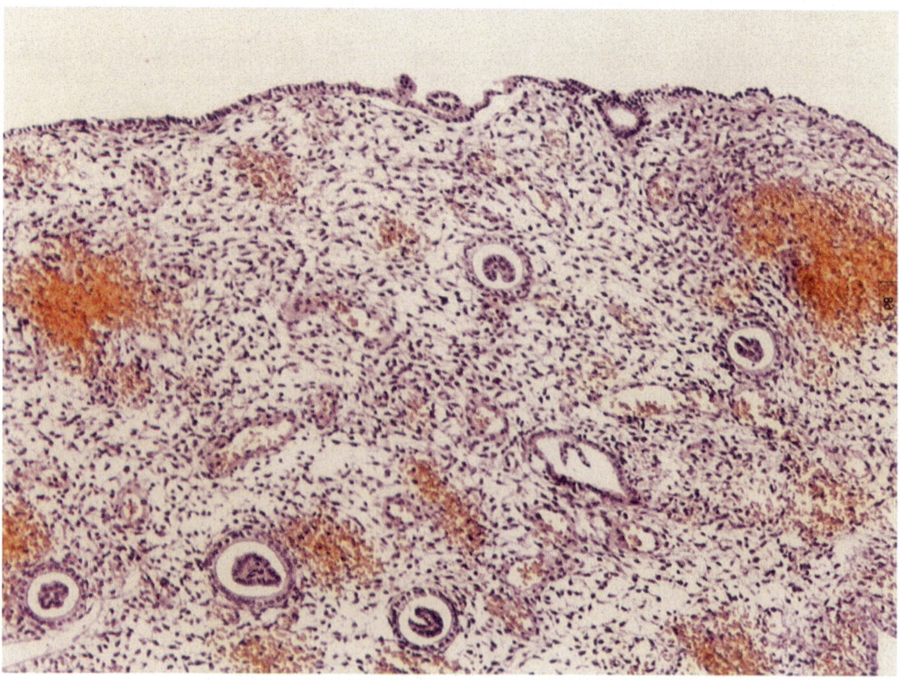

Fig. 7.13 Abortive secretion after combined hormonal therapy, late stage. H & E, ×100

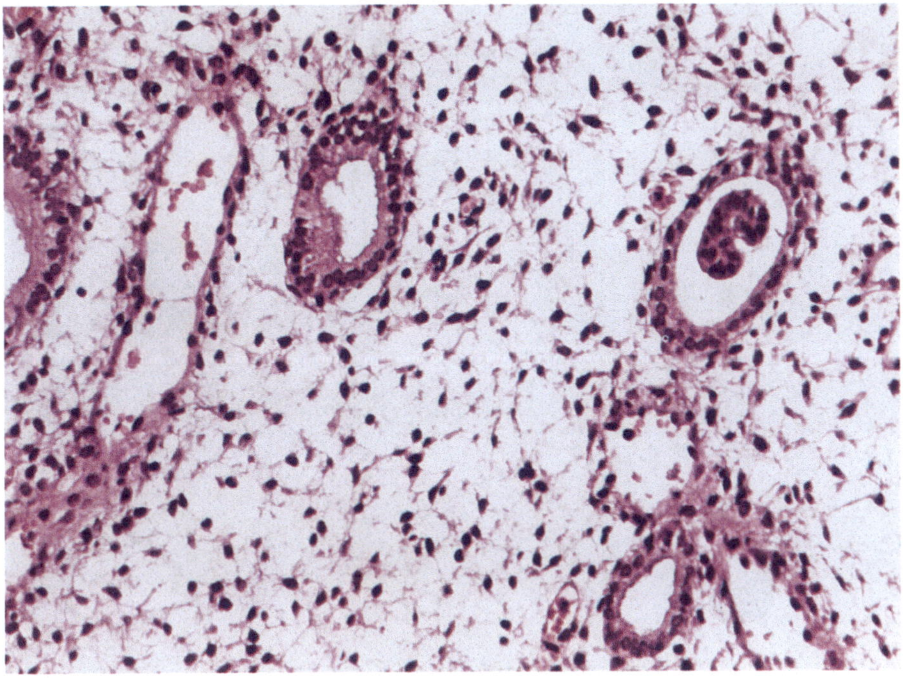

Fig. 7.14 Abortive secretion after combined hormonal therapy. H & E, ×250

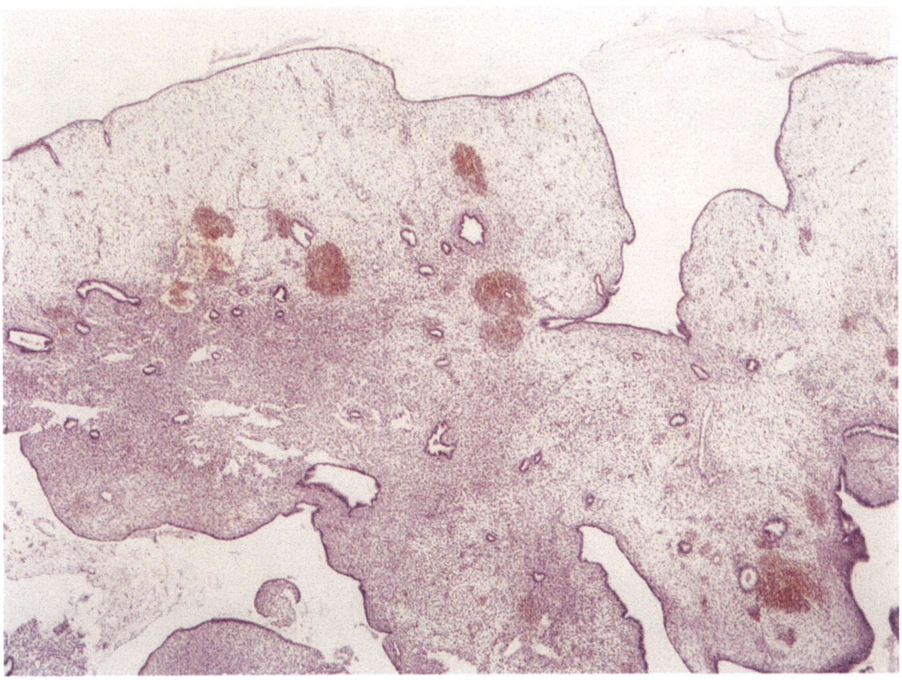

Fig. 7.15 Breakthrough bleeding in irregular atrophy. H & E, ×25

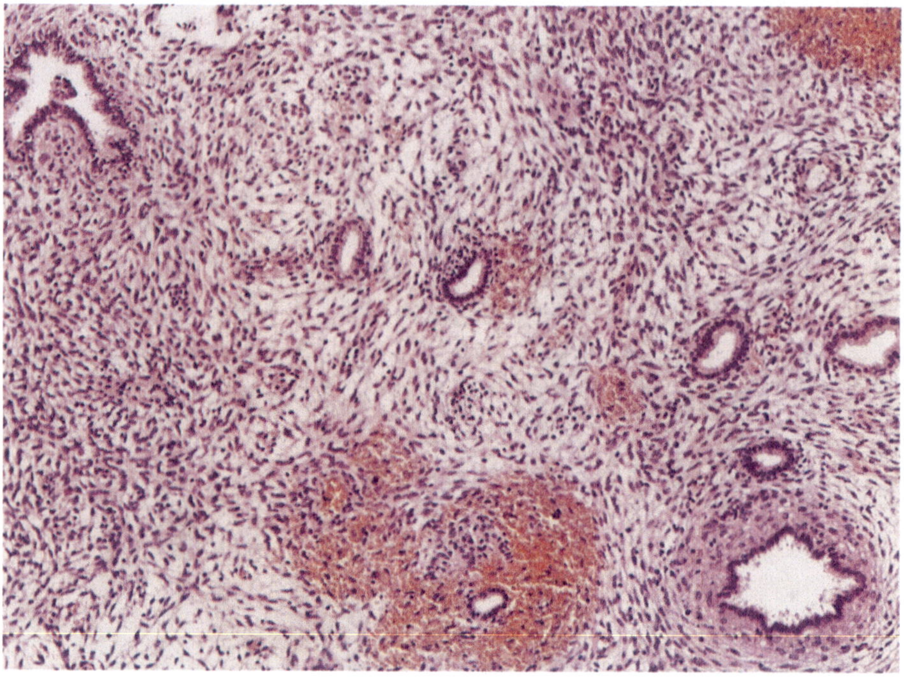

Fig. 7.16 Breakthrough bleeding in irregular atrophy. H & E, ×100

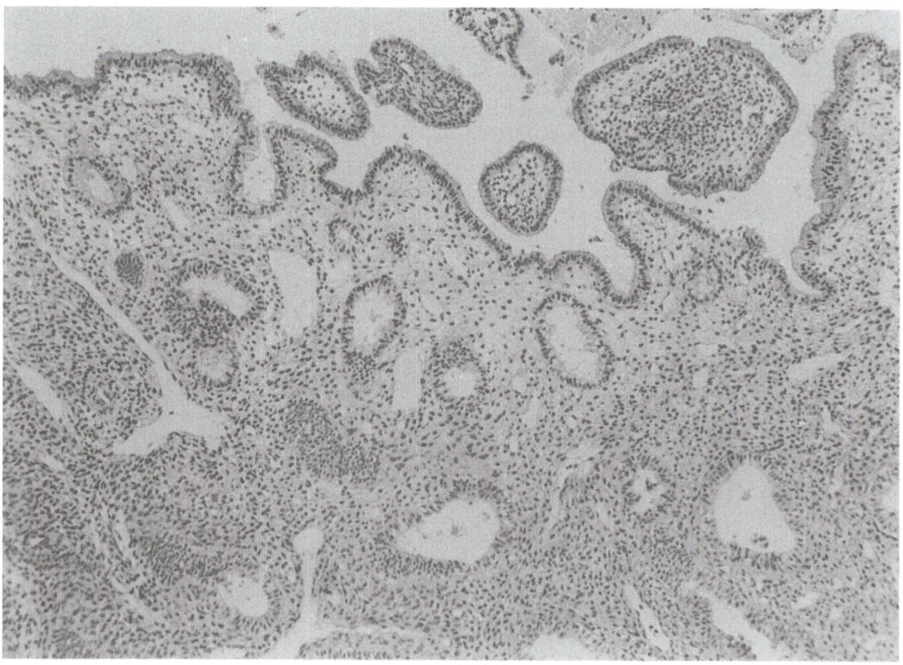

Fig. 7.17 Irregular regeneration following oral contraceptives. H & E, ×100

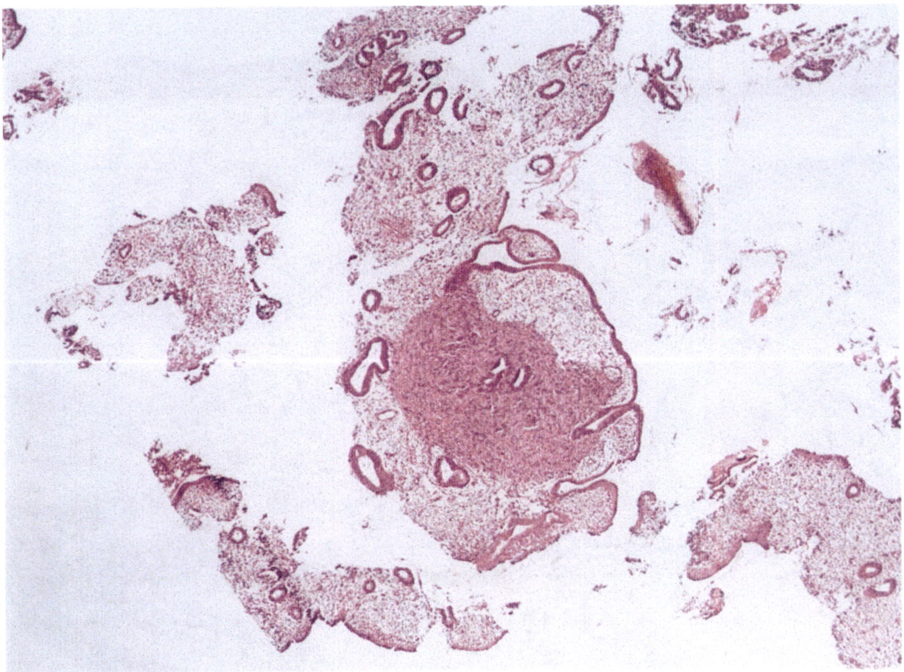

Fig. 7.18 Focal stromal hyperplasia. H & E, ×25

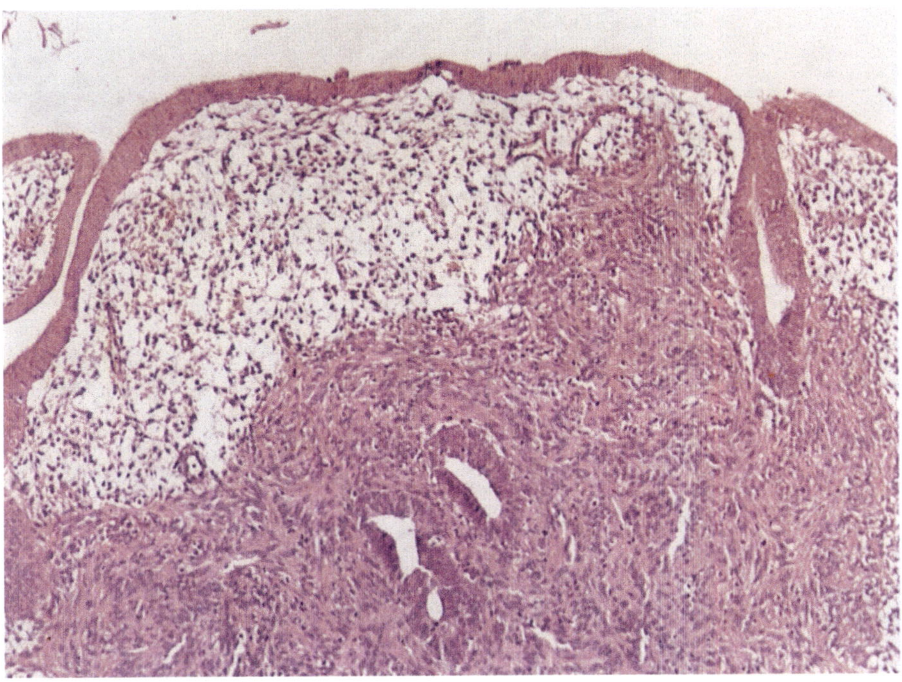

Fig. 7.19 Focal stromal hyperplasia. H & E, ×100

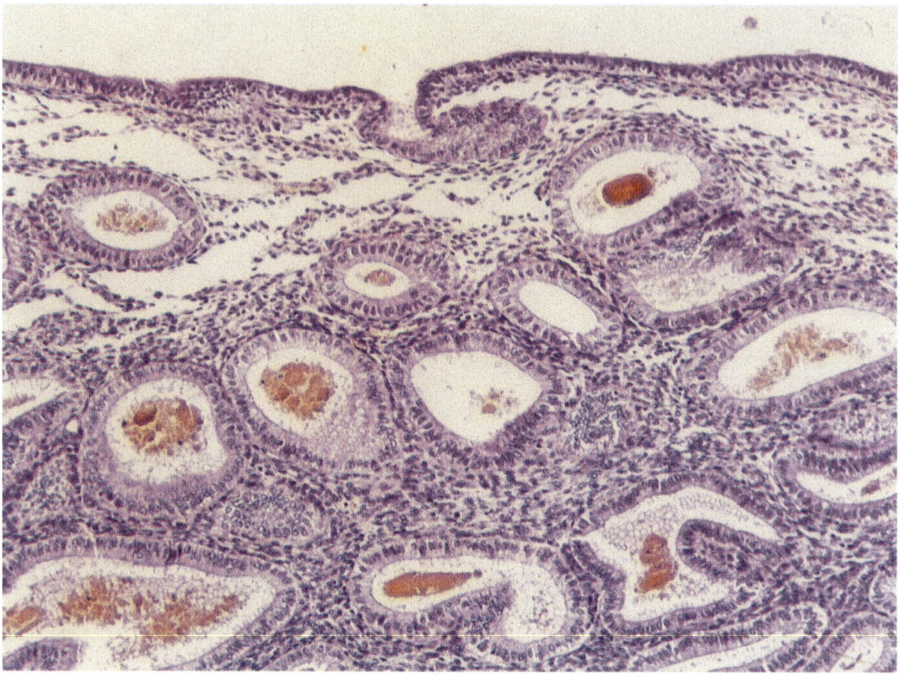

Fig. 7.20 Pseudomelanosis following oral contraceptives. H & E, ×100

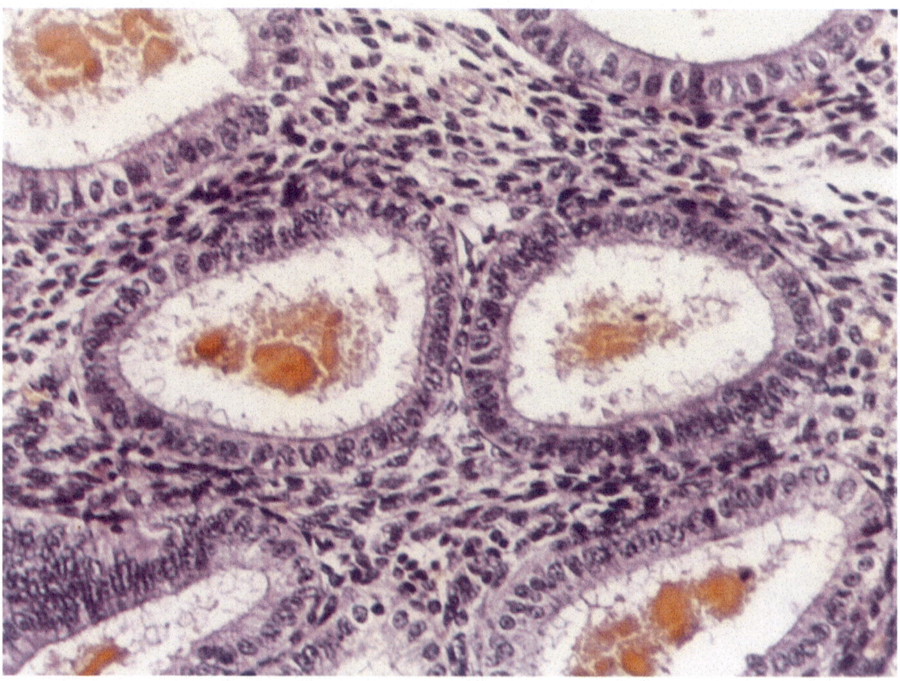

Fig. 7.21 Pseudomelanosis following oral contraceptives. H & E, ×250

dense nuclei in sparse eosinophilic cytoplasm, only occasionally containing tiny vacuoles of glycogen not indicative of ovulation (Fig. 7.14). Protein synthesis is reduced (Verhagen and Themann 1970; Toth et al. 1972). The stromal cells are mostly spindle shaped, incompletely differentiated, and separated by edema.

Clinical Possibilities and Differential Diagnosis. (a) Combined hormone therapy with functional predominance of gestagen; (b) sporadic luteinization in an insufficient follicle (see p. 59).

Distinction is possible only by evaluating the clinical history.

7.1.4.2 Irregular Atrophy

Irregular atrophy (Figs. 7.15, 7.16) develops from abortive secretion when hormone therapy is continued for many months. Groups of glands become quite narrow and lined by atrophic epithelium until they disappear completely, whereas neighboring glands still remain in abortive secretion. The undifferentiated stroma is focally dense. The general height of the endometrium is decreased and the endometrial surface is irregular.

Clinical Possibilities. Irregular atrophy is characteristic of long-term hormone combination therapy. Rare endogenous causes (e.g., sudden cessation of estrogen secretion following irregular proliferation) must be excluded by the clinical history.

7.1.4.3 Breakthrough Bleeding

Breakthrough bleeding (Figs. 7.15, 7.16) results from focal dissolution of reticulin fibers due to the variations in hormone deficiency from area to area caused by an insufficient blood supply. Spiral arterioles fail to develop, but small or dilated capillaries proliferate in areas of incomplete stromal differentiation (Ober 1966, 1967). Together with vascular breakage, the regional drop in hormone supply results in spotty, round hemorrhages characteristic of the artificial cycle.

Clinical Possibilities. The round circumscribed hemorrhages in an atrophic endometrium are characteristic of breakthrough bleeding under hormonal therapy. Anovulatory withdrawal bleeding from endogenous sources is more diffuse (see Figs. 6.13, 6.14).

7.1.4.4 Irregular Regeneration

Irregular regeneration (Fig. 7.17) occurs when oral contraceptives are discontinued. While some glands remain atrophic, others regenerate as in a normal cycle, but their shape and location vary. The stroma is densely cellular. The surface epithelium is focally low or cuboidal, but in neighboring areas it is tall and columnar. The general height is quite irregular.

Clinical Possibilities and Differential Diagnosis. (a) Discontinuation of hormone therapy; (b) resumption of cyclic function following abortion or pregnancy.

Distinction is possible by evaluation of the clinical history.

7.1.4.5 Focal Stromal Hyperplasia

Focal stromal hyperplasia (Figs. 7.18, 7.19) develops on rare occasions as an individual reaction to combined treatment with hormones. In these foci the stromal cells have hyperchromatic enlarged nuclei, and there is excessive formation of reticulin fibers. The number and the structure of the endometrial glands in these foci remain unaltered.

Morphologic Differential Diagnosis. These foci of iatrogenic stromal hyperplasia must be differentiated from the rare stromal nodule, which is a circumscribed stromal proliferation (see p. 173).

7.1.4.6 Pseudomelanosis

On gross examination in pseudomelanosis (Figs. 7.20, 7.21) the endometrial surface is sprinkled with tiny, grayish-black dots caused by the inspissation of blood in the slightly dilated glandular lumina. This change indicates that the endometrium has not been shed with menstruation. The glands have merely regenerated and been incorporated in the next cycle.

Clinical Possibilities and Differential Diagnosis. Incomplete or absent menstrual shedding with inspissation of menstrual blood from the uterine cavity into the regenerating glands due to: (a) hormone therapy, or (b) endogenous disturbance such as insufficient stromal differentiation with absence of granular endometrial stromal cells.

Distinction is possible by evaluation of the clinical history.

7.1.4.7 Focal Complex Hyperplasia

Focal adenomatous hyperplasia may develop after prolonged treatment with agents that contain predominantly estrogen, particularly after sequential oral contraceptive agents, or after metabolic conversion of gestagens into compounds with estrogenic action (Charles 1964; Henzl et al. 1964). Structurally, these foci are identical with those of complex hyperplasia (see Figs. 6.27, 6.28).

The *early structural changes following sequential therapy* are identical to those of the deficient secretory phase with coordinated true delay of maturation (see p. 96).

7.1.5 Hormones for Inducing Ovulation

7.1.5.1 Therapy with Gonadotropins

Treatment with *gonadotropins* (human menopausal and chorionic gonadotropin, HMG/HCG) to induce ovulation may result in irregular secretory changes of the endometrium, whereby the nuclei of many overstimulated glandular epithelial cells become large and pleomorphic like those in an Arias-Stella reaction (see Figs. 6.64, 6.65).

7.1.5.2
Therapy with Clomiphen

Clomiphen, on the other hand, because of its antiestrogenic effect, acts on the endometrium as synthetic gestagens do, causing premature abortive secretory transformation of endometrial glands.

7.1.6
Therapy with Tamoxifen

Tamoxifen has an even stronger antiestrogenic, gestagen-like action; by binding to the estrogen receptor (ER), it inhibits the replenishment of ER, but increases the concentration of progesterone receptor (PR) and thereby its own gestagen-like effect (Horwitz et al. 1989). Consequently, tamoxifen causes endometrial atrophy and often endocervical-type mucinous, serous papillary or clear cell metaplasias in the endometrial glands (see p. 48). Such metaplasias may be precursors of mucinous or clear cell adenocarcinomas of the endometrium (see p. 165; Dallenbach-Hellweg and Hahn 1995; Dallenbach-Hellweg and Schmidt 1998; Dallenbach-Hellweg et al. 2000). Endometrial polyps are also often observed under tamoxifen therapy (see p. 91; Nuovo et al. 1989; Cohen et al. 1994; Ismail 1994; Schlesinger et al. 1998). Their glands are typically cystic, but lined by flat atrophic, metaplastic (Fig. 6.48) or abortively secreting epithelium, indicating previous focal estrogenic stimulation preceding the tamoxifen therapy.

7.2
After Intrauterine Contraceptive Devices

The histologic reaction of the endometrium to an intrauterine contraceptive device varies with the type used (Fig. 7.22) and with the stage of endometrial function before insertion.

7.2.1
Mechanical Decidualization

With the inert device, mechanical pressure or injury of the endometrium results in early decidualization of the surrounding stroma (Figs. 7.23, 7.24), a change that can be observed shortly after ovulation (Wynn 1968). The endometrium directly beneath the device may show pressure atrophy with focal fibrosis and occasional ulceration with perifocal inflammatory infiltrates (Fig. 7.23). The decidualization is limited to small foci and is surrounded by nondecidualized endometrium corresponding to the day of the cycle (Fig. 7.24).

Morphologic Differential Diagnosis. Mechanical decidualization must be distinguished from early decidua of intra- or extrauterine pregnancy.

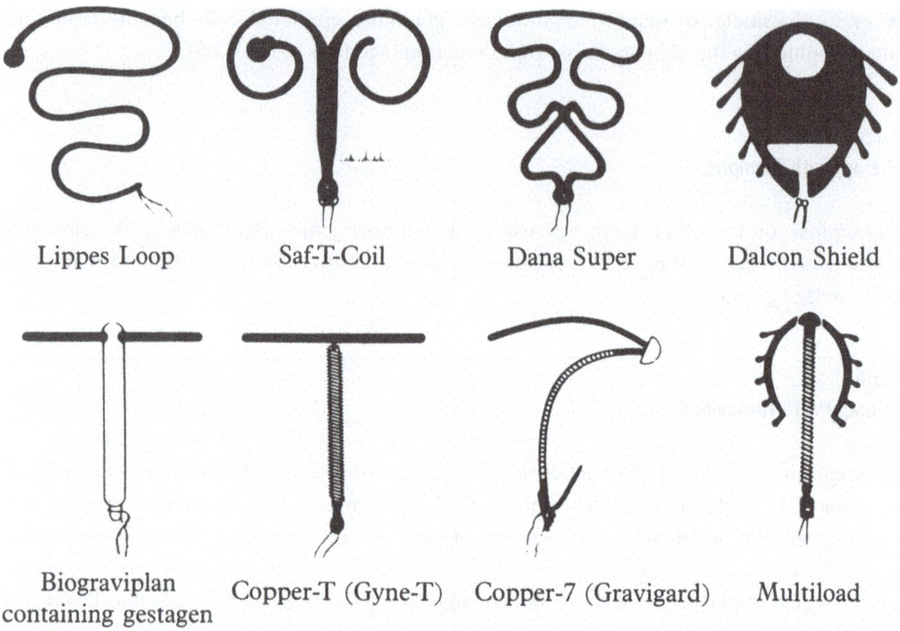

Fig. 7.22 The various generations of intrauterine devices. The shape of a recently developed and now frequently used device containing gestagen (Mirena) is very similar to Biograviplan

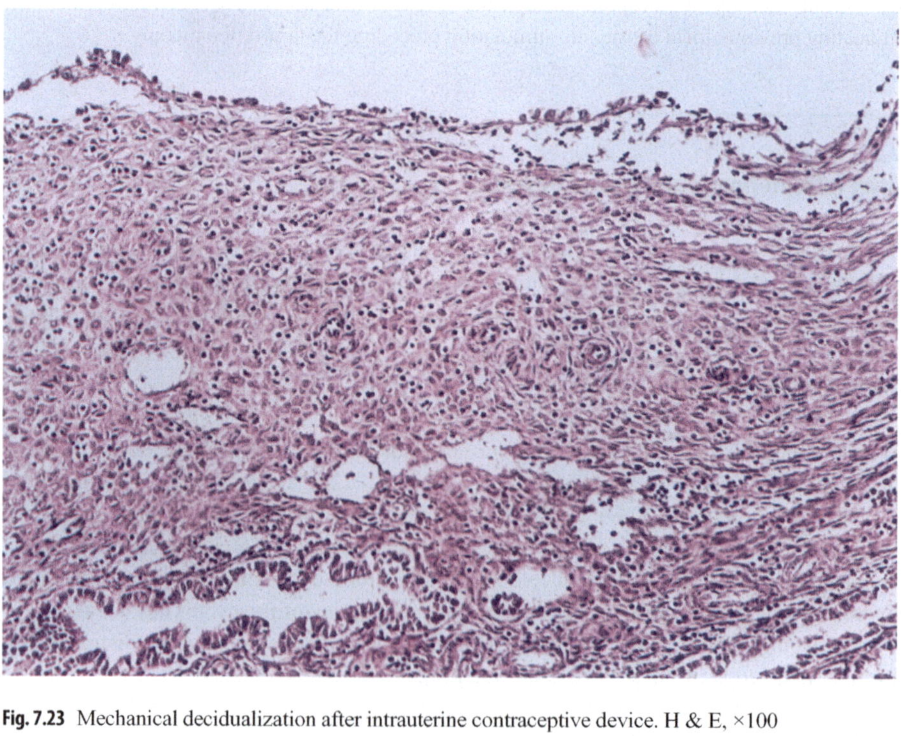

Fig. 7.23 Mechanical decidualization after intrauterine contraceptive device. H & E, ×100

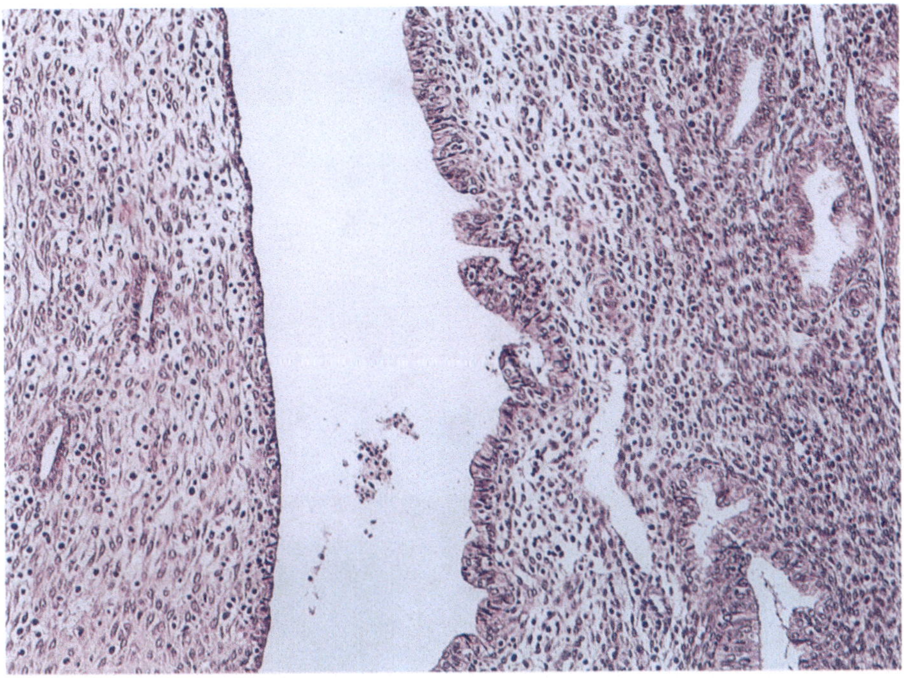

Fig. 7.24 Mechanical decidualization (left side) after intrauterine contraceptive device. H & E, ×100

Distinction is possible if previous insertion of IUD is known or if neighboring nondecidualized endometrium is found, proving the focal character of the decidual change. Arrested secretion can be excluded by the atrophy of the glands (see Figs. 7.6, 7.7).

7.2.2 Perifocal Arrested Secretion

Progesterone-medicated devices release small amounts of the hormone from the depot into the uterine cavity. Gestagen penetrates into the endometrium and acts locally in a paracrine manner. The diffusion only reaches the superficial layers and ends with a discrete horizontal line which can be seen on histologic examination (Fig. 7.25). The upper compact layer shows very sparse, narrow, atrophic glands surrounded by decidualized stroma (Fig. 7.26). Sinusoidal spaces are cystically dilated. Surface indentations indicate pressure exerted by the device (Fig. 7.25). This perifocal arrested secretion presents the same morphologic and histochemical changes as diffuse arrested secretion (Johannisson et al. 1977; see Figs. 7.6, 7.7), but without systemic effects (Wan et al. 1977). Beneath the decidualized layer one finds unaffected endometrial glands and stroma corresponding to the day of the cycle.

Morphologic Differential Diagnosis. It is possible to distinguish perifocal arrested secretion from: (a) arrested secretion induced by administration of gestagens orally or parenterally, which involves the entire endometrium; (b) mechanical decidualization

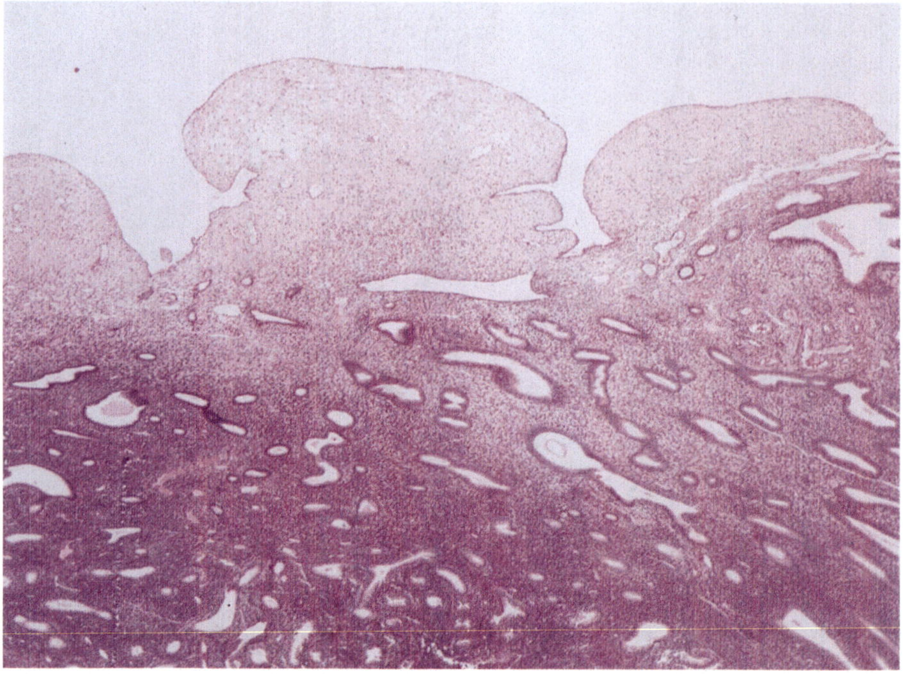

Fig. 7.25 Perifocal arrested secretion following gestagen-laden device. H & E, ×25

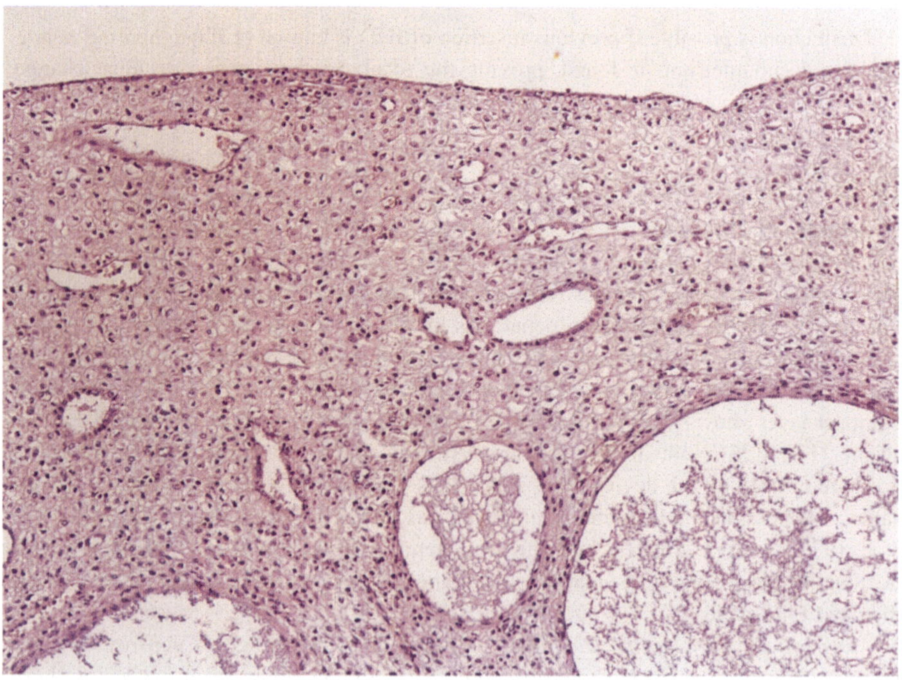

Fig. 7.26 Perifocal arrested secretion following gestagen-laden device. H & E, ×100

brought about by pressure or trauma of a mechanical device; this condition resembles a normal decidua with secretory glands but is focally limited.

7.2.3 Surface Reaction Following Copper Devices

The devices entwined with a copper wire cause regular pressure indentations in the endometrium, the size of the wire used resulting in a corrugated endometrial surface (Figs. 7.27, 7.28). There is slight pressure atrophy directly underneath the wire, but the surface epithelium generally remains intact (Fig. 7.28). Except for a dysfunctional endometrium (Fig. 7.30), no inflammatory changes are found with normal endometrial function. The endometrium of uteri bearing this type of device remains morphologically unchanged, presenting a normal secretory and proliferative phase (Fig. 7.27). The contraceptive action apparently comes about by biochemical changes (Rosado et al. 1976; Wilson 1977).

Clinical Correlation. The corrugated endometrial surface is seen only after insertion of a copper device.

Leukocytes in glandular lumina (Fig. 7.29) indicate that a copper device has been inserted. They are pushed into the glandular mouth of normally secreting glands. There is no inflammatory reaction of the glandular epithelium or stroma. Note the intact surface epithelium. These leukocytes are thus of no clinical importance.

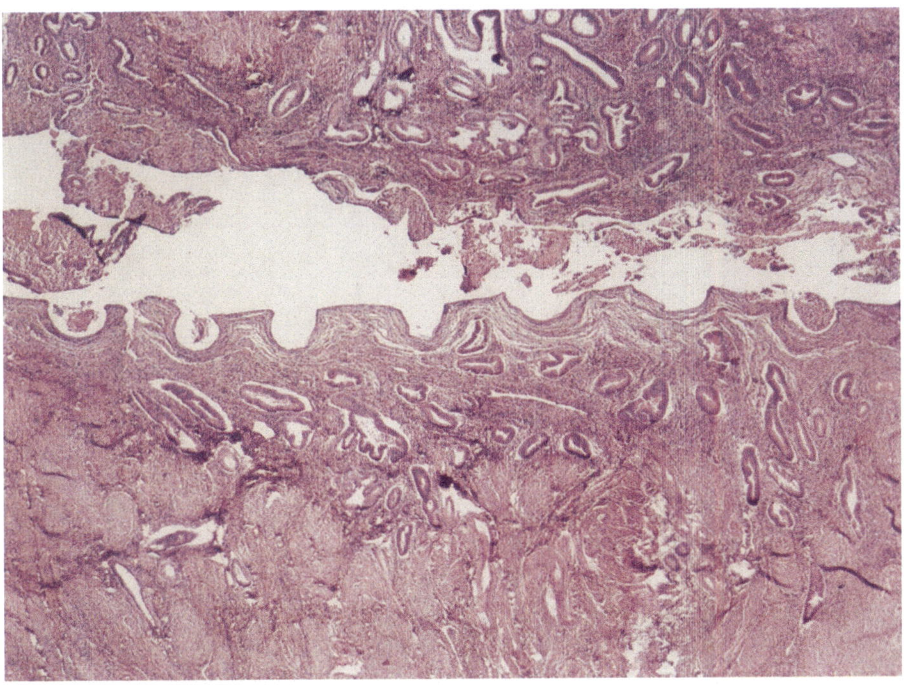

Fig. 7.27 Surface reaction following copper device. H & E, ×25

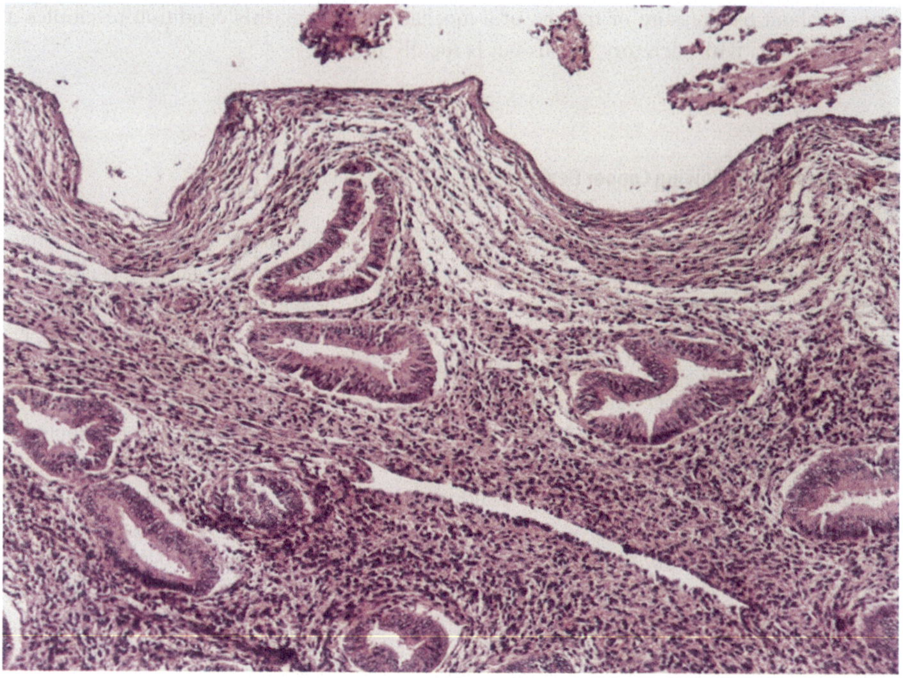

Fig. 7.28 Surface reaction following copper device. H & E, ×100

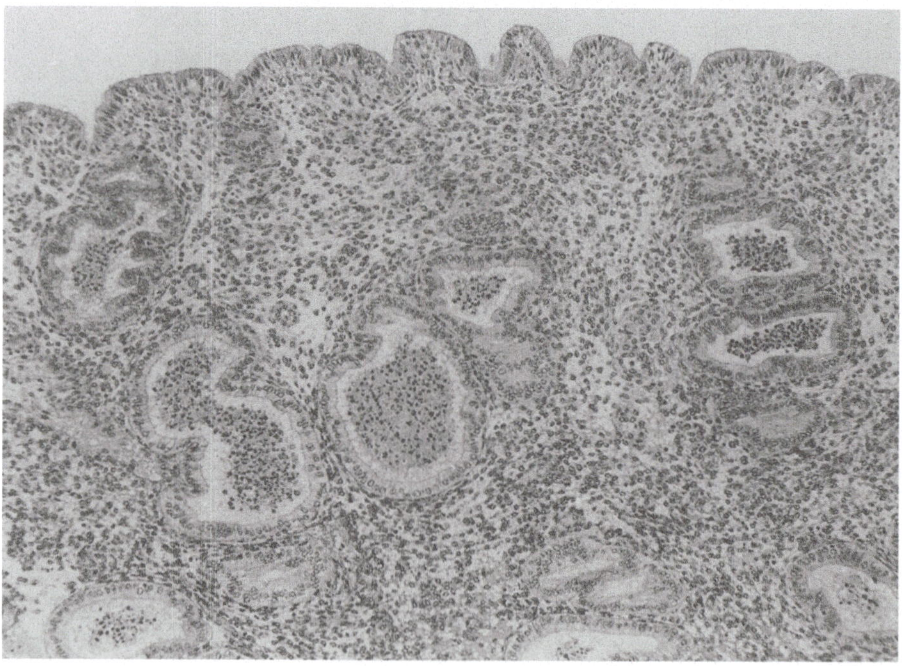

Fig. 7.29 Leukocytes in glandular lumina following copper device. H & E, ×100

Morphologic Differential Diagnosis. It is necessary to distinguish these intraglandular leukocytes from endometritis, which shows glandular and stromal infiltration by inflammatory cells.

7.2.4 Endometritis

A focal, erosive, or even diffuse endometritis may develop with any type of IUD if the endometrium is atrophic or deficiently proliferated (Fig. 7.30), as with previous use of oral contraceptives or endogenous hormone deficiency. A nonfunctioning endometrium acts as a "locus minoris resistentiae" with infection caused by ascending bacteria, whereas normal, functional endometrium is resistant to infection even under local pressure.

7.3 After Intrauterine Instillation

When a contrast medium (for hysterosalpingography) or a liquid adhesive (for permanent sterilization) is instilled into the uterine cavity, various histologic changes may develop.

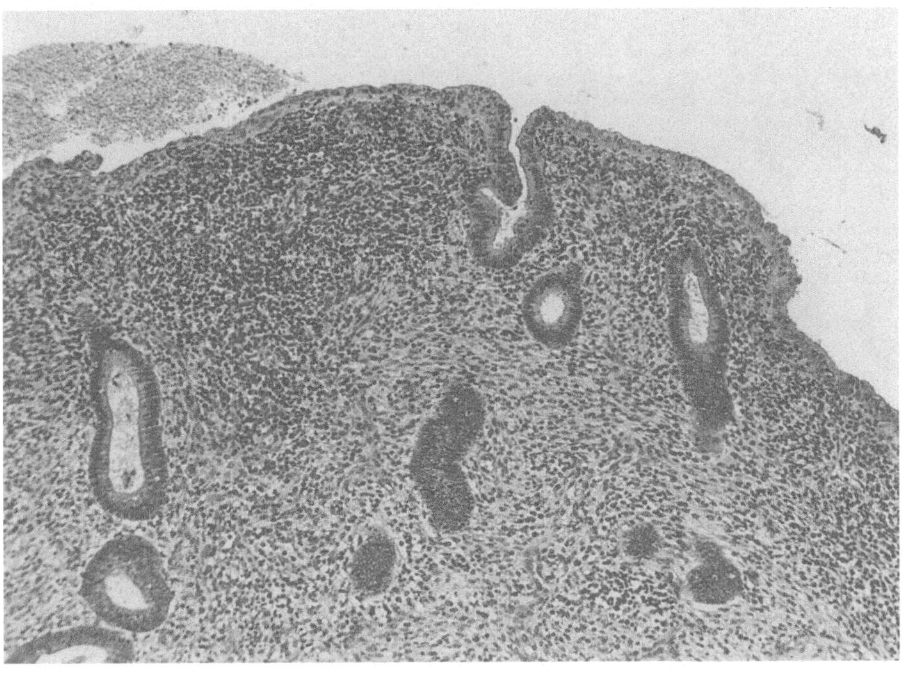

Fig. 7.30 Deficient endometrial proliferation with slight superficial (perifocal) chronic endometritis following copper device. H & E, ×100

7.3.1 Histiocytic Storage Reaction

A histiocytic storage reaction (Figs. 7.31, 7.32) may occur in hyperplastic endometria that do not shed cyclically, as histiocytes may incorporate the material that has been pressed into the superficial stroma. Patches of necrotic material can be seen in the stroma between cystically dilated glands and surrounded by small histiocytes, and partly incorporated by large macrophages laden with a foamy substance which displaces their nuclei (Fig. 7.32).

Morphologic Differential Diagnosis. It is necessary from: (a) foci of epithelial or stromal metaplasia; (b) neoplastic cells.

Distinction is possible by careful examination of these foci and by applying special stains to identify cells and accumulations.

Clinical Correlation. Since this storage is usually an incidental finding, it may be difficult to explain clinically.

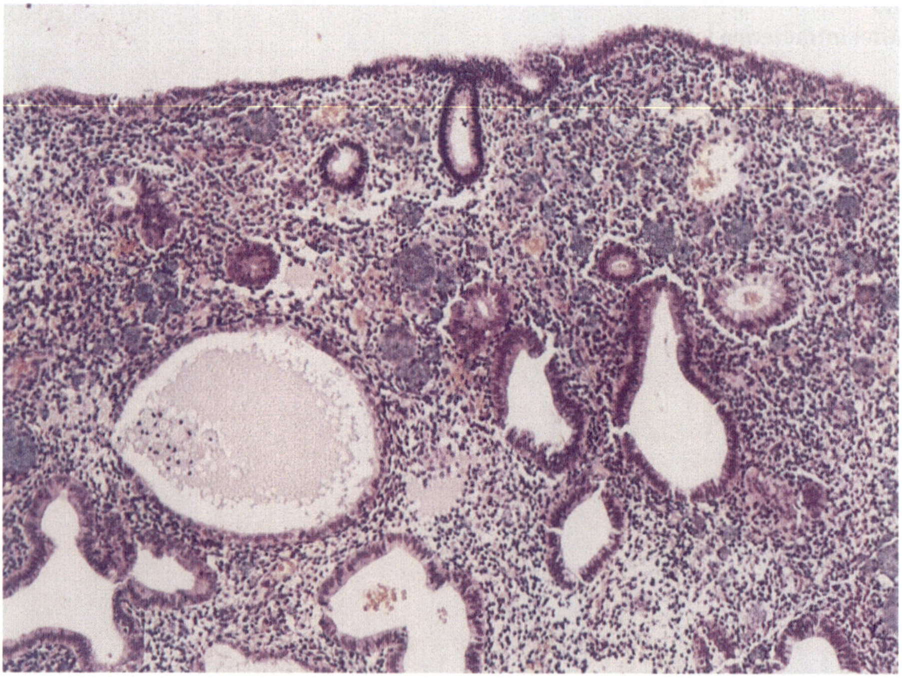

Fig. 7.31 Histiocytic storage reaction. H & E, ×100

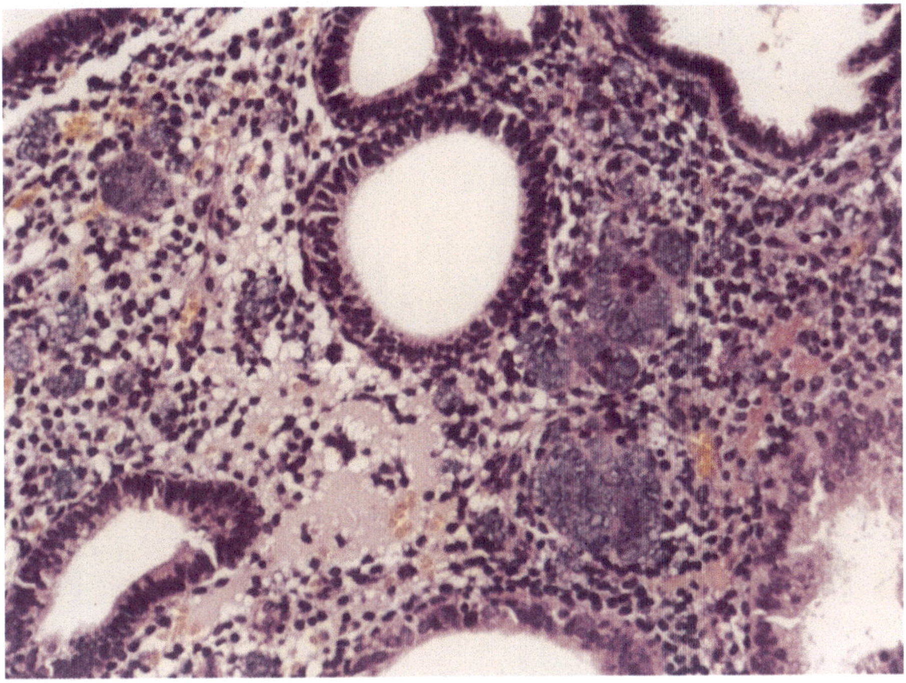

Fig. 7.32 Histiocytic storage reaction. H & E, ×250

Endometritis

8

With normal endometrial function, endometritis is rare. If not severely injured, normal endometrium is resistant against acute infection, and since it is regularly shed every 4 weeks, there is little time for a chronic infection to develop. Endometritis should be diagnosed only if either the glandular epithelium is destroyed by inflammatory cells or if plasma cells are present in addition to neutrophils and lymphocytes.

8.1 Acute Endometritis

Although the causative agents of acute endometritis (Figs. 8.1, 8.2) are numerous, the inflammatory reactions to them are generally the same. Stroma and glands are diffusely or focally infiltrated with polymorphonuclear leukocytes intermixed with lymphocytes and occasional plasma cells. The surface and glandular epithelia are more or less destroyed by the heavy infiltrates, and the reticulin fibers of the stroma disintegrate. There are areas of hemorrhage or edema in the stroma. The cyclic function of the endometrium is often preserved. The infected portions of the endometrium may be shed with the next menstruation unless the basal layer is also involved.

Morphological Differential Diagnosis. Distinction of the inflammatory infiltrates from granular endometrial stromal cells is necessary; the granular stromal cells, which closely resemble polymorphonuclear leukocytes in shape, do not destroy the glandular epithelium. Furthermore, areas of hemorrhagic necrosis, occurring in endometria with protracted shedding in functional disorders, should not be misinterpreted as signs of endometritis.

Clinical Possibilities and Differential Diagnosis. Acute endometritis occurs as an ascending infection when the cervical barrier is damaged: (a) most frequently in abortion; (b) following menses, delivery, curettage, or insertion of an IUD. Endometritis post abortum can be recognized from the characteristic changes of the endometrial glands (irregular shedding; see Figs. 6.58–6.61), remnants of decidua, and possibly placental villi or trophoblasts.

G. Dallenbach-Hellweg et al., *Atlas of Endometrial Histopathology*,
DOI: 10.1007/978-3-642-01541-0_8, © Springer-Verlag Berlin Heidelberg 2010

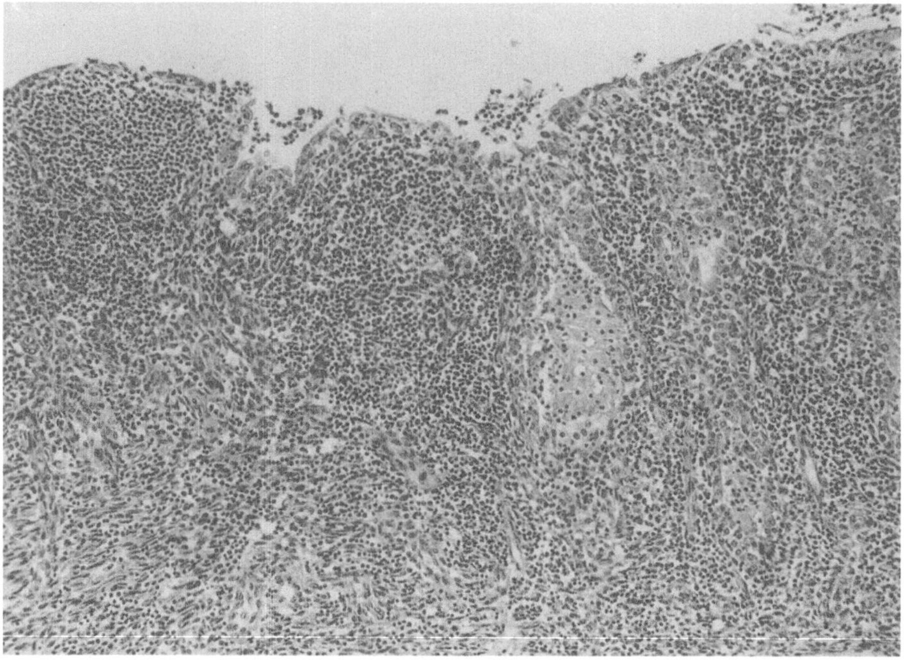

Fig. 8.1 Acute endometritis. H & E, ×100

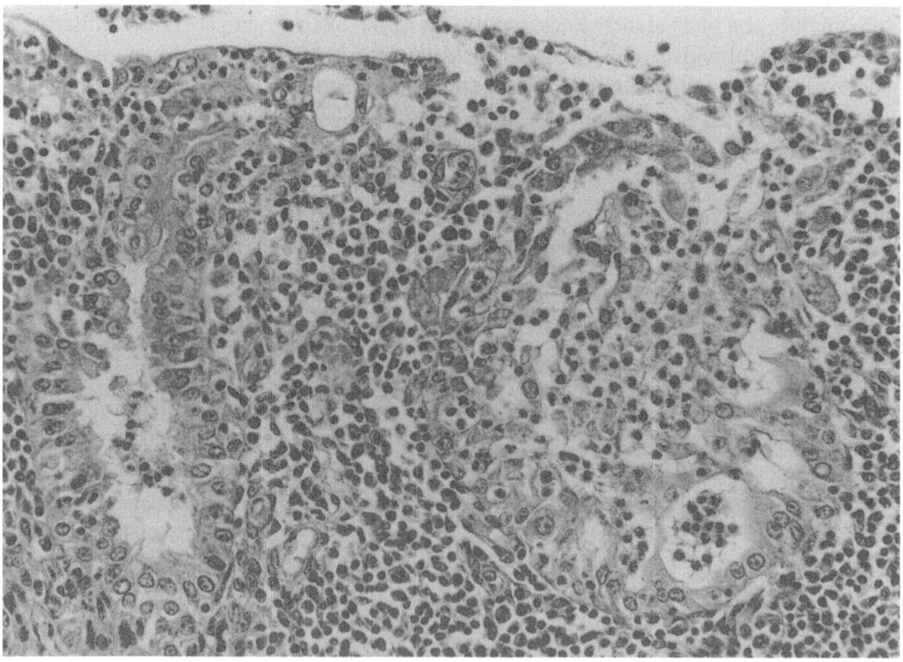

Fig. 8.2 Acute endometritis. H & E, ×250

8.2 Chronic Endometritis

Endometritis can only become chronic (Figs. 8.3–8.5) if the endometrium is not shed with menstruation. Hence, the endometrial glands are hyperplastic, irregularly or insufficiently proliferated, resting or atrophic, and the stromal cells are spindle shaped. The inflammatory infiltrates mainly consist of lymphocytes and plasma cells, which are scattered diffusely throughout the stroma or aggregated focally. They also infiltrate and destroy the glandular and surface epithelium. There is, however, no destruction of reticulin fibers, and the endometrial architecture is preserved.

Morphologic Differential Diagnosis. Lymphocytic infiltrates or lymph follicles without glandular involvement in the absence of plasma cells are not indicative of chronic endometritis, but may occur physiologically. On the other hand, chronic endometritis must be differentiated from tuberculous endometritis, which may have lost most of its characteristic granulomatous reaction with Langhans giant cells. A careful search for epithelioid tubercles is necessary to exclude such a possibility.

Distinction is also necessary from lymphomatous infiltrations (see Chap. 9.5), which are rather uniform in contrast to the heterogeneous admixture of lymphoid cells with neutrophils and plasma cells in endometritis (Young et al. 1985). Very occasionally, a subacute and chronic immunoreactive endometritis may develop (Skensved et al. 1991); such cases may be caused by infection with *Chlamydia trachomatis* (Winkler et al. 1984).

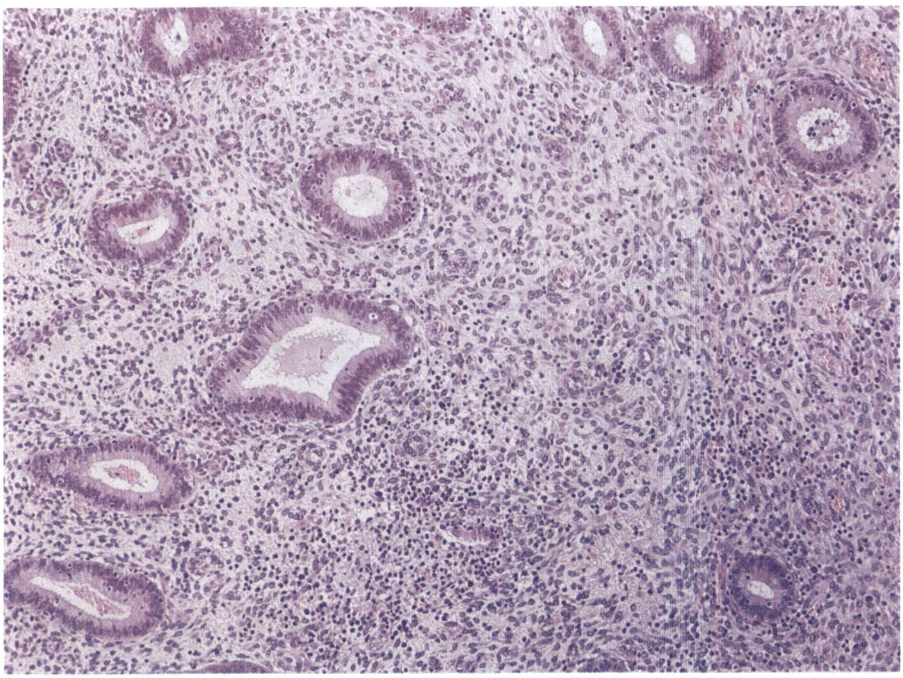

Fig. 8.3 Chronic endometritis. H & E, ×100

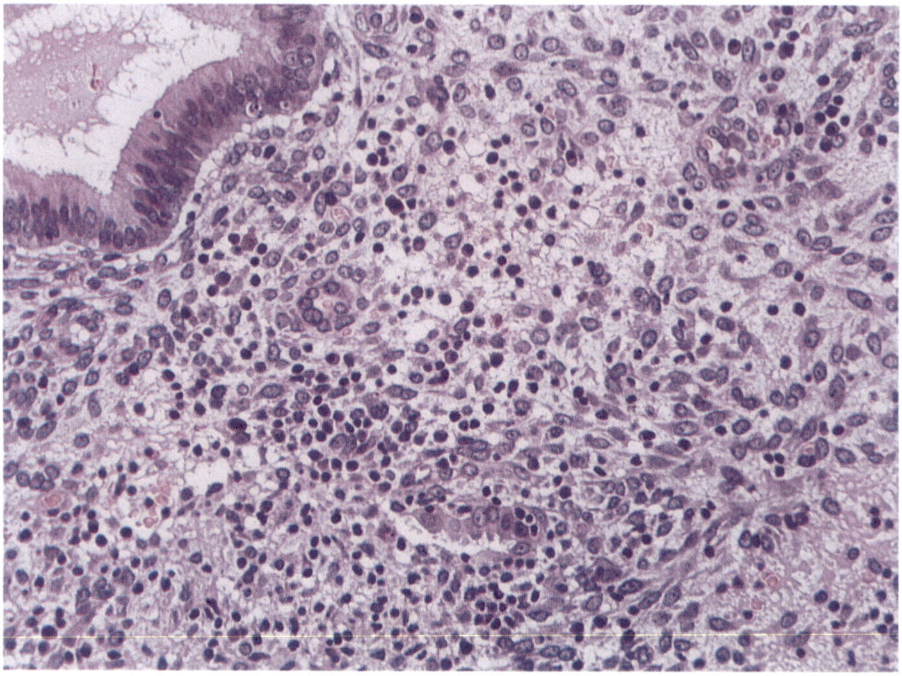

Fig. 8.4 Chronic endometritis. H & E, ×250

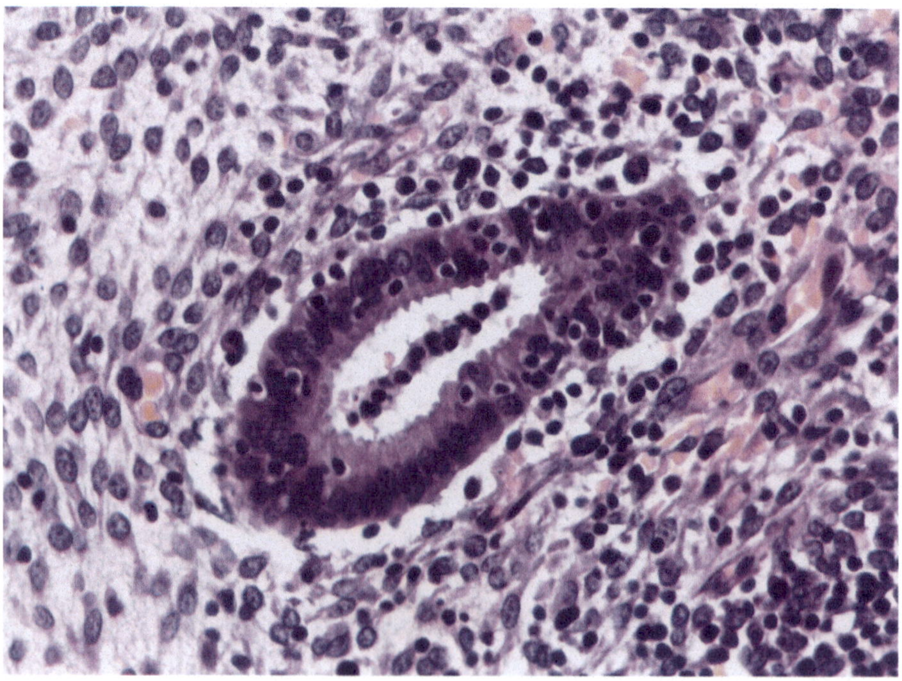

Fig. 8.5 Chronic endometritis. H & E, ×400

Clinical Correlation and Differential Diagnosis. The causative agents are the same as in acute infection. In senile patients chronic endometritis easily develops in low resistant atrophic endometrium and may be associated with necrotic polyps or carcinoma.

8.3 Tuberculous Endometritis

In tuberculous endometritis, the extent of the involvement of the endometrium may vary greatly. In severe infection, typical granulomas with Langhans giant cells and epithelioid cells surrounded by lymphocytes are crowded together to varying extents, filling large portions of the stroma (Figs. 8.6, 8.7) and protruding into glandular lumina. There may be caseous necrosis and ulceration of the endometrial surface. The glandular epithelium often responds by atypical proliferation, stratification, metaplasia, or new gland formation. The endometrial function is disturbed, and the peritubercular fibrosis inhibits endometrial shedding.

Morphologic Differential Diagnosis. Tuberculous endometritis must be distinguished from similar specific granulomas, such as sarcoidosis and mycotic infections, and from foreign body granuloma. Sarcoidosis contains no acid-fast bacteria and shows no caseation. In mycotic granulomas, fungal organisms can often be found by special stains. Foreign body granulomas often can be recognized by their birefringent material under polarizing illumination (Fig. 8.12).

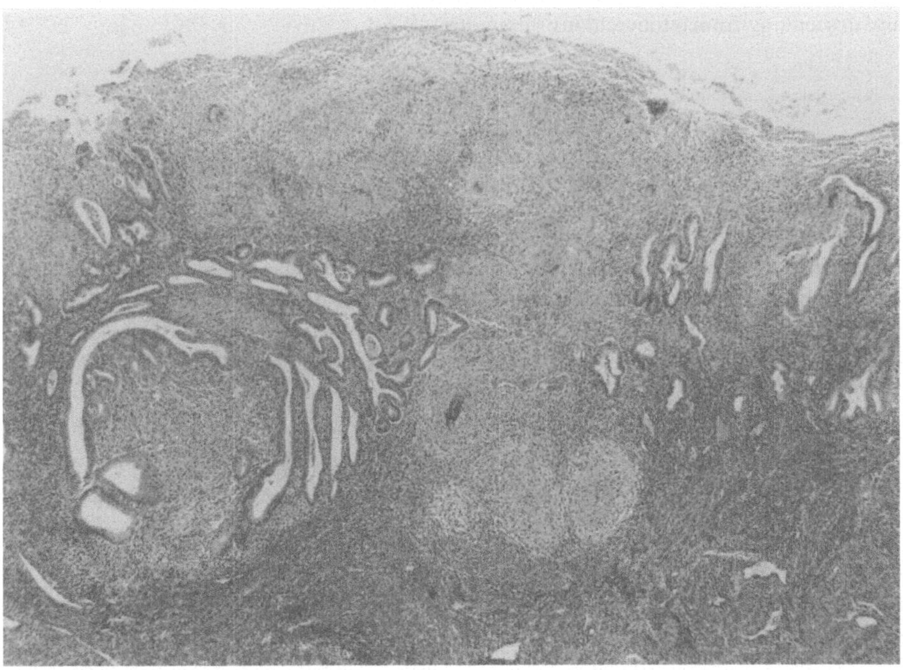

Fig. 8.6 Tuberculous endometritis. H & E, ×25

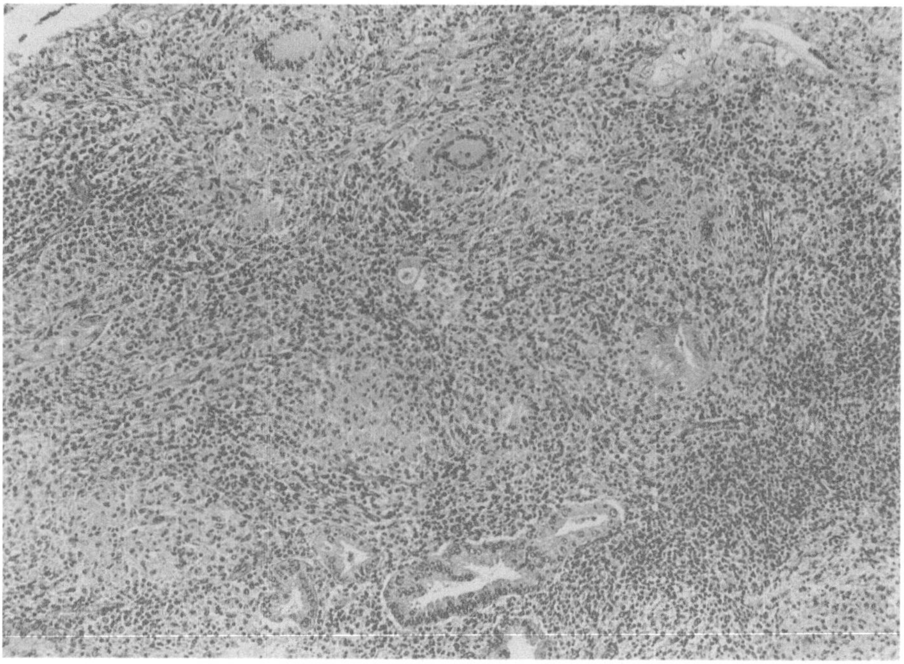

Fig. 8.7 Tuberculous endometritis. H & E, ×100

Clinical Correlation. Endometrial involvement occurs from tuberculous bacteria, usually descending from a tuberculous salpingitis.

8.4 Sarcoidosis

In sarcoidosis (Figs. 8.8, 8.9) granulomas consisting of epithelioid cells and usually multinucleated giant cells closely resembling tuberculous granulomas occupy areas of the endometrial stroma. In contrast to tuberculosis, there is no caseation, and glandular involvement or reactive epithelial proliferation is very rare. The endometria involved are often diffusely hyperplastic (Fig. 8.8), since they do not shed with menstruation.

Morphologic Differential Diagnosis. Tuberculous or related granulomas.

Clinical Correlation and Differential Diagnosis. Endometrial involvement in a systemic sarcoidosis is rare, but differentiation from tuberculosis is of clinical importance.

8.5 Actinomycosis

In actinomycosis (Fig. 8.10), characteristic radiating particles of various sizes can be found between endometrial fragments disintegrated by inflammatory infiltrates.

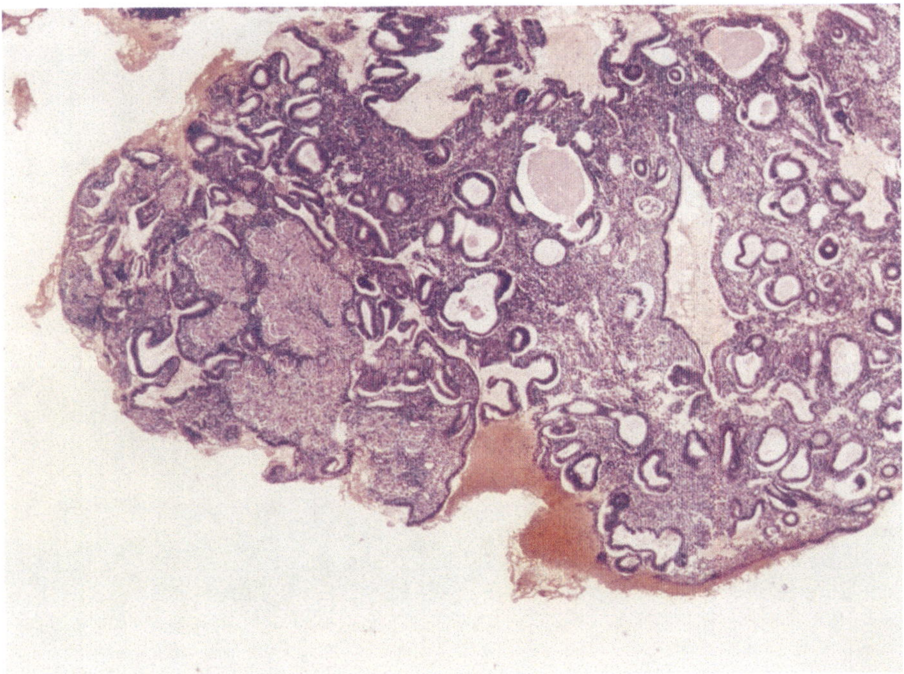

Fig. 8.8 Sarcoidosis. H & E, ×25

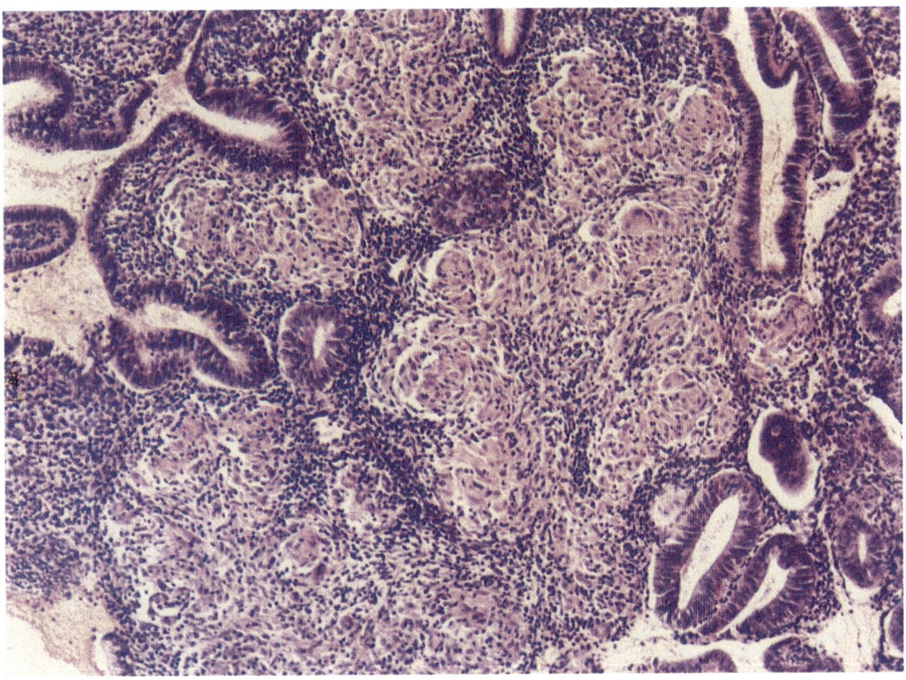

Fig. 8.9 Sarcoidosis. H & E, ×100

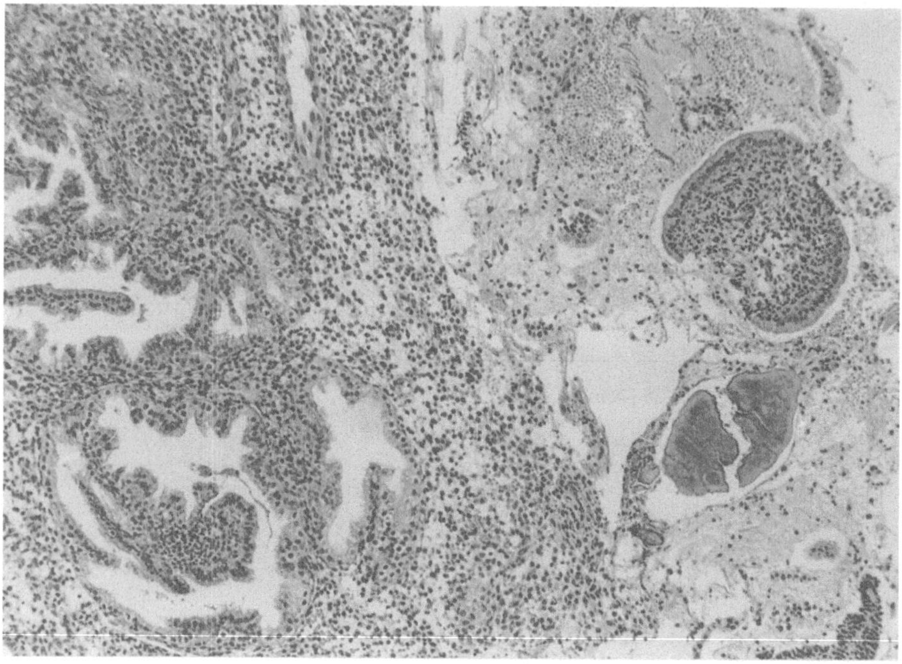

Fig. 8.10 Actinomycosis. H & E, ×100

Clinical Correlation. Actinomyces infection of the endometrium is a rare complication after insertion of an IUD (Lomax et al. 1976).

8.6 Foreign Body Granuloma

Resting or cystic atrophic endometria that are not shed may harbor foreign body granulomas (Figs. 8.11–8.13), preferably in the basal layer (Fig. 8.11), consisting of multinucleated foreign body giant cells surrounded by chronic inflammatory infiltrates. The giant cells may contain variously shaped birefringent crystals (Fig. 8.12) which they have phagocytized (Fig. 8.13).

Morphologic Differential Diagnosis. Similar granulomas (see above). The presence of birefringent inclusions under polarized light is diagnostic.

Clinical Correlation. Talcum granulomas may develop after intrauterine procedures. Foreign body granulomas caused by other materials are rare in the endometrium.

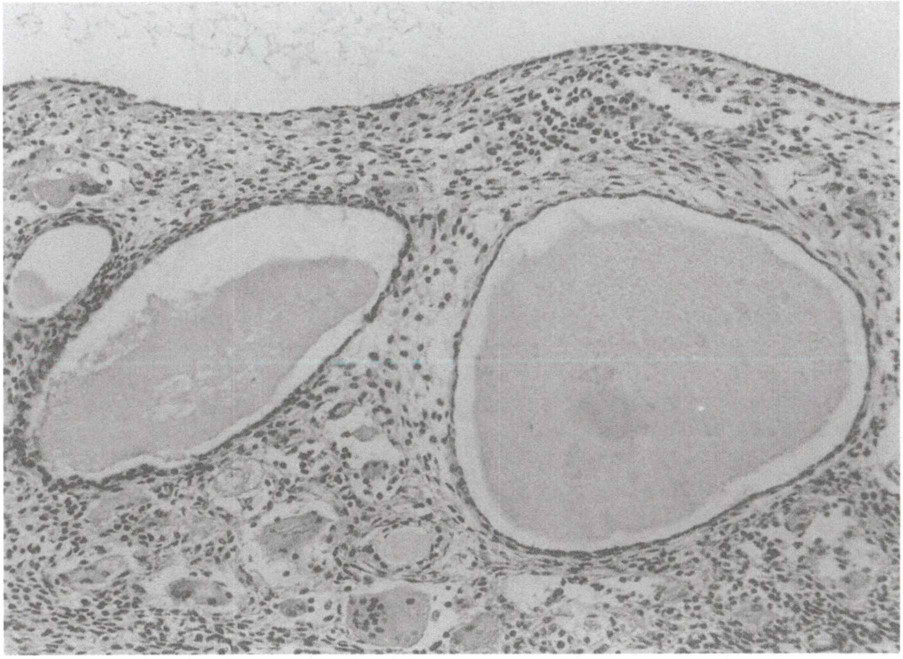

Fig. 8.11 Foreign body granuloma. H & E, ×100

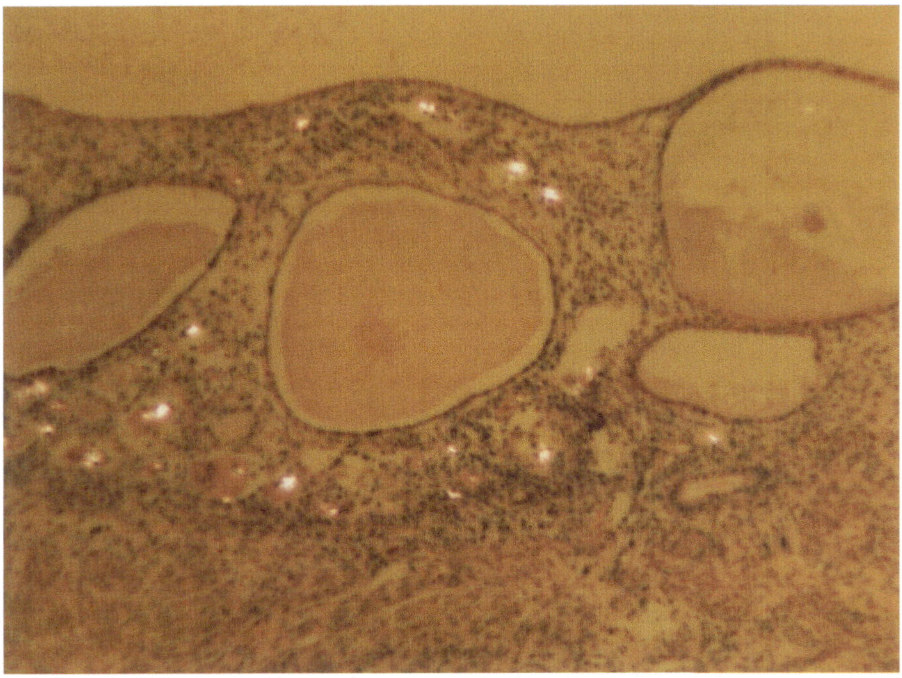

Fig. 8.12 Foreign body granuloma (same as Fig. 8.11) under polarized light, showing birefringent crystalline inclusions. H & E, ×75

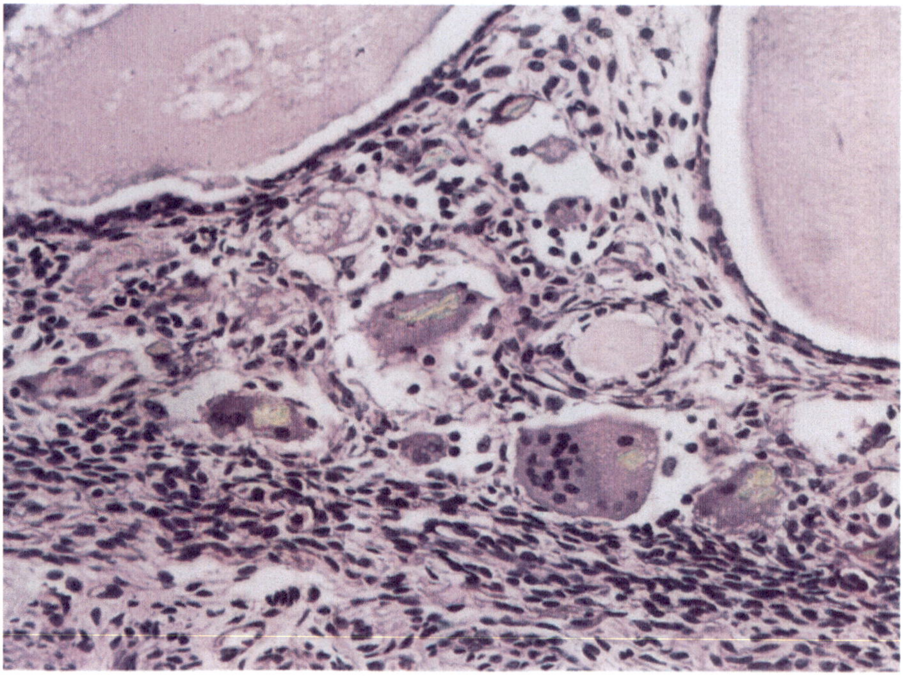

Fig. 8.13 Foreign body granuloma. H & E, ×250

Neoplasms 9

9.1 Carcinomas

In the characterization of endometrial carcinomas there are three possibilities: histologic typing, grading of differentiation, and staging (Poulsen et al. 1975).

Histologic Typing. According to histogenetic principles, carcinomas of the endometrium can be subdivided into those of endometrioid origin under estrogenic hyperstimulation (adenocarcinoma; adenocarcinoma with squamous differentiation or glandular variants), and those from estrogen-independent pluripotential Müllerian epithelium (carcinomas of endocervical type: mucinous and mucoepidermoid adenocarcinoma; clear cell; serous; squamous cell; transitional cell; small cell carcinomas; see Table 9.1). Both major types, the endometrioid and the nonendometrioid carcinomas also differ considerably at their molecular level: endometrioid carcinomas and their precursors show LOH mainly at 10q23.3 (PTEN) (in 40%, Velasco et al. 2008) as well as MMR deficiency with microsatellite instability (MSI) and hypermethylation of MLHA as early events in carcinogenesis in 20–30% of all carcinomas of this type (Karamurzin and Rutgers 2009). In contrast, nonendometrioid carcinomas and their precursors often present LOH at 17p13 resulting in mutations with overexpression of p53 (Velasco et al. 2008) and p16 mutations.

Histologic Grading. This should be based on the degree of structural differentiation and cytologic atypia. In accordance with FIGO (1988) and WHO (2003), three grades can be distinguished (Table 9.2).

The following should be noted concerning pathologic grading:

- Notable nuclear atypia, inappropriate for the architectural grade, raises the grade of a grade 1 or 2 tumor by 1.
- In serous adenocarcinomas, clear cell adenocarcinomas, and squamous cell carcinomas, nuclear grading takes precedence.
- Adenocarcinomas with squamous differentiation are graded according to the nuclear grade of the glandular component.

Surgical Staging. According to FIGO 1988 (refer to Creasman 1989), carcinomas of the endometrium can be staged as shown in Table 9.3.

G. Dallenbach-Hellweg et al., *Atlas of Endometrial Histopathology*,
DOI: 10.1007/978-3-642-01541-0_9,

Table 9.1 Carcinomas of the endometrium, histological classification

Structure and grading	Survival rate (%)	Relative frequency (%)
Endometrioid adenocarcinoma		40
Grade 1 (glandular)	93	
Grade 2 + 3 (dedifferentiated)	61	
Villoglandular variant	76	
Secretory variant	87	
Ciliated cell variant		
With squamous differentiation		30
Grade 1	87	
Grade 2 + 3	47	
Mucinous adenocarcinoma	47	18
With squamous differentiation		
Grade 1–3		
Serous adenocarcinoma	44–11	6
Clear cell adenocarcinoma	59–15	4
Squamous cell carcinoma		
Small cell carcinoma		
Undifferentiated carcinoma		

Table 9.2 Histologic grading according to the degree of glandular differentiation

Grade	Degree of differentiation
G1	5% or less of a nonsquamous or nonmorular solid growth pattern
G2	6–50% of a nonsquamous or nonmorular solid growth pattern
G3	More than 50% of a nonsquamous or nonmorular solid growth pattern

Table 9.3 Staging of endometrial cancer

Stage	Grade	Surgical/pathologic spread
IA	G123	Tumor limited to the endometrium
IB	G123	Invasion to less than one half of the myometrium
IC	G123	Invasion to more than one half of the myometrium
IIA	G123	Endocervical glandular involvement only
IIB	G123	Cervical stromal invasion
IIIA	G123	Positive peritoneal cytology and/or tumor invades serosa and/or adnexa
IIIB	G123	Vaginal metastases
IIIC	G123	Metastases to pelvic and/or para- aortic lymph nodes
IVA	G123	Tumor invasion of bladder and/or bowel
IVB		Distant metastases including intraabdominal and/or inguinal lymph nodes

9.1.1 Adenocarcinomas of the Endometrioid Type

9.1.1.1 Early Adenocarcinoma

Early carcinomatous changes (Figs. 9.1–9.4) may develop focally or multicentrically within an atypical hyperplasia. They are always limited to the endometrium (Fig. 9.1). Within these foci, groups of glands are lined by multilayered, atypical epithelial cells which have depolarized, enlarged nuclei containing prominent nucleoli. They are frequently in mitosis. Their cytoplasm is pale or vacuolated (Fig. 9.4). The stroma is rarefied and focally scant, particularly in regions with microalveolar change. The early carcinomatous foci have compressed borders and may be surrounded by lymphocytic infiltrates indicating stromal invasion (Fig. 9.3). Most of these early carcinomas are glandular grade 1 carcinomas, but occasionally grade 2 or even grade 3 changes may be seen.

Morphologic Differential Diagnosis. Early adenocarcinoma must be differentiated from atypical hyperplasia (see Figs. 6.31–6.34). The most important criterion for the beginning of carcinomatous growth is stromal invasion (Kurman and Norris 1982). According to Kurman and Norris, the main criteria for invasion are: a desmoplastic stromal reaction around irregularly infiltrating glands, a confluent glandular pattern with microalveolar proliferation and loss of stroma, and an extensive papillary pattern or large areas of squamous

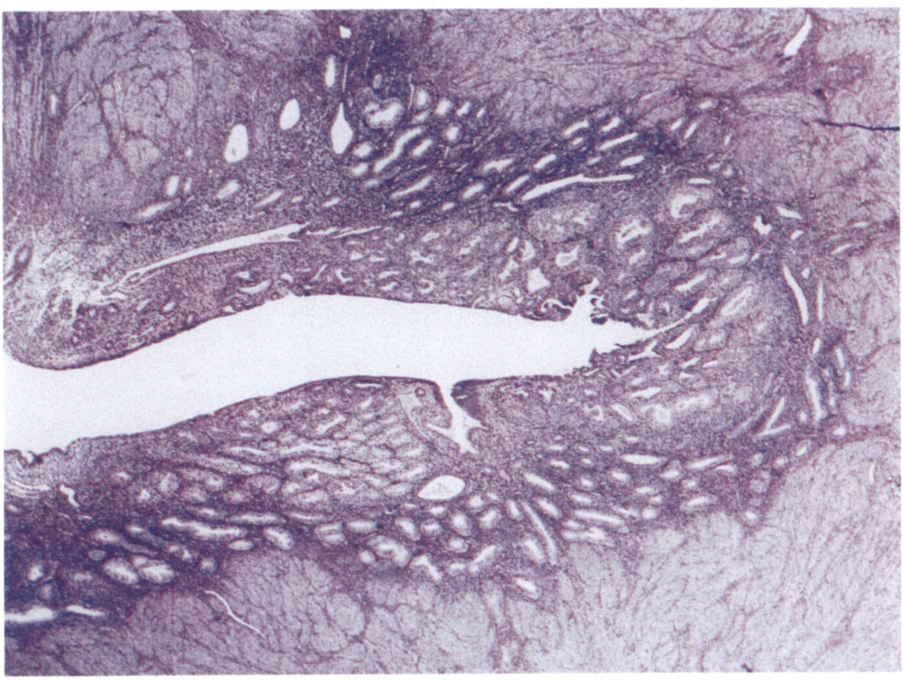

Fig. 9.1 Early adenocarcinoma, grade 1. H & E, ×25

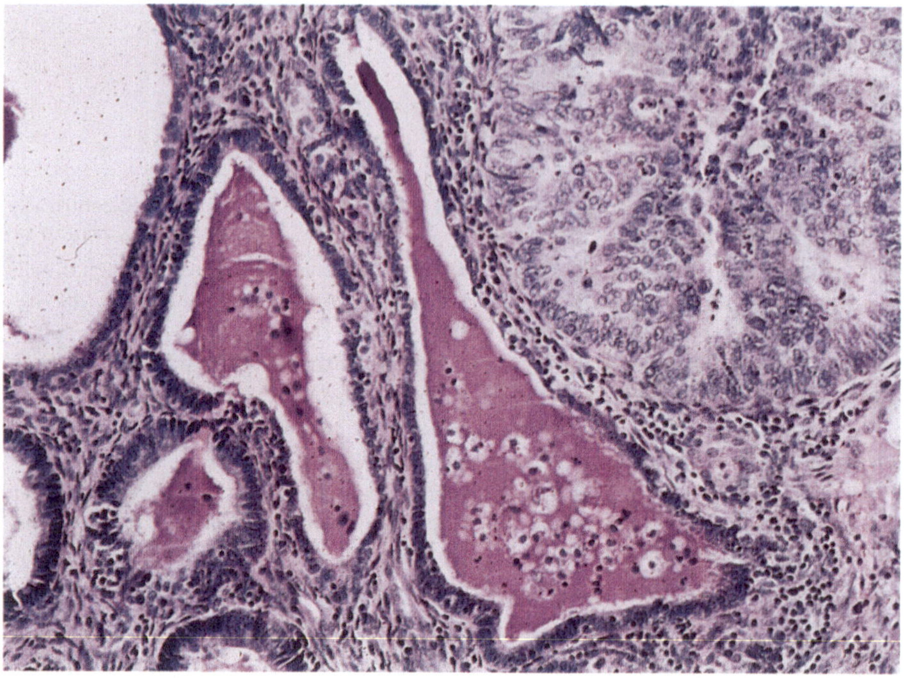

Fig. 9.2 Early adenocarcinoma, grade 1, endometrioid type. Periodic acid-Schiff (PAS) reaction, ×150

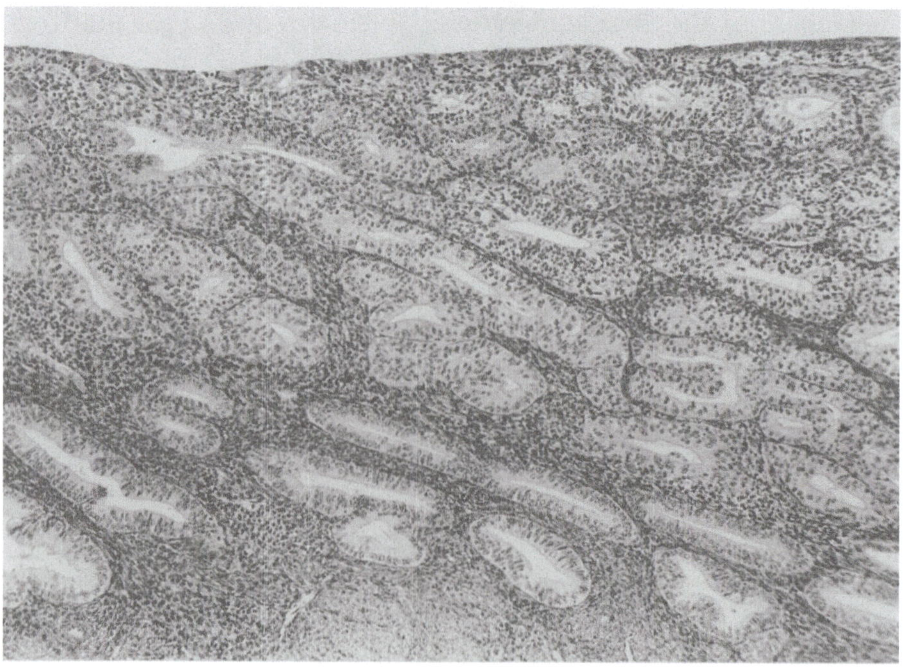

Fig. 9.3 Early adenocarcinoma, grade 1. H & E, ×100

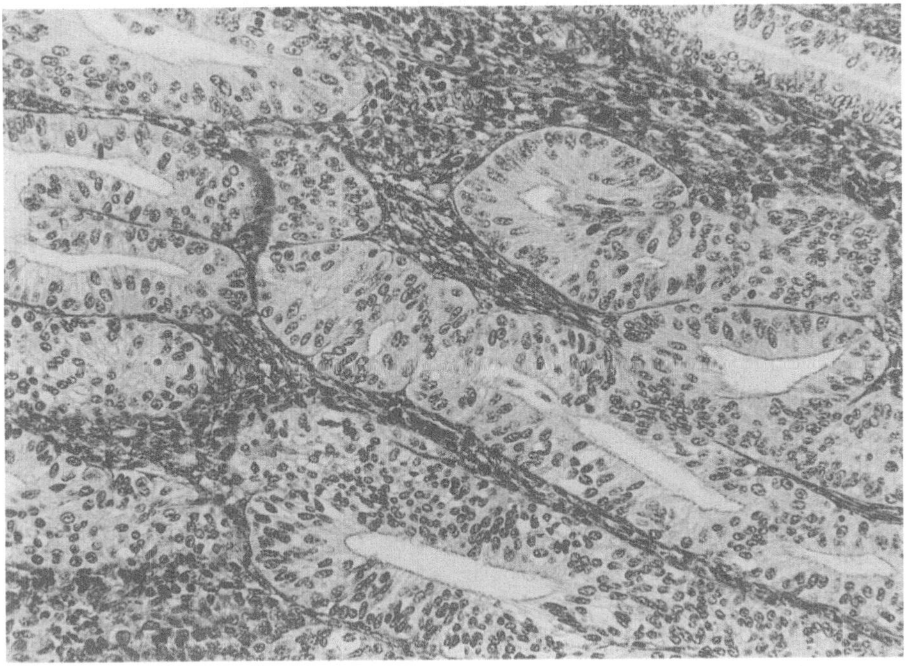

Fig. 9.4 Early adenocarcinoma, grade 1. H & E, ×250

metaplasia. One of these criteria, if it occupies one half of a low-power field 4.2 mm in diameter, would be sufficient for a diagnosis of stromal invasion.

9.1.1.2 Well-Differentiated Adenocarcinoma

In well differentiated adenocarcinoma (FIGO grade 1, 5% or less solid growth pattern; Figs. 9.5–9.7), the well differentiated tubular glands appear slender, contain little or no mucus (Fig. 9.5), and are lined by pseudostratified or stratified epithelial cells with elongated large nuclei, prominent nucleoli, and frequent mitoses. Their cytoplasm is sparse. A few long and thin papillary structures may be seen in the villoglandular variant (Fig. 9.6). The stroma between the glands is reduced to scanty fibers of collagen and thin capillaries.

Morphologic Differential Diagnosis. The villo-glandular type of endometrioid adenocarcinoma must be distinguished from serous adenocarcinoma (Fig. 9.30) which is much more aggressive. Serous adenocarcinoma is nearly always strongly positive for p16 (Chiesa-Vottero et al. 2007), whereas endometrioid adenocarcinoma contains few small patches of positive cells only.

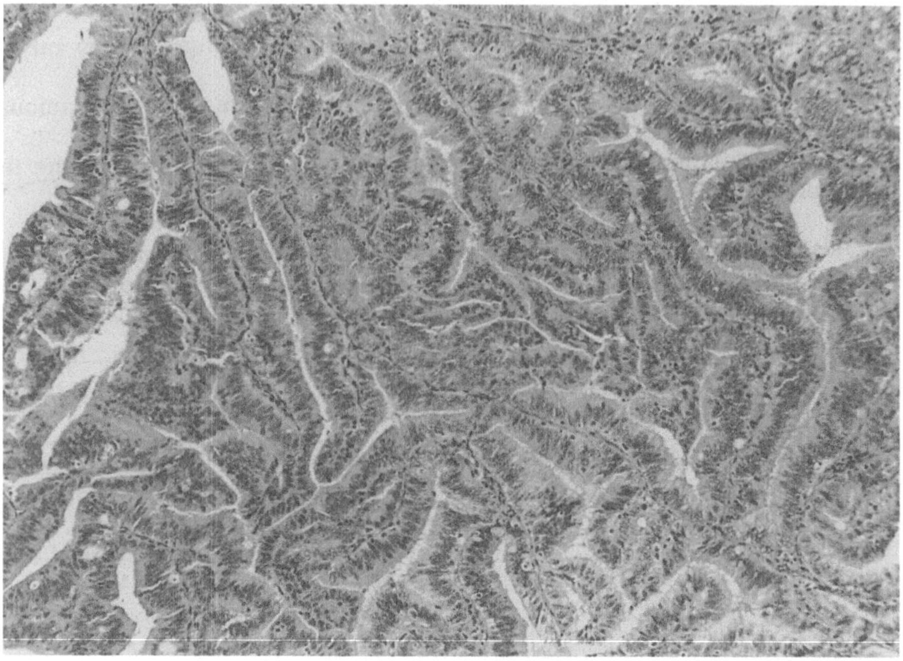

Fig. 9.5 Well differentiated adenocarcinoma, glandular (grade 1, endometrioid type). H & E, ×100

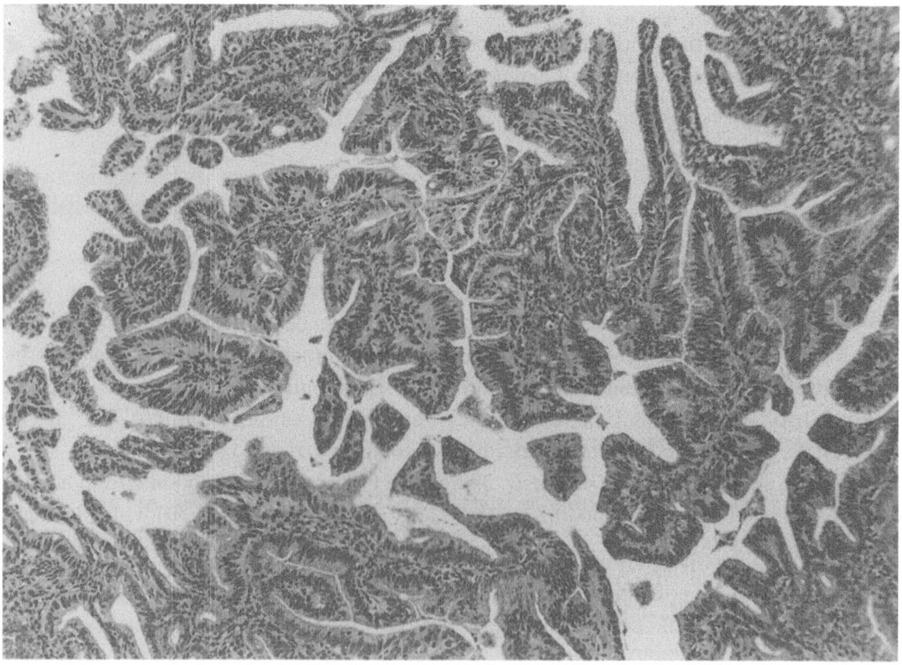

Fig. 9.6 Well differentiated adenocarcinoma, villo-glandular variant (grade 1, endometrioid type). H & E, ×100

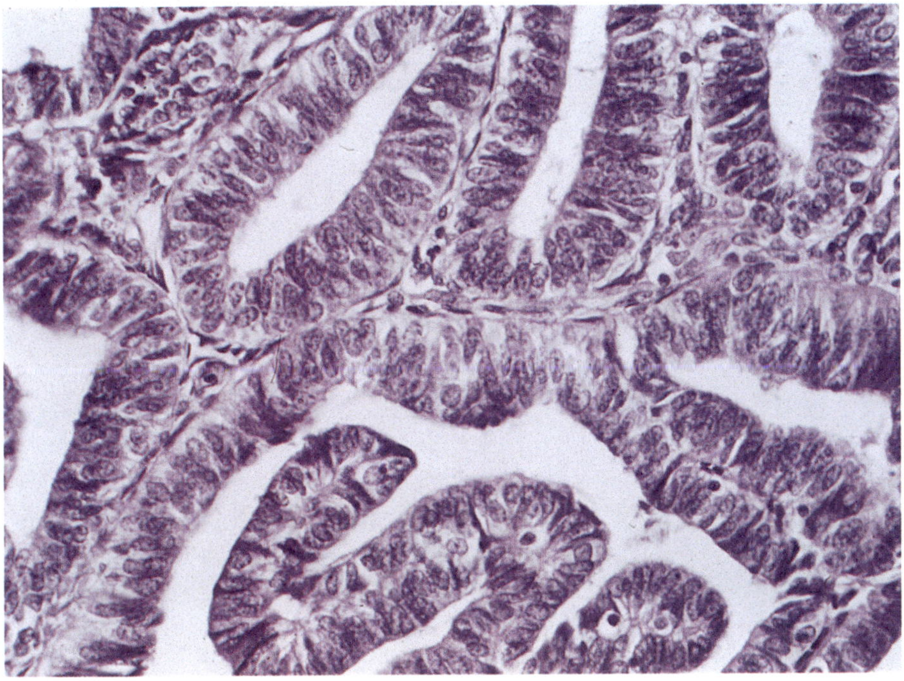

Fig. 9.7 Well differentiated adenocarcinoma (grade 1, endometrioid type). H & E, ×350

9.1.1.3
Dedifferentiated Adenocarcinoma

Dedifferentiated adenocarcinomas include grade 2 tumors with poorly differentiated glands (Fig. 9.8) as well as grade 3 tumors with more than 50% solid growth pattern (Figs. 9.9, 9.10). There may be a sharp line between well-differentiated and dedifferentiated carcinomatous areas (Fig. 9.9), or early stages of microglandular formation may be poorly recognized between strands of glandular cells (Fig. 9.8). The grading is nevertheless determined by the solid component. In grade 3 adenocarcinomas consisting mainly or only of solid areas of disorderly arranged undifferentiated carcinomatous cells (Fig. 9.10) pseudorosettes may be distinguished, indicating the adenomatous nature of the tumor. This criterion and immunohistochemical stains for cytokeratin 13 (squamous) and 18 (glandular epithelium) can be used to differentiate the solid adenocarcinoma from an undifferentiated squamous cell carcinoma.

Clinical Correlations. Endometrioid adenocarcinomas with MSI are often less well differentiated and occur in non-obese patients with a lower average age than the carcinomas of mainly obese patients with endogenous hyperestrogenism.

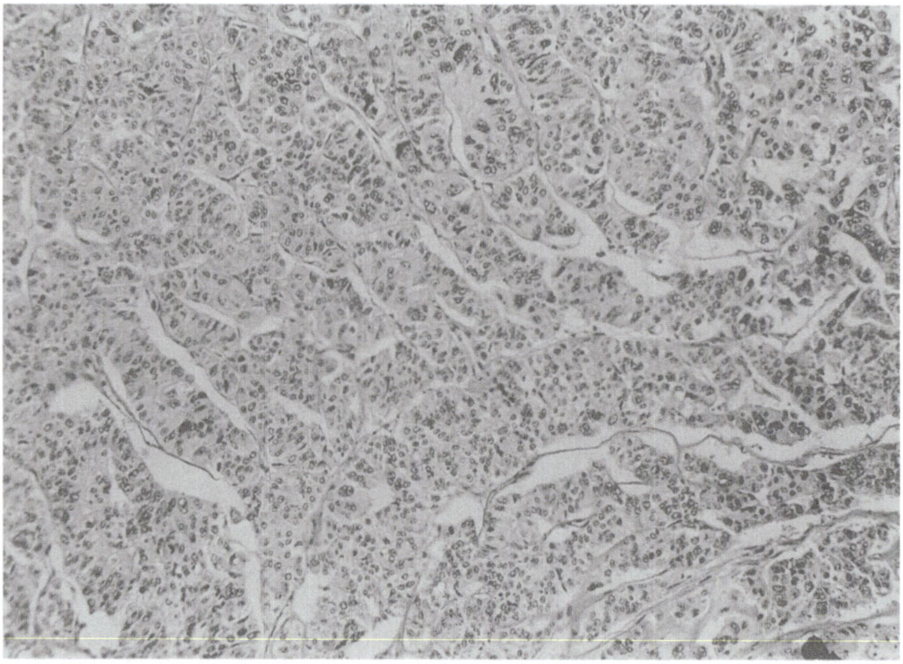

Fig. 9.8 Poorly differentiated adenocarcinoma (grade 2, endometrioid type). H & E, ×100

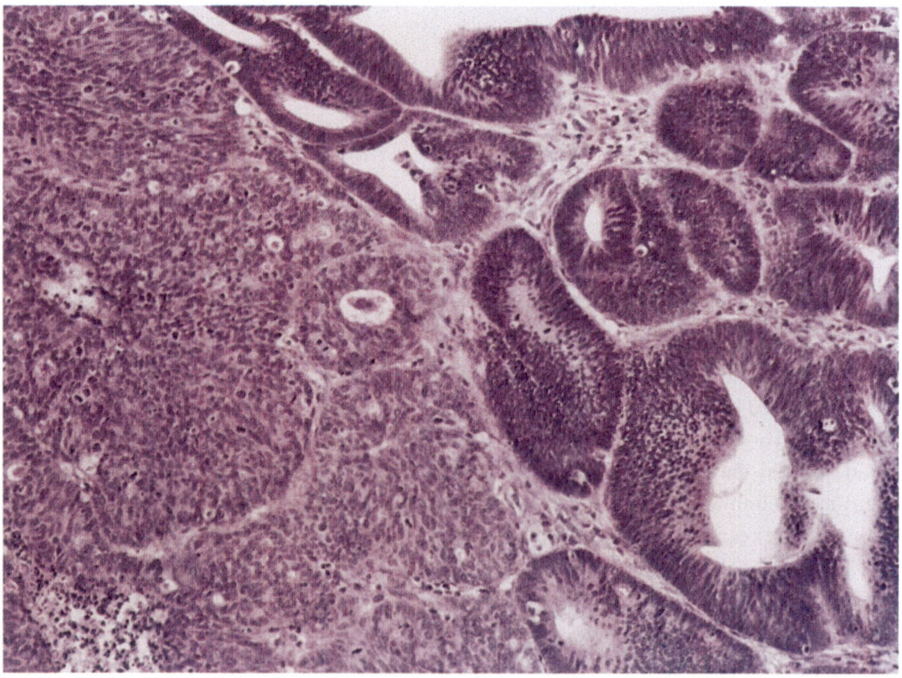

Fig. 9.9 Partly dedifferentiated adenocarcinoma (grade 3, endometrioid type). H & E, ×100

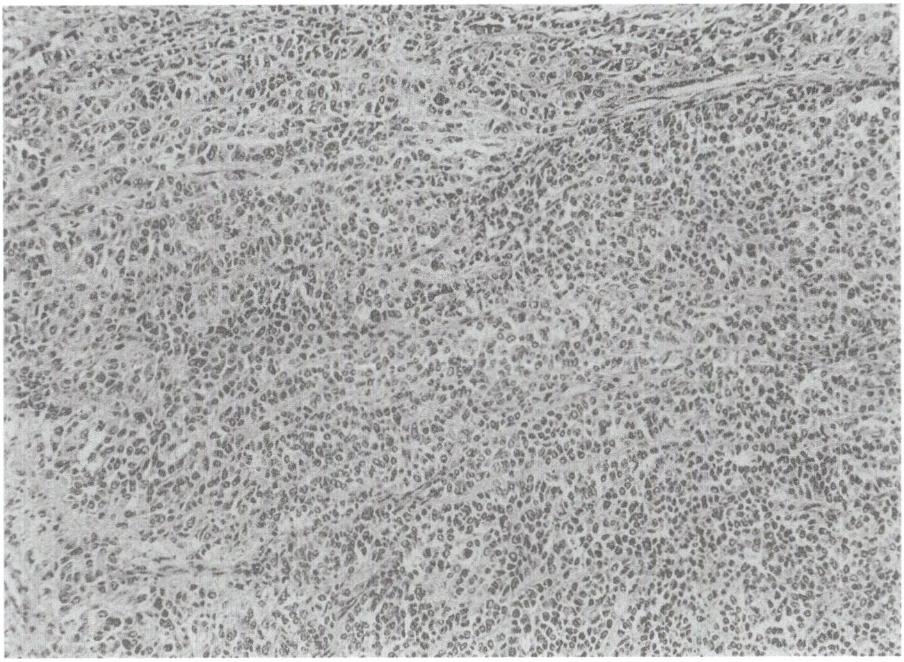

Fig. 9.10 Dedifferentiated solid adenocarcinoma (grade 3, endometrioid type). H & E, ×100

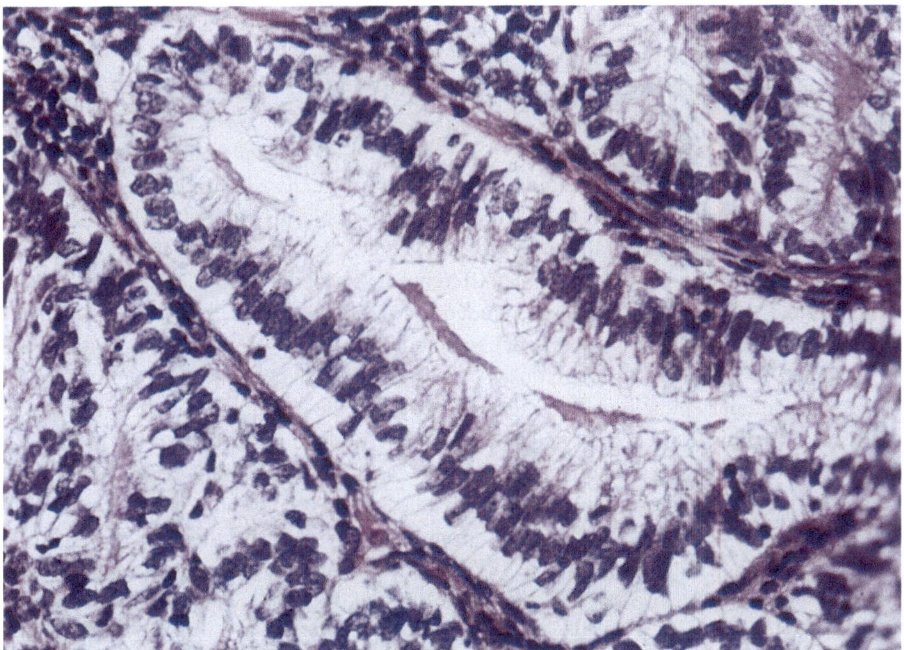

Fig. 9.11 Secretory adenocarcinoma, grade 1. H & E, ×350

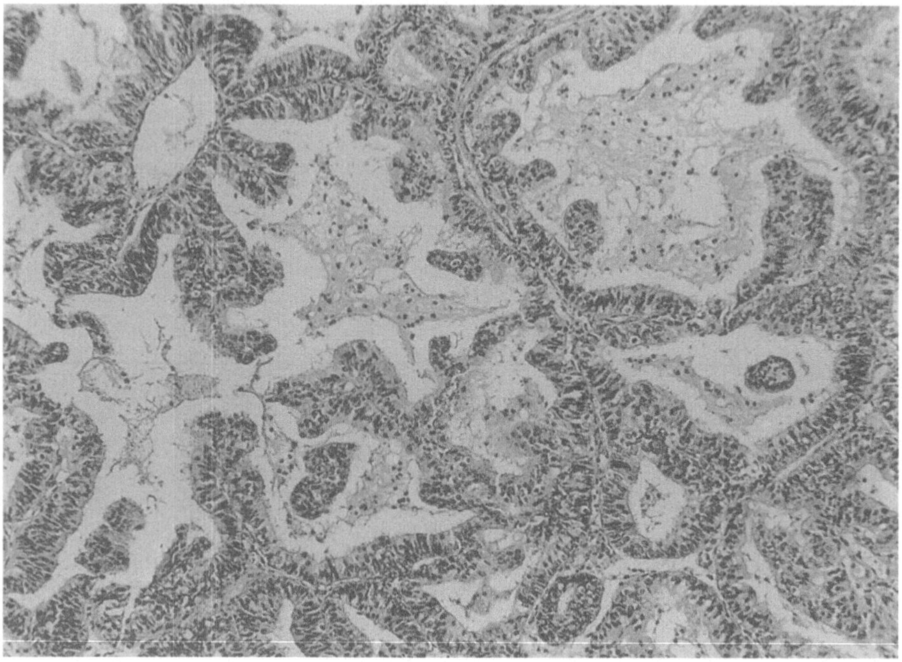

Fig. 9.12 Secretory adenocarcinoma, grade 1. H & E, ×100

9.1.1.4 Secretory Adenocarcinoma

Secretory adenocarcinoma (Figs. 9.11, 9.12) is a well-differentiated adenocarcinoma of the endometrioid type with convoluted glands containing cells with irregular, depolarized nuclei often in a single row in abundant secreting cytoplasm with subnuclear vacuoles (Fig. 9.11), or producing intraluminal secretion (Fig. 9.12). Except for this pronounced secretory change, there is no remarkable difference between this type of carcinoma and the non-secretory well-differentiated type of adenocarcinoma (see Figs. 9.5, 9.6).

Clinical Correlation. Secretory adenocarcinoma is rare. Some patients with these tumors have been treated with high doses of gestagen, which explains the secretory activity of the glandular epithelium (see Figs. 7.9, 7.10). In the remaining patients, the source of this progestational effect may be difficult to clarify, since most of them are in the late postmenopausal period (Christopherson et al. 1982a). In those very rare cases encountered in premenopausal women who have not received gestagen therapy a corpus luteum is usually found (Kurman and Scully 1976). Approximately 50% of those premenopausal patients have microsatellite - instable (MSI-positive) carcinomas, often combined with hereditary colorectal carcinomas (Sutter et al 2003; cf. to p. 84). The rare occurrence of endometrial carcinomas with intrauterine pregnancy has been reviewed by Schammel et al. (1998).

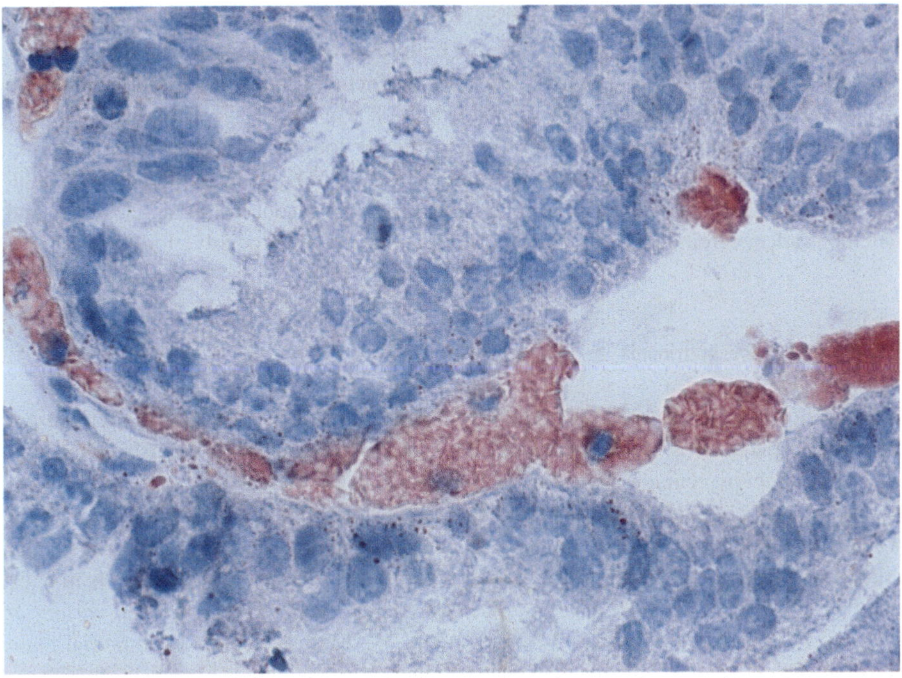

Fig. 9.13 Endometrioid adenocarcinoma with foam cells. Cryostat section, Sudan red, ×400

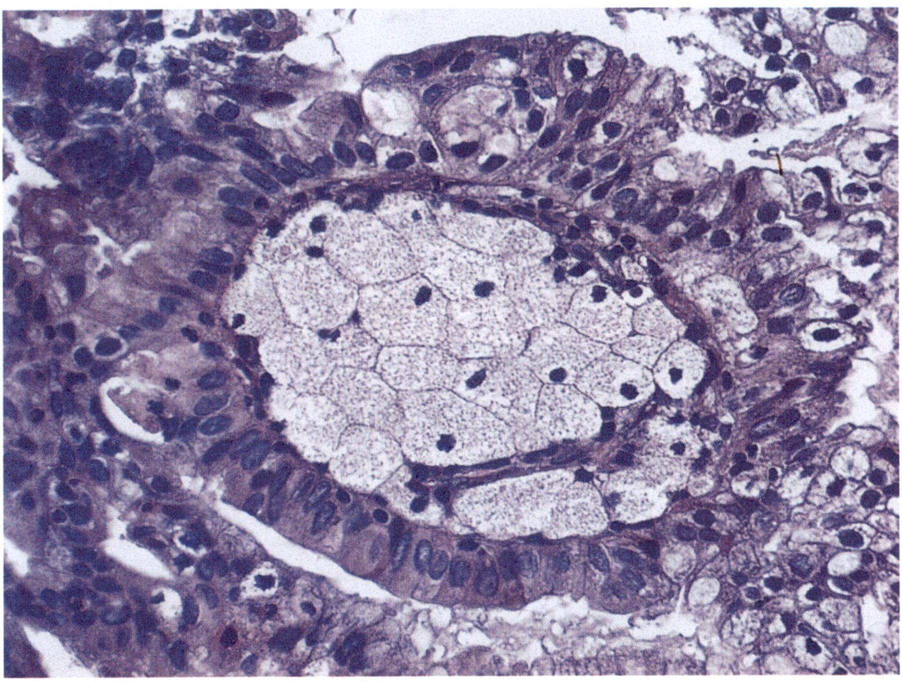

Fig. 9.14 Foam cells in endometrioid adenocarcinoma. PAS, ×350

Morphologic Differential Diagnosis. Secretory adenocarcinoma must be differentiated from clear cell carcinoma, because of its much more favorable prognosis, and from mucinous adenocarcinoma (mucin stains). The latter distinction is clinically important because the adjuvant hormonal therapy differs considerably. The mucopolysaccharides of secretory (endometrioid) adenocarcinoma differ histochemically and in their composition of cytokeratin filaments from those of mucinous (endocervical-type) adenocarcinoma (Moll et al. 1983; Czernobilsky et al. 1980). In contrast to secretory adenocarcinoma, clear cell and mucinous adenocarcinomas are negative for vimentin and often positive for CEA.

9.1.1.5
Estrogen Type of Adenocarcinoma

The adenocarcinomas developing under the influence of exogenous estrogen often present a characteristic pattern, which inspired the name "estrogen carcinomas" (Gusberg and Hall 1961). A high percentage of these carcinomas contain nodules or accumulations of squamous epithelium (Robboy and Bradley 1979). Most of the carcinomatous glands are well differentiated, but may vary in their structure from area to area, some being cystically dilated with branching intraluminal epithelial papillae. Large parts of the glands may be lined by ciliated cells, which develop under estrogen stimulation (*ciliated cell variant of adenocarcinoma*; Hendrickson and Kempson 1983). Accumulations of endometrial foam cells between the carcinomatous glands are frequently encountered (Figs. 9.13, 9.14).

9.1.1.6
Sertoliform Variant of Adenocarcinoma

In rare instances, a sertoliform variant of endometrioid adenocarcinoma can be observed (Eichhorn et al 1996) with focal formation of sertoliform tubules positive for vimentin, EMA and CD99 (Liang et al. 2007). This rare variant can be distinguished from stromal sarcomas with sexcord-like differentiation and from uterine tumors resembling ovarian sexcord tumors by neighboring foci of typical endometrioid adenocarcinoma.

9.1.1.7
Adenocarcinoma with Squamous Differentiation

The term adenocarcinoma with squamous differentiation includes endometrioid adenocarcinomas with both mature and immature squamous metaplasia.

Well differentiated (Adenoacanthoma)

Well differentiated endometrioid adenocarcinoma with squamous differentiation (formerly adenoacanthoma; Figs. 9.15, 9.16) contains nodules as well as islets of mature squamous epithelium. Some nodules contain parakeratotic horn pearls; others reveal intercellular bridges.

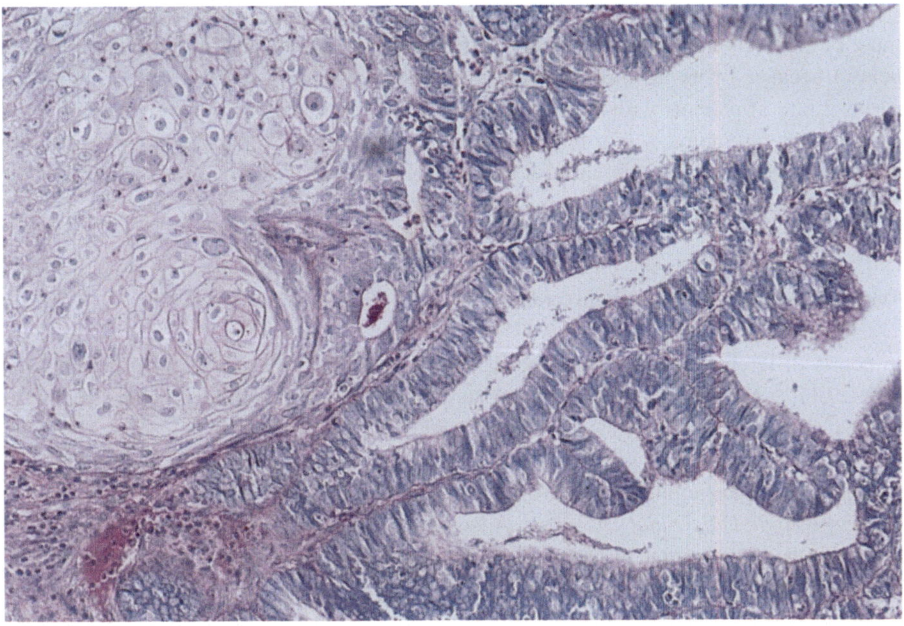

Fig. 9.15 Well-differentiated adenocarcinoma with squamous differention (adenoacanthoma grade 1). Periodic acid-Schiff (PAS) reaction, ×150

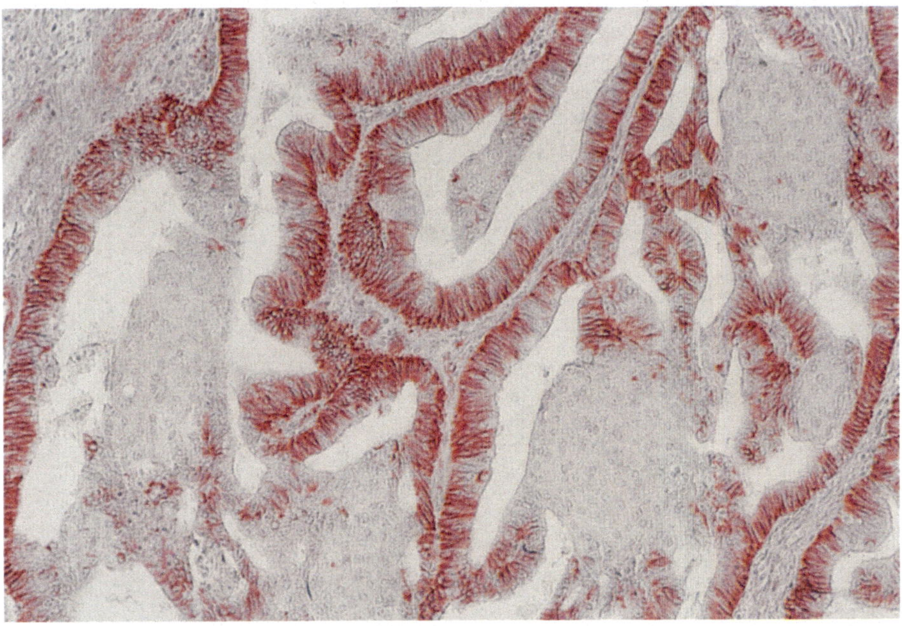

Fig. 9.16 Well-differentiated adenocarcinoma with squamous differention (adenoacanthoma grade 1). Immunohistochemical stain for vimentin, ×150

Morphologic Differential Diagnosis. This well differentiated type (adenoacanthoma) must be differentiated from the poorly differentiated (adenosquamous) carcinoma (see below) because of its far more favorable prognosis (Connelly et al. 1982). The 5-year survival rate of patients with adenoacanthoma is 87%, whereas that of patients with adenosquamous carcinoma is only 47%. Intermediary stages, however, do occur. In such cases it is usually the squamous component that worsens prognosis and is responsible for early deep myometrial invasion (Demopoulos et al. 1986).

Poorly Differentiated (Adenosquamous Carcinoma)

In poorly differentiated (adenosquamous) adenocarcinoma with squamous differentiation (Figs. 9.17, 9.18), there is an intimate mixture of glandular and solid epithelial structures. Some glands are more or less well differentiated, while others are microalveolar. The solid areas consist of immature squamous elements with atypical nuclei, frequent mitoses, and fairly abundant eosinophilic cytoplasm.

Morphologic Differential Diagnosis. Adenoacanthoma: The most important clue for distinction is the irregularity in distribution and the immaturity of the squamous component; only carcinomas with nodules of mature squamous metaplasia should be diagnosed as well differentiated (adenoacanthoma). The nuclei of the squamous cells in adenoacanthoma reveal diploid

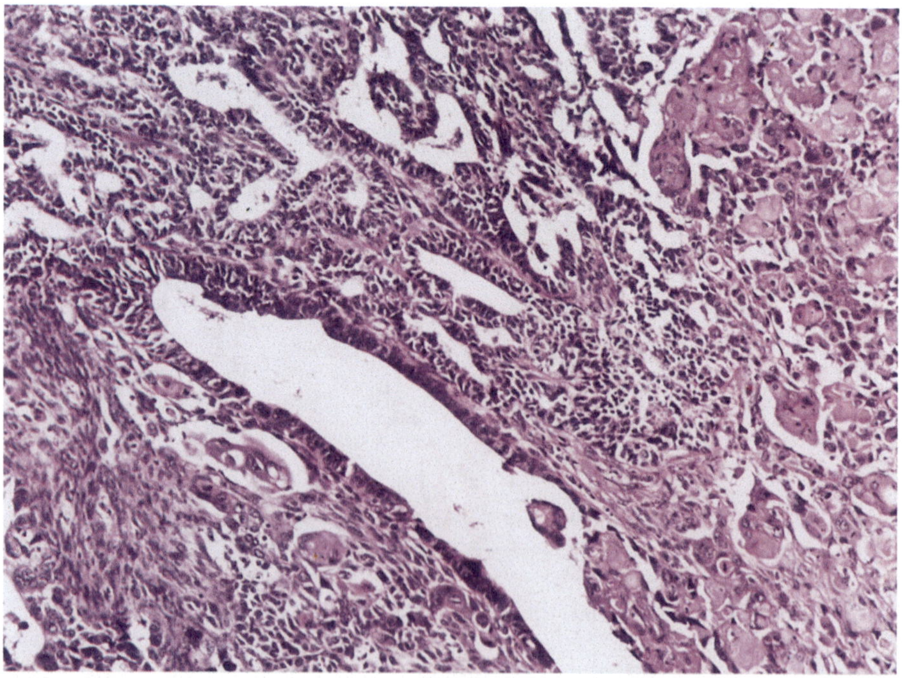

Fig. 9.17 Poorly differentiated adenocarcinoma with squamous differentiation (adenosquamous carcinoma, grade 2). H & E, ×100

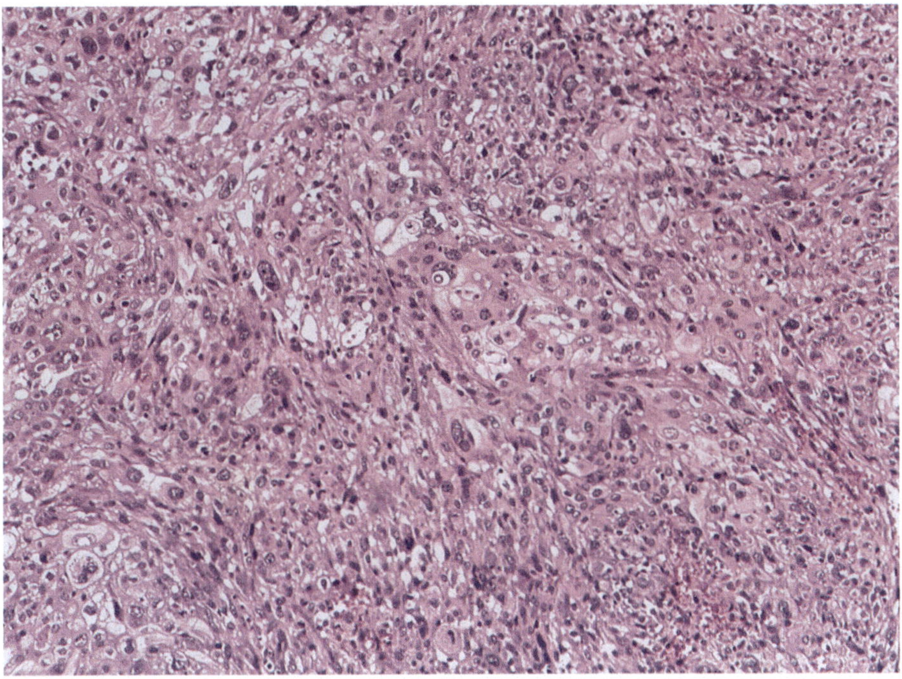

Fig. 9.18 Poorly differentiated adenocarcinoma with squamous differentiation (adenosquamous carcinoma, grade 3). H & E, ×100

DNA measurements, whereas those in poorly differentiated (adenosquamous) carcinoma have aneuploid values. In addition, the glandular component in adenosquamous carcinoma is usually much less well differentiated than in adenoacanthoma. The lack of intracytoplasmic mucin can help to distinguish the adenosquamous type from the mucoepidermoid variant of mucinous adenocarcinoma. The poorly differentiated squamous component must be distinguished from solid glandular foci in a poorly differentiated adenocarcinoma; squamous epithelial foci do not show nuclear palisading, usually have sharp cell margins and more eosinophilic or glassy cytoplasm, and differ in their cytokeratin expression (see p. 151).

9.1.2 Carcinomas of the Nonendometrioid Müllerian Type

This group of endometrial carcinomas is not preceded by a typical (endometrioid) hyperplasia. In stead, their precursors may be various types of metaplasia within a resting or atrophic endometrium (see Table 9.4). They also differ in their immunohistochemical reactions (Table 9.5) and their mutational changes (Table 9.6).

Table 9.4 Various types of endometrial carcinomas and their possible precursors under different hormonal stimulation

Estrogen:	
Atypical hyperplasia → with squamous metaplasia →	endometrioid adenocarcinoma with squamous differentiation
Gestagen/Tamoxifen:	
Mucinous metaplasia → Clear cell metaplasia → Serous papillary metaplasia →	mucinous adenocarcinoma clear cell carcinoma serous carcinoma

Table 9.5 Immunohistochemistry in endometrial hyperplasia and carcinoma

	CK 13	CK 8, 18, 19	Vim	CEA	p16	p53
Hyperplasia	–	+	+	–	–	–
Endometrioid carcinoma	–	+	+	–	–	–
With squamous metapl.	–/+	+/–	+/–	–	–	–
Mucinous carcinoma	–	+	–	+	+	–
Clear cell carcinoma	(+)	(+)	+	+	+	+
Serous carcinoma	–	+	(+)	–	+	+

Table 9.6 Mutations in endometrial carcinomas

	p53	p16	Ki-ras	erbB2	MSI	PTEN
Endometrioid	–	–	11–13%	–	20–30%	40%
Mucinous	–	+	–	–	–	–
Clear cell	47%	+	–	20%	–	–
Serous	80–90%	+	–	9%	–	–

9.1.2.1 Mucinous Adenocarcinoma

Mucinous adenocarcinoma of the endometrium (Figs. 9.19–9.23) structurally and histochemically closely resembles the mucinous adenocarcinoma of the endocervical mucosa. Similar to its endocervical counterpart, it may be well, moderately, or poorly differentiated (Ross et al. 1983; Melhem and Tobon 1987). The carcinomatous glands are generally cystic, filled with mucus, and lined by a tall, mucus-secreting epithelium with atypical nuclei (Fig. 9.19). Branching intraluminal papillae may develop. Poorly differentiated types contain microglandular and solid areas (Fig. 9.21). At the margins of the carcinoma, foci of endocervical metaplasia may be found.

Morphologic Differential Diagnosis. Since the immunohistochemical reactions are almost identical (contents of sulfated and nonsulfated acid MPS; positive reaction for carcinoembryonic antigen, CEA), its morphologic distinction from a primary endocervical adenocarcinoma is virtually impossible from curettings (Czernobilsky et al. 1980; Azumi et al. 1991). The distinction from an adenocarcinoma of the endometrioid type can be made in most cases with

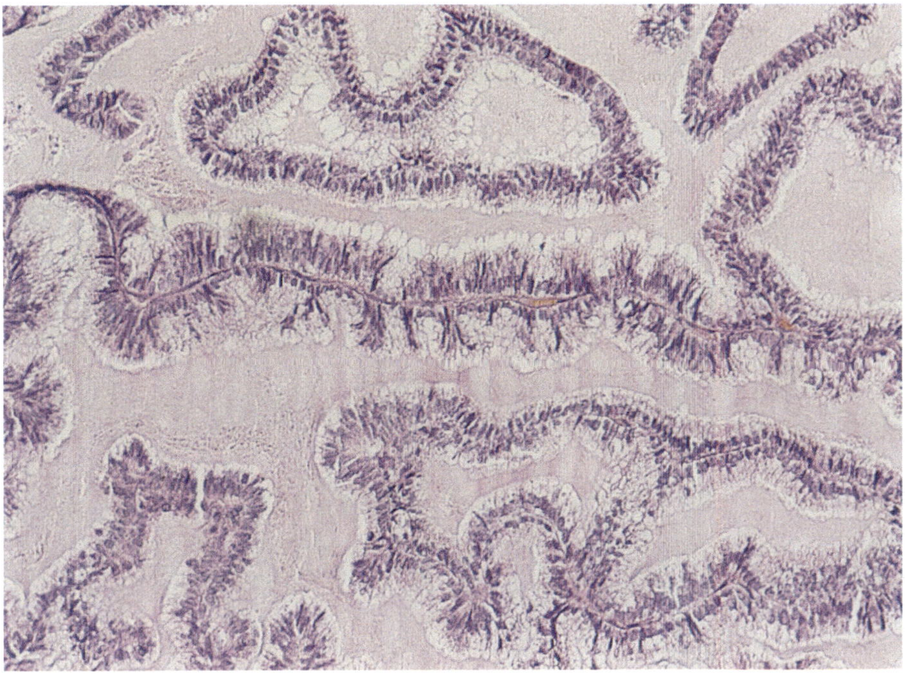

Fig. 9.19 Mucinous adenocarcinoma, grade 1. H & E, ×100

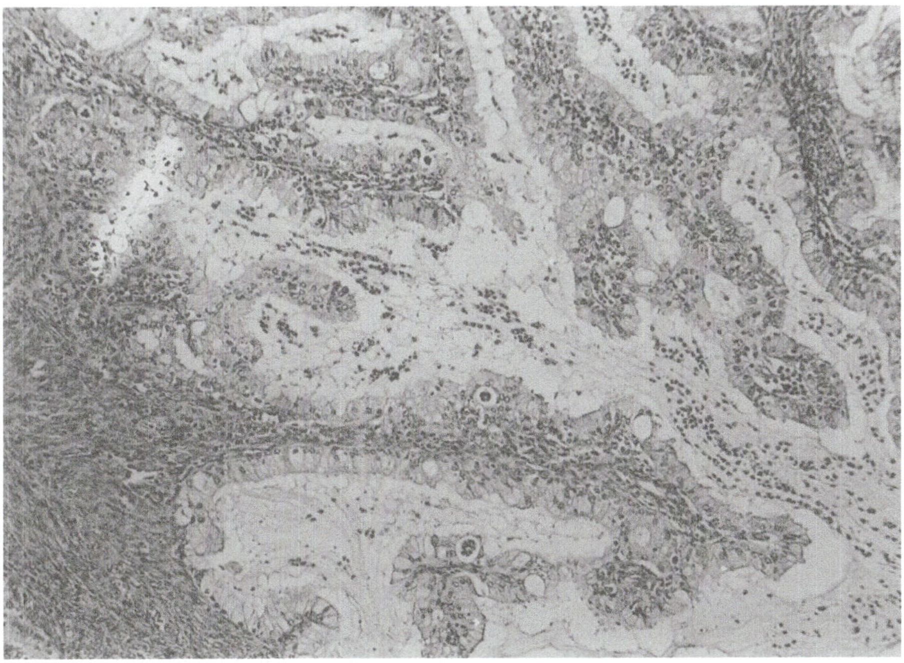

Fig. 9.20 Mucinous adenocarcinoma, grade 2. H & E, ×100

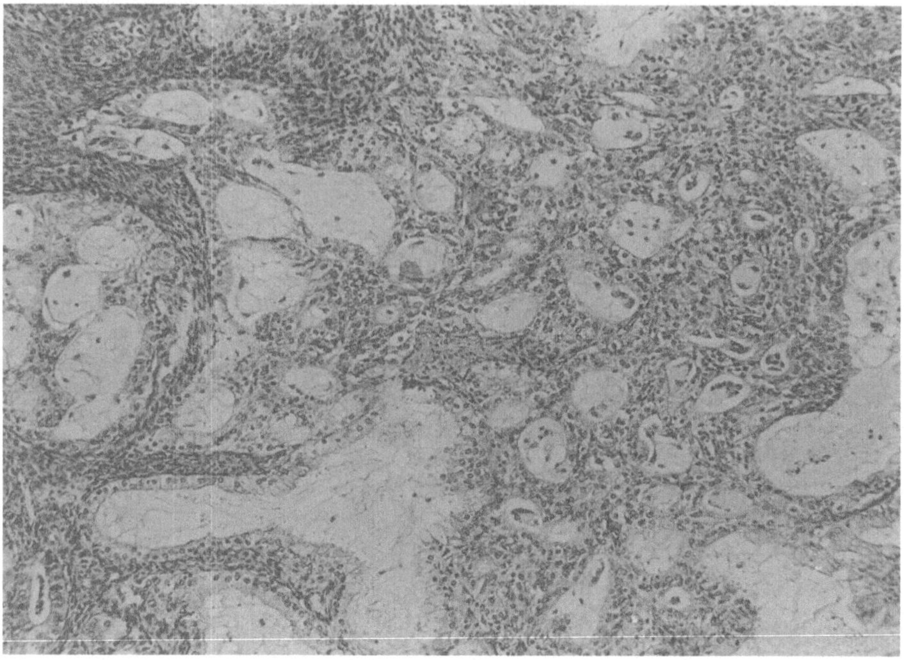

Fig. 9.21 Mucinous adenocarcinoma, grade 2. H & E, ×100

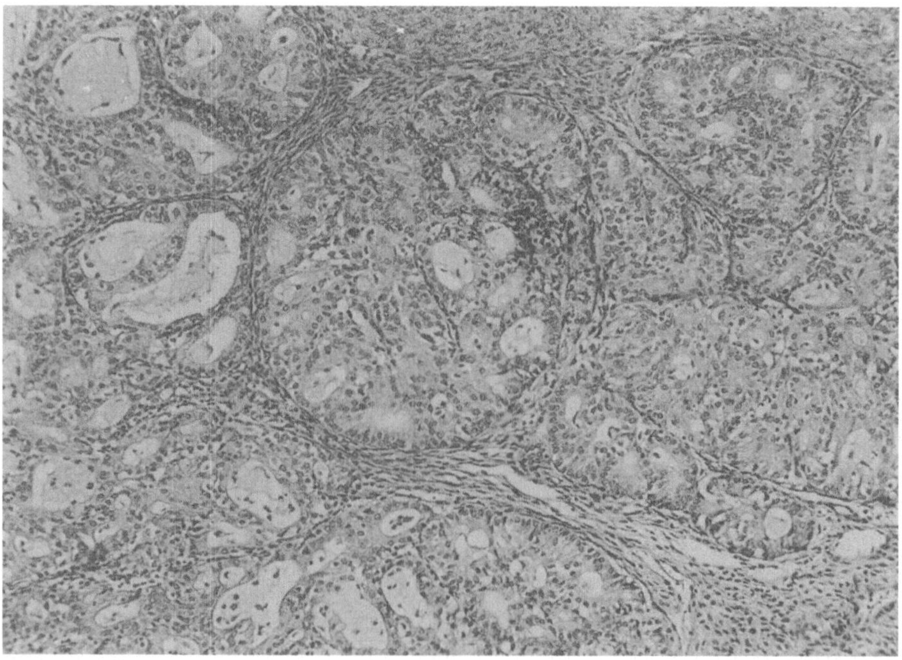

Fig. 9.22 Mucinous adenocarcinoma, grade 2. H & E, ×100

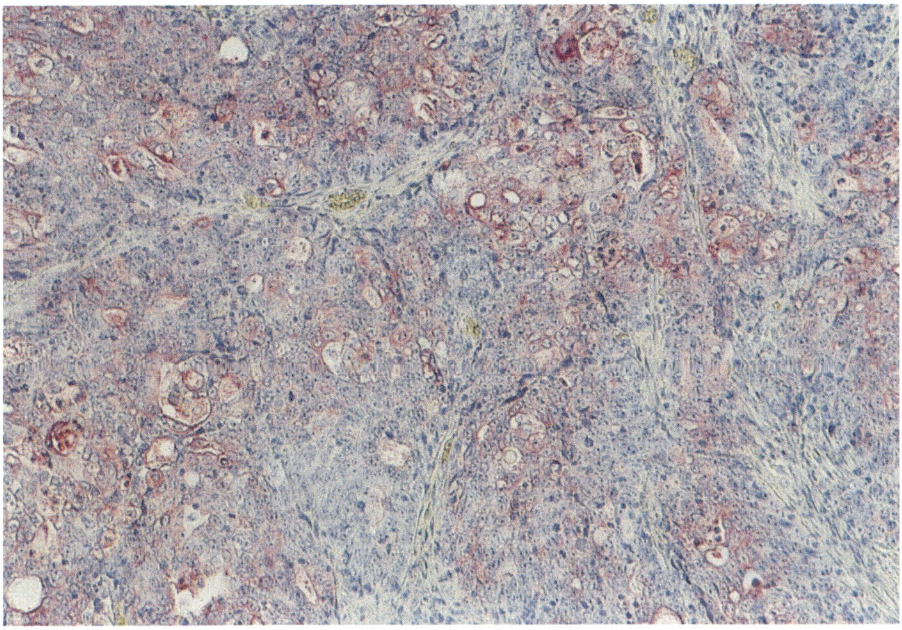

Fig. 9.23 Mucinous adenocarcinoma, grade 3. Immunohistochemical stain with carcinoembryonic antigen (CEA), ×100

CEA, as the reaction is positive in mucinous (Fig. 9.23) and negative in endometrioid carcinoma, and with vimentin, as the reaction is positive in endometrioid and negative in mucinous carcinoma (Dabbs et al. 1986; Dallenbach-Hellweg et al. 1991). This distinction is important, since mucinous adenocarcinomas with very little mucin formation in the glandular epithelial cells may mimic endometrioid-type adenocarcinoma, and vice versa. In addition, mucinous carcinomas are often positive for p16, whereas endometrioid carcinomas are usually negative (Velasco et al. 2008), or contain only occasional positive cells in small patches. A positive reaction for p16 can also help to differentiate microglandular forms of mucinous adenocarcinoma of the endometrium from particles of benign microglandular hyperplasia of the endocervix which may be constituents of endometrial curettings, and which are p16 negative (Chekmareva et al. 2008). Since, however, reserve cells and metaplastic cells in cervical microglandular hyperplasia may react positively with p16 (Roh et al. 2009), they must be distinguished from carcinomatous cells by a double stain with Ki-7. The antiproliferative tumor suppressor gene p16 is overexpressed in proliferating metaplastic cells as well as in tumor cells where its cycle control mechanism is by-passed through inactivation of pRb. In both instances the p16 reaction is positive, but only the carcinoma cells also overexpress Ki-7.

Clinical Correlations. We have observed a relative increase in the frequency of mucinous adenocarcinomas in comparison to endometrioid adenocarcinoma. This parallels the change in HRT from unopposed estrogen to combined therapy with added synthetic gestagens (see also Young and Scully 1992). In addition, many endometrial carcinomas developing during or after treatment with tamoxifen for breast carcinoma are of the mucinous (approximately 60%), clear cell or serous (35%) type (Dallenbach-Hellweg and Hahn 1995; Dallenbach-Hellweg and Schmidt 1998; Schlesinger et al 1998; Dallenbach-

Hellweg et al. 2000). If an endometrioid adenocarcinoma is histologically discovered during tamoxifen therapy, it most likely preexisted before the onset of that treatment and was caused by the same hyperestrogenic stimulus that fostered the development of the breast cancer (e.g., metabolic syndrome, see also Schlesinger et al. 1998).

9.1.2.2 Mucinous Adenocarcinoma with Squamous Differentiation (Mucoepidermoid Adenocarcinoma)

This tumor (Figs. 9.24, 9.25) shows mucus formation in some of the glands, which may be cystically dilated. Occasionally intracellular mucin is also found. The squamous areas may contain horn pearls or develop monocellular keratinization or mucus formation and, in addition, show a general cellular pleomorphism.

Morphologic Differential Diagnosis. Mucoepidermoid adenocarcinoma of the endocervix. This distinction may prove to be extremely difficult, if not impossible, from curettings consisting of only carcinomatous tissue. A fractionated abrasio may help, but it is not fully reliable. An important factor may be the age of the patient: mucoepidermoid adenocarcinoma of the endometrium occurs predominantly in old age, often beyond the age of 70, whereas mucoepidermoid carcinoma of the endocervix is found in women with an average age of 39 years (Dallenbach-Hellweg 1982). The distinction can be made with much more accuracy if a hysterectomy specimen is available for examination. Sheets of dysplastic squamous epithelium found in curettings of postmenopausal or senile patients are always highly suspicious of an underlying mucoepidermoid carcinoma. That possibility should therefore be mentioned in the diagnostic report to the gynecologist.

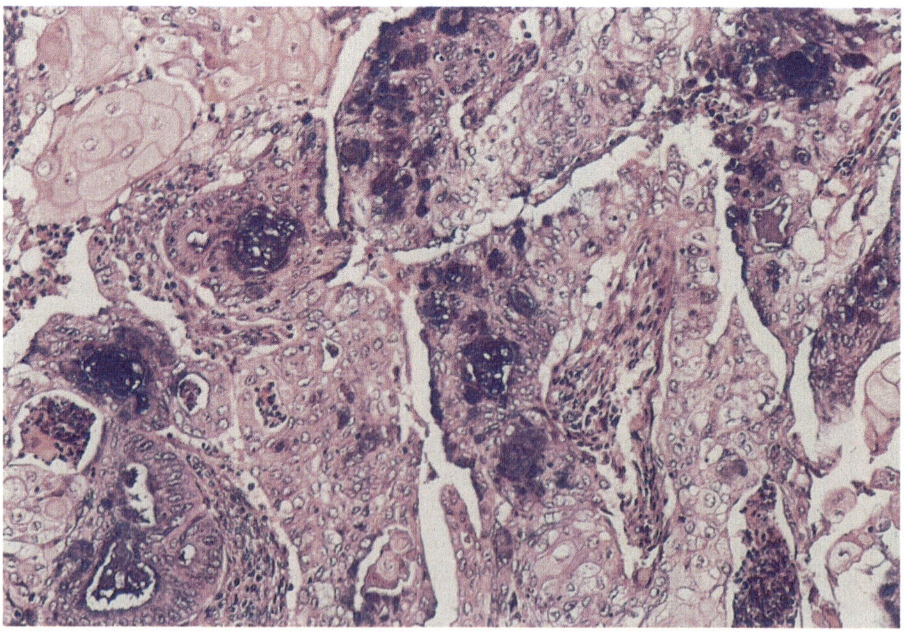

Fig. 9.24 Mucinous adenocarcinoma with squamous differentiation (mucoepidermoid adenocarcinoma), grade 3. H & E, ×100

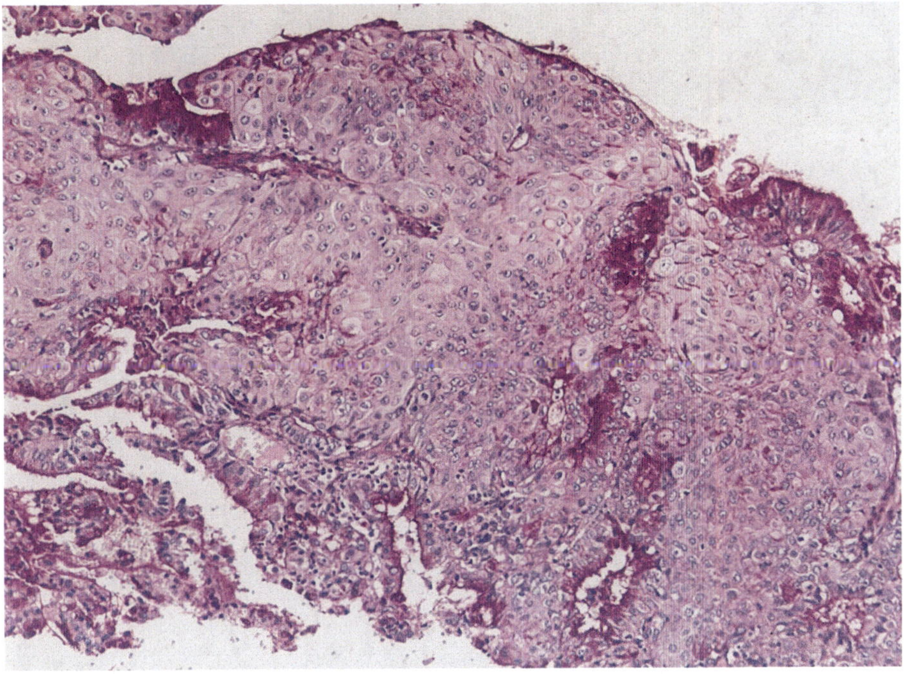

Fig. 9.25 Mucinous adenocarcinoma with squamous differentiation (mucoepidermoid adenocarcinoma), grade 3. Periodic acid-Schiff (PAS) reaction, ×100

9.1.2.3
Clear Cell Adenocarcinoma

Clear cell adenocarcinoma (Figs. 9.26–9.29) of the endometrium looks very much like the clear cell adenocarcinomas of the ovary, cervix, and vagina (Rorat et al. 1974; Roth 1974; Kurman and Scully 1976; Horie et al. 1977; Abeler and Kjorstad 1991). The clear cells may be arranged in solid sheets (Figs. 9.26, 9.27), or may form cystic and tubular glands or papillae (Figs. 9.28, 9.29). The large nuclei have irregular shapes and chromatin densities. Mitoses are frequent, but vary from region to region. The clear cytoplasm may contain glycogen or round PAS-positive and diastase-resistant hyaline inclusions (Christopherson et al. 1982a), or, rarely, may be diffusely eosinophilic (Fig 9.29). The cells forming papillae are often hobnail in shape (Fig. 9.29).

Morphologic Differential Diagnosis. Differentiation from clear cell adenocarcinoma of the endocervix may be impossible. For this distinction, the same criteria as for adenosquamous carcinoma are valid (see above).

Occasionally, an Arias-Stella reaction may be misinterpreted as clear cell adenocarcinoma. The distinction is usually, but not always (see p. 103) possible based on the age of the patient and the focal character of the Arias-Stella reaction with perifocal, decidualized stroma, or irregular shedding. On the other hand, the distinction should not be based solely on the presence or absence of mitoses, since these may also be found in the Arias-Stella reaction (Arias-Stella et al. 1994).

Clinical Correlation. Histologic grading is of no importance, since all grades have an equally poor clinical prognosis (Christopherson et al. 1982a). The 5-year survival rate

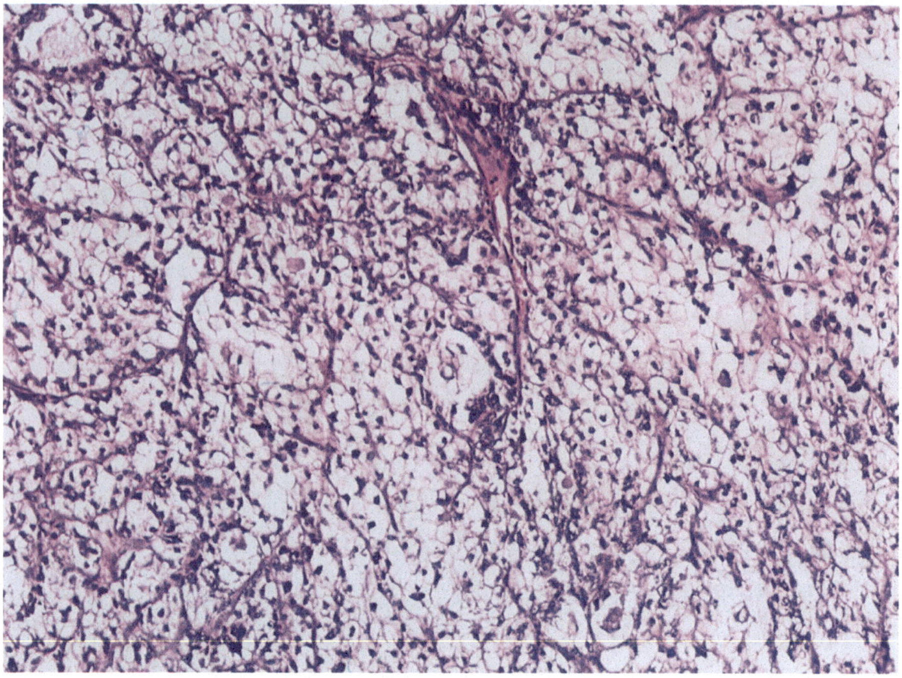

Fig. 9.26 Clear cell adenocarcinoma, solid pattern. H & E, ×100

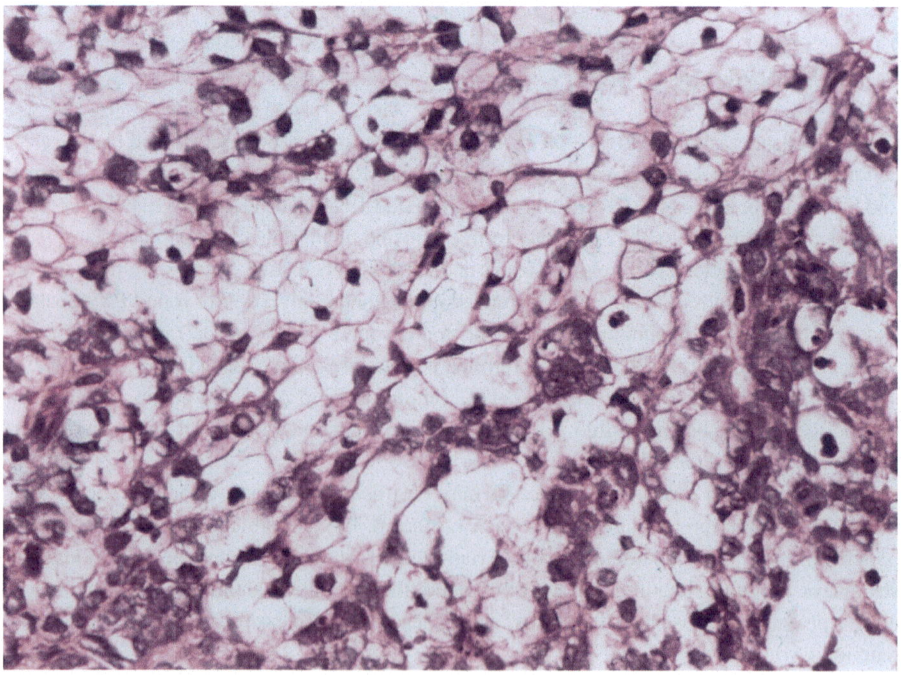

Fig. 9.27 Clear cell adenocarcinoma, solid pattern. H & E, ×250

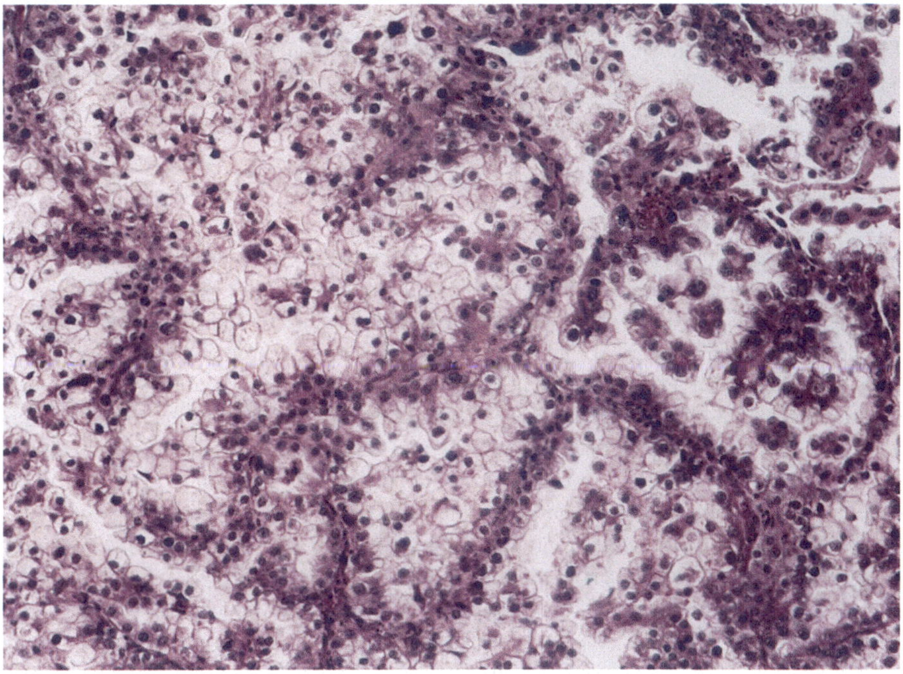

Fig. 9.28 Clear cell adenocarcinoma, glandular papillary pattern. H & E, ×100

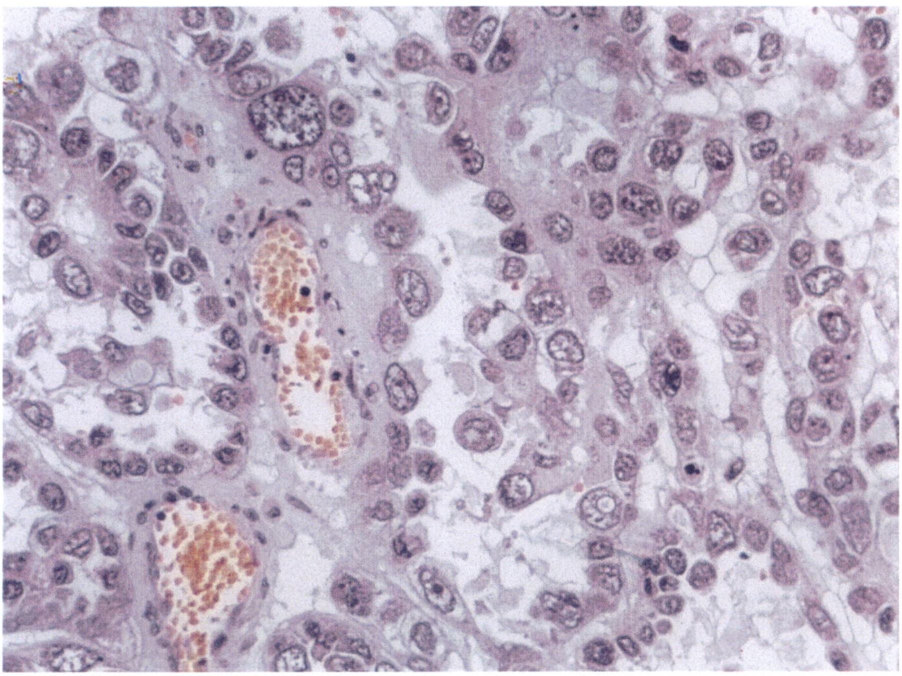

Fig. 9.29 Clear cell adenocarcinoma, eosinophilic type. H & E, ×250

depends on the stage at diagnosis, averaging 59% at stage II (Carcangiu and Chambers 1995), but dropping down to 15% in cases with deep myometrial invasion (Abeler and Kjorstad 1991).

9.1.2.4 Serous Adenocarcinoma

Serous adenocarcinoma (Figs. 9.30–9.35) closely resembles the serous type of ovarian carcinoma. It consists almost exclusively of complex branching papillae with central stalks of connective tissue. The lining epithelial cells are round to columnar and contain elongated or rounded, usually highly atypical nuclei with varying densities of chromatin in an eosinophilic cytoplasm (Fig. 9.32). Progressive dedifferentiation may also produce solid types of serous carcinoma (Fig. 9.34) with identical nuclear atypia and small foci of glandular remnants (Fig. 9.33). These tumors generally grow expansively into the uterine cavity, may originate from a carcinomatous intraepithelial surface lesion without stromal invasion (Fig. 9.30), often develop in polyps, but infiltrate the myometrium early and extensively, mainly by lymphatic or hematogenous spread. Their prognosis is even less favorable than that for the clear cell type of carcinoma (Christopherson et al. 1982b; Hendrickson et al. 1982); in other series, 44% survival rates for stage I, 32% for stage II (Carcangiu and Chambers 1995), and 11% and 2% for stages III and IV, respectively (Chambers et al. 1987) were found. In contrast to the endometrioid type of carcinoma, serous carcinoma develops without preceding endometrial hyperplasia, usually in atrophic endometria. Also in contrast to the endometrioid type, there is c-*myc* amplification and strong overexpression of p53 (Fig. 9.35) in many and of

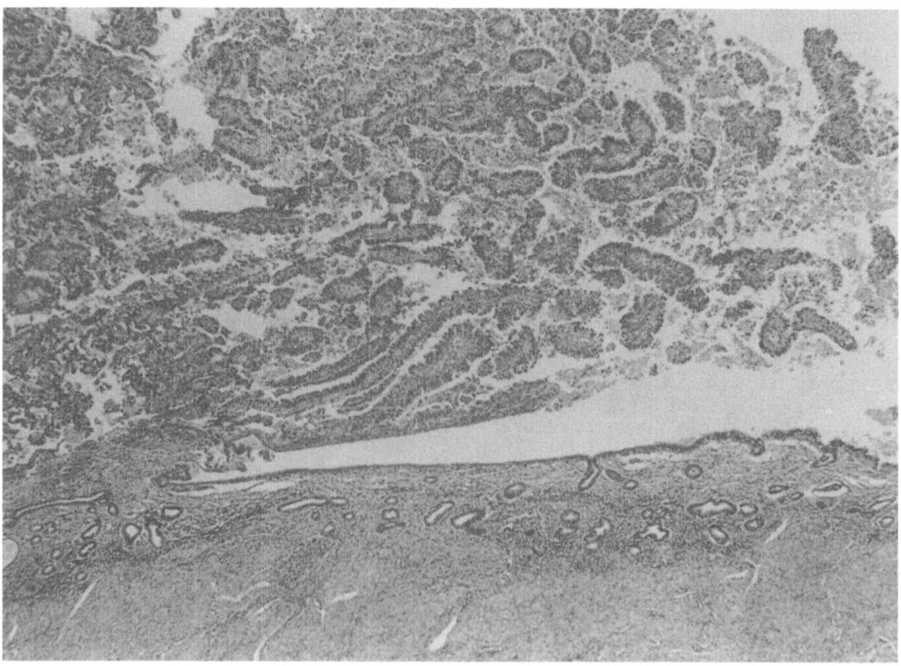

Fig. 9.30 Serous adenocarcinoma. H & E, ×25

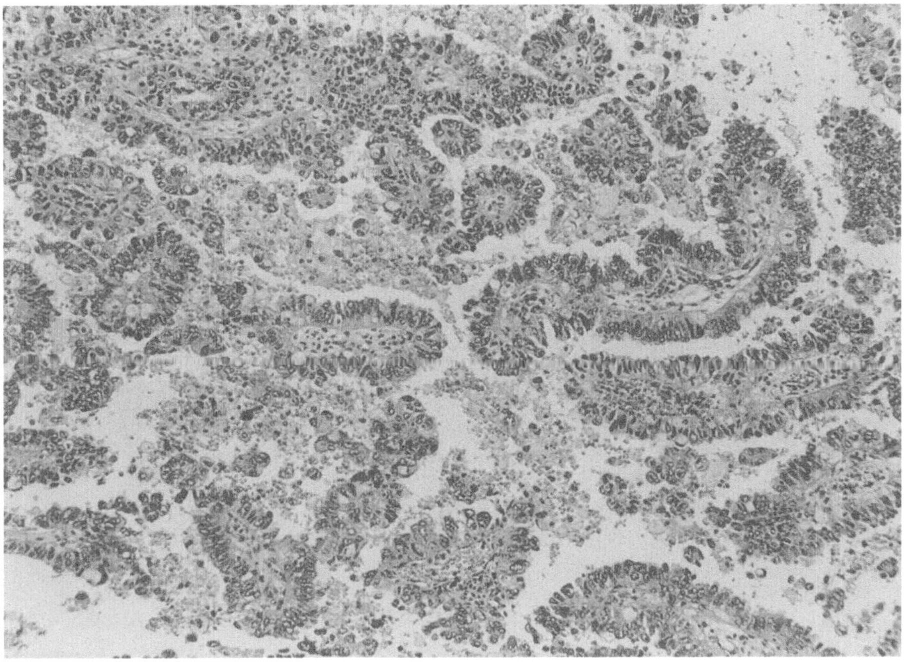

Fig. 9.31 Serous adenocarcinoma. H & E, ×100

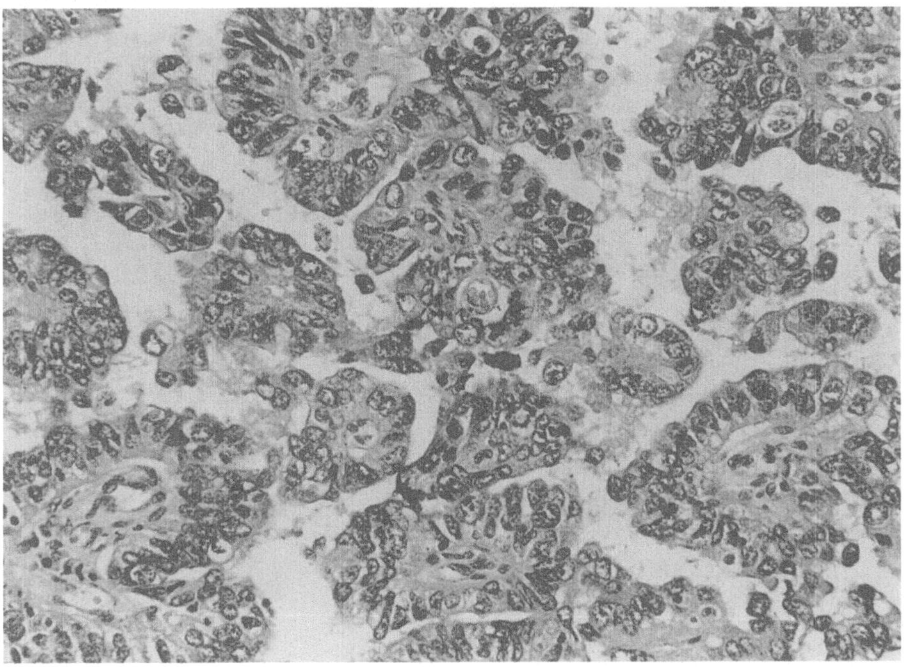

Fig. 9.32 Serous adenocarcinoma. H & E, ×250

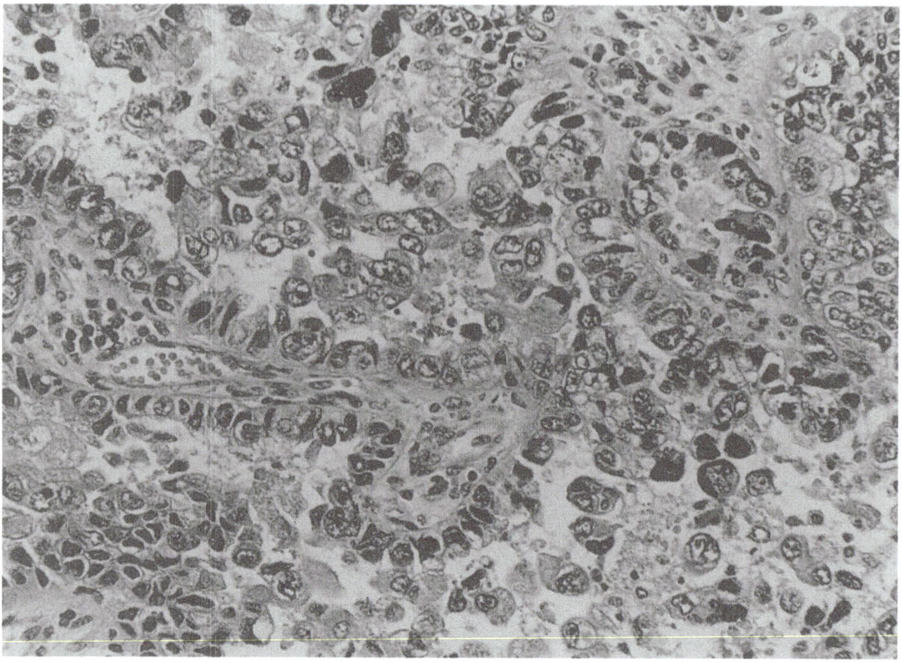

Fig. 9.33 Serous adenocarcinoma. H & E, ×250

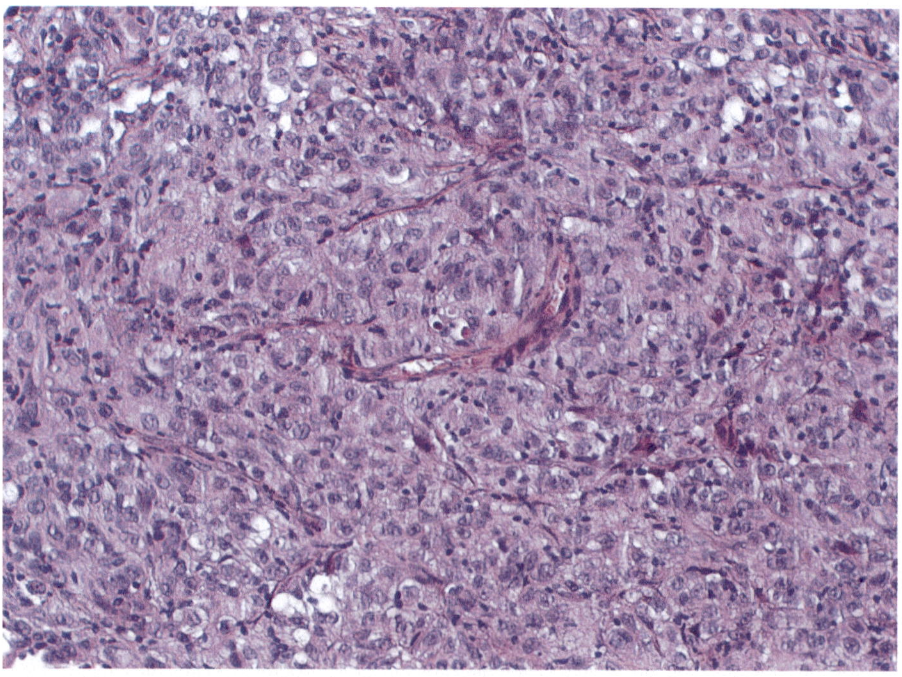

Fig. 9.34 Serous adenocarcinoma, solid area. H & E, ×150

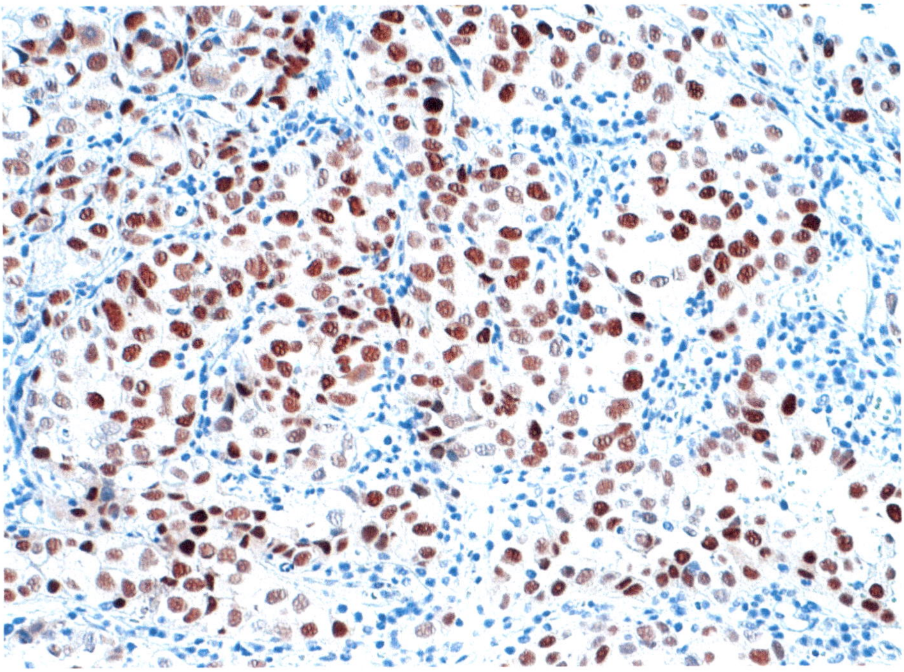

Fig. 9.35 Serous adenocarcinoma. Immunostaining for p53: strong over-expression in most of the nuclei. H & E, ×150

p16 in nearly 100% (Chiesa-Vottero et al. 2007) of serous carcinomas, whereas estrogen receptors are positive in approximately 50% (Reid-Nicholson 2006).

Morphologic Differential Diagnosis. This is of clinical importance from (a) papillary formations in the well-differentiated villo-glandular type of endometrioid adenocarcinoma, in which the papillae are elongate, and the cells are regularly arranged, and (b) the papillary type of clear cell carcinoma, which presents a hobnail formation of nuclei and intracytoplasmic hyalin inclusions. For the distinction from endometrioid carcinoma p16 is a helpful marker. As to origin of the neoplasm, a metastatic spread from an extrauterine serous adenocarcinoma ought to be considered (Baergen et al. 2001).

9.1.2.5
Squamous Cell Carcinoma

Squamous cell carcinoma is very rare, seldom primary (only 31 cases were collected from the literature; Abeler and Kjorstad 1990), and nearly always secondary (see Fig. 9.76).

9.1.2.6
Small Cell Neuroendocrine Carcinomas of the Endometrium

Small cell neuroendocrine carcinomas of the endometrium are very rare (Schmidt 1997). Except for single case reports (Hendrickson and Scheithauer 1986), only a few larger series have been published (Huntsman et al. 1994, van Hoeven et al. 1995, Katahira et al. 2004).

Histogenetically, they most likely derive from endocervical reserve cells like their more frequent counterparts in the cervix, or from local neuroendocrine cells. They are not seldom associated with other endometrial carcinomas especially adenocarcinomas and adenosquamous carcinomas. Both components of these neoplasms have been shown to be genetically similar indicating a common origin (Mhawech-Fauceglia et al. 2008). Histologically, the tumor cells have round monomorphic hyperchromatic nuclei with frequent mitoses (Fig. 9.36). They react positively with cytokeratins and with most neuroendocrinic markers: NSE, Chromogranin, CD 56, S 100, and with p16, but negative with HPV tests (Melgoza et al 2006; Albores-Saavedra et al. 2008). The highly malignant small cell carcinomas have a very poor prognosis.

Morphologic Differential Diagnosis. The distinction from undifferentiated components of endometrioid carcinoma, endometrial stromal sarcoma, malignant lymphoma and embryonal rhabdomyosarcoma is possible with the relevant immunohistochemical markers, and by its neuroendocrine differentiation with markers for chromogranin, synaptophysin, Leu-7 (CD57) or NSE (van Hoeven et al. 1995). Stromal sarcoma also differs from small cell neuroendocrine carcinoma by its bland nuclei, low mitotic activity and large number of reticulum fibrils. The primitive neuroectodermal tumor (PNET) often demonstrates glial, ependymal and medulloepithelial differentiation with a positive reaction for glial fibrillary acidic protein (Daya et al. 1993), and it reacts negatively with markers for cytokeratins, CEA and S100. The distinction from a primary endocrine small cell carcinoma of the cervix may raise problems that can only be solved by their different location, from small cell non-keratinizing carcinomas by their lack of neuroendocrine differentiation (Fujii et al. 1986; Ueda et al. 1989).

The *large cell variant of neuroendocrine carcinoma* consists of solid sheets of cells with large vesicular nuclei and prominent nucleoli, whereas all other features are identical with the small cell variant (Gilks et al. 1997).

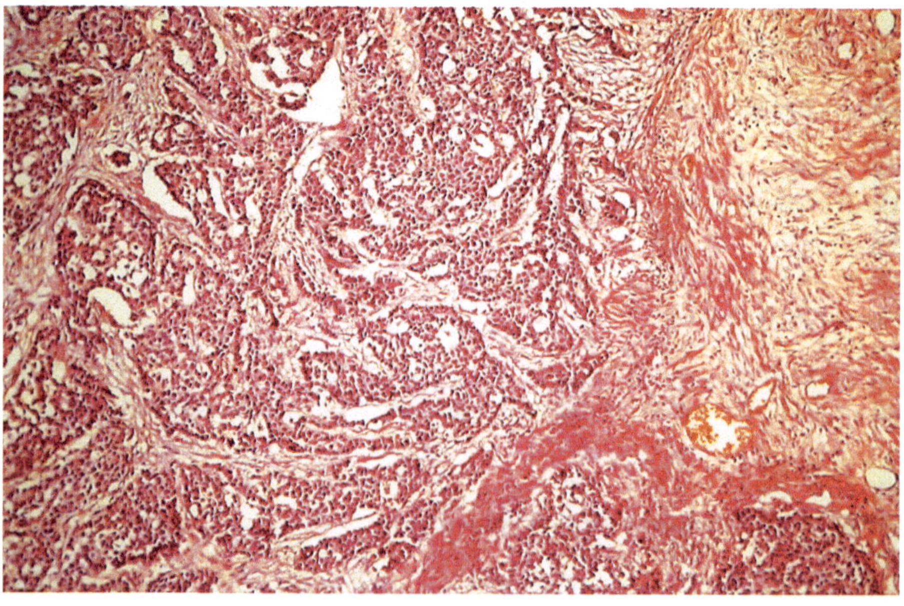

Fig. 9.36 Small cell neuroendocrine carcinoma. H & E, ×75

9.1.2.7 Mixed Carcinomas

Under the influence of various endogenous or exogenous hormones, mixed types of carcinoma may develop. If one component clearly predominates, the carcinoma should be classified accordingly, e.g., endometrioid adenocarcinoma with focal mucinous differentiation. The term mixed carcinomas is correct if one or more additional types exceed 10% of the entire tumor. In such cases, the major and minor tumor types should be specified and added to the diagnosis, e.g., mixed carcinoma with mucinous and clear cell differentiation.

9.1.2.8 Undifferentiated Carcinoma

With minimal or no differentiation of carcinoma cells, typing is not possible. Such cases are rare, accounting for less than 2% of endometrial carcinomas. They may be of large or small cell type. Their distinction from small cell neuroendocrine carcinomas, primitive neuroectodermal tumors with argyrophilic cells and from stromal sarcomas or lymphomas may require immunohistochemical stains (neuron-specific enolase, NSE; chromogranin, CR; cytokeratin, CK; vimentin; see p. 187). They should be requested before diagnosing a carcinoma as undifferentiated.

9.2 Stromal Tumors

9.2.1 Endometrial Stromal Nodule

Endometrial stromal nodule (Fig. 9.37) is a rare, well-circumscribed tumor that may be located in the endometrium or myometrium; about 5% are multiple (Tavassoli and Norris 1981). Histologically, these tumors are composed of uniform cells closely resembling normal endometrial stromal cells. Mitotic activity is usually low, but may be high in exceptional cases. Individual cells are enveloped by a dense reticulin network and occasionally by ribbons of hyalinized collagen. The cells are diffusely arranged (Fig. 9.37) or form small cords which may have a gland-like appearance. There are no glands, however. The nodules have rather sharp borders compressing the adjacent endometrium or myometrium. They are claimed to be benign, independent of their mitotic rate.

Morphologic Differential Diagnosis. Differentiation between endometrial stromal nodule and stromal sarcoma is necessary. Since both tumors have an equally low mitotic rate and lack nuclear pleomorphism, the distinction can only be safely made by observing the interface with the myometrium; stromal sarcomas permeate the myometrium in irregular tongues and extend into lymphatic spaces (see below). In most cases, the distinction can only be safely made on the hysterectomy specimen.

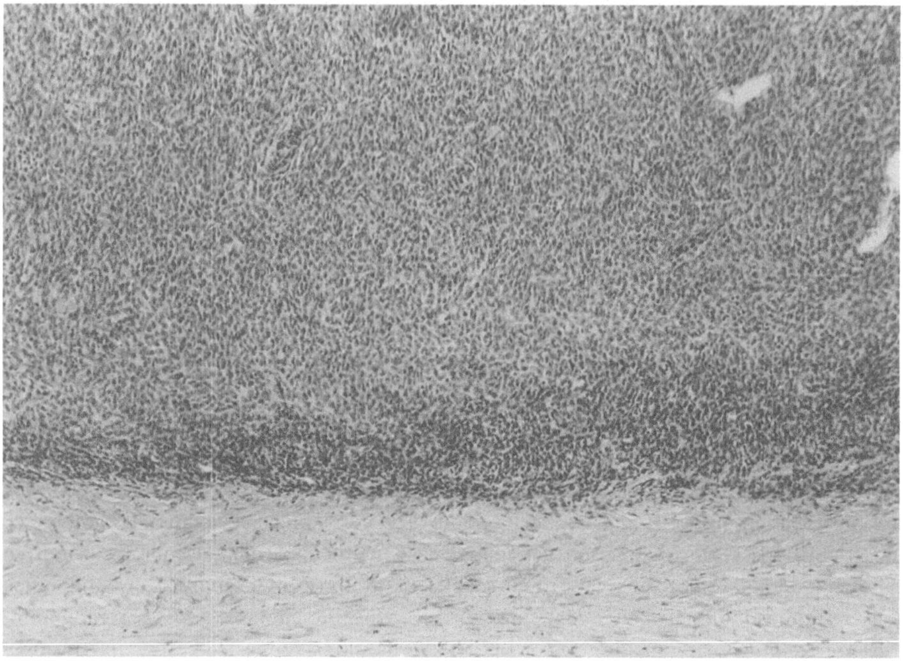

Fig. 9.37 Endometrial stromal nodule. H & E, ×100

9.2.2 Endometrial Stromal Sarcoma, Low Grade

Endometrial stromal sarcoma (ESS) (Figs. 9.38–9.44) has the same cellular structure as the endometrial stromal nodule. Characteristic of endometrial stromal sarcoma is an early and extensive invasion of the lymphatic vascular spaces of the myometrium and penetration into tissue clefts of the myometrium without destruction and necrosis (Zaloudek and Norris 1982; Chang et al. 1990) (Figs. 9.38, 9.39). Ultrastructurally the uniform tumor cells resemble the stromal cells of the early proliferative phase (Komorowski et al. 1970; Akhtar et al. 1975). Mitotic activity is low (Fig. 9.40) but may also be moderate (Fig. 9.41) to pronounced (Fig. 9. 42). Plaques of hyalinized collagen between the tumor cells may be prominent (Fekete and Vellios 1984), in addition to a dense reticular network. Whereas most of these stromal sarcomas have a uniform pattern, a plexiform sex-cord like arrangement is occasionally seen (Figs. 9.43, 9.44) (Clement and Scully 1976). In some cases tubular differentiation can be found. Focally, papillary structures may also be observed (McCluggage and Young 2008).

Morphologic Differential Diagnosis. (a) Stromal nodule according to the criteria described above. (b) Undifferentiated endometrial sarcoma. This tumor consists of cells with marked cellular atypia and numerous mitoses. The growth pattern is destructive and infiltrative. (c) Leiomyoma with or without intravenous spread (Bohr and Thomsen 1991). In contrast to ESS the neoplastic cells are positive with markers for h-caldesmon and oxytocin receptor (Loddenkemper et al. 2003, 2005). (d) Low-grade adenosarcoma (see p. 182). Finally, the formation of papillae in ESS may require their distinction from papillary structures of serous carcinomas: the sarcomatous papillae express CD10 and no cytokeratins, they also lack an epithelial covering.

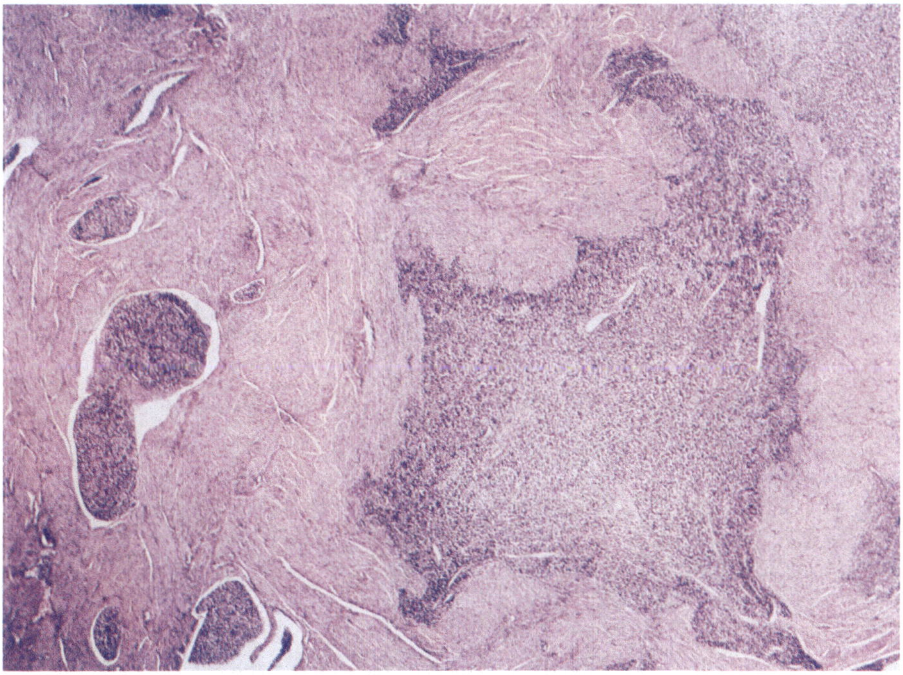

Fig. 9.38 Endometrial stromal sarcoma, worm-like growth pattern. H & E, ×25

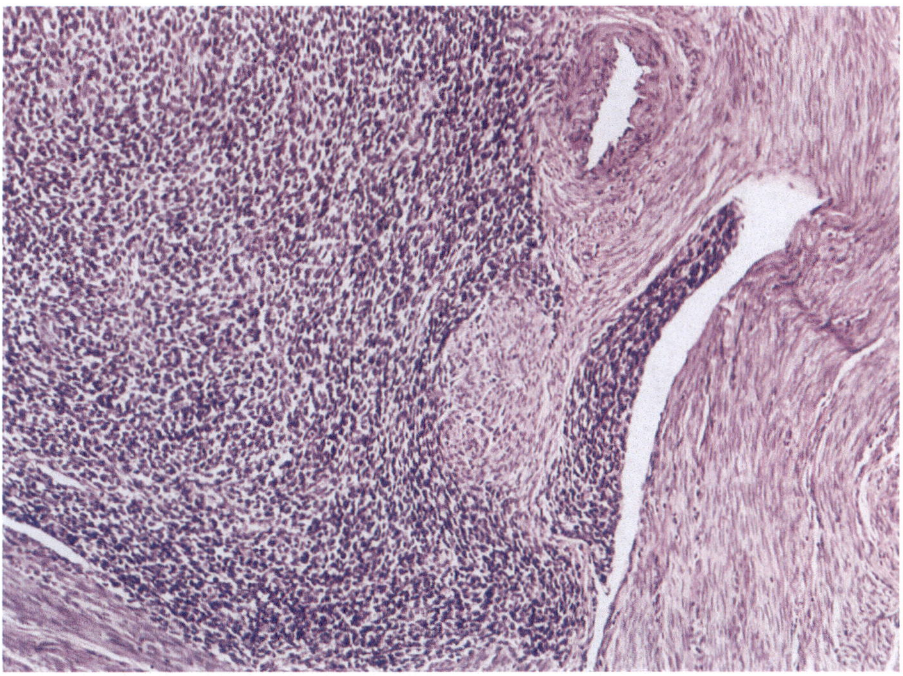

Fig. 9.39 Endometrial stromal sarcoma, cells resemble endometrial stromal cells of proliferative phase. H & E, ×100

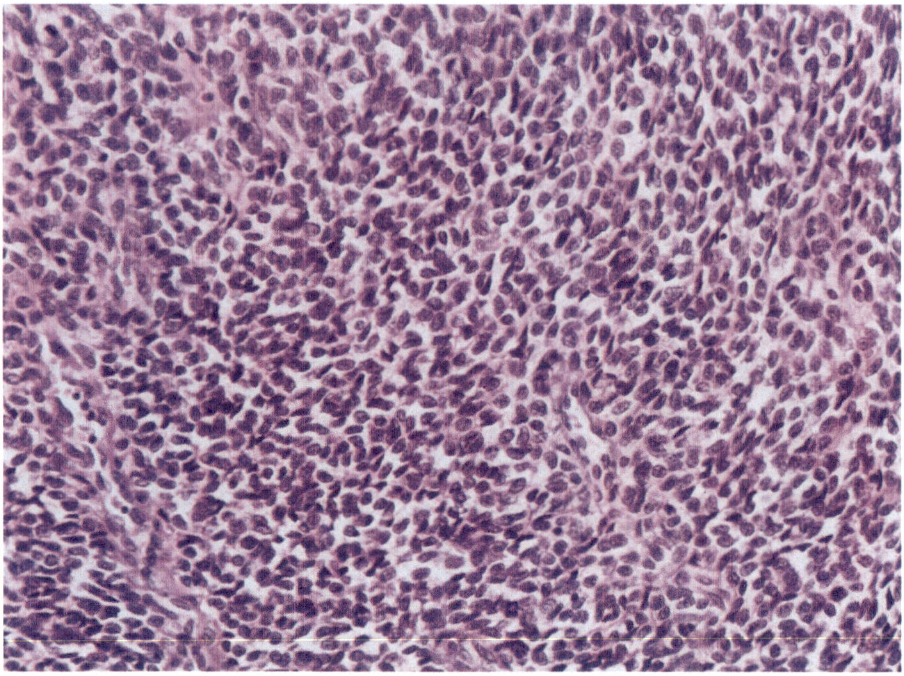

Fig. 9.40 Endometrial stromal sarcoma. Several thin-walled blood vessels. H & E, ×250

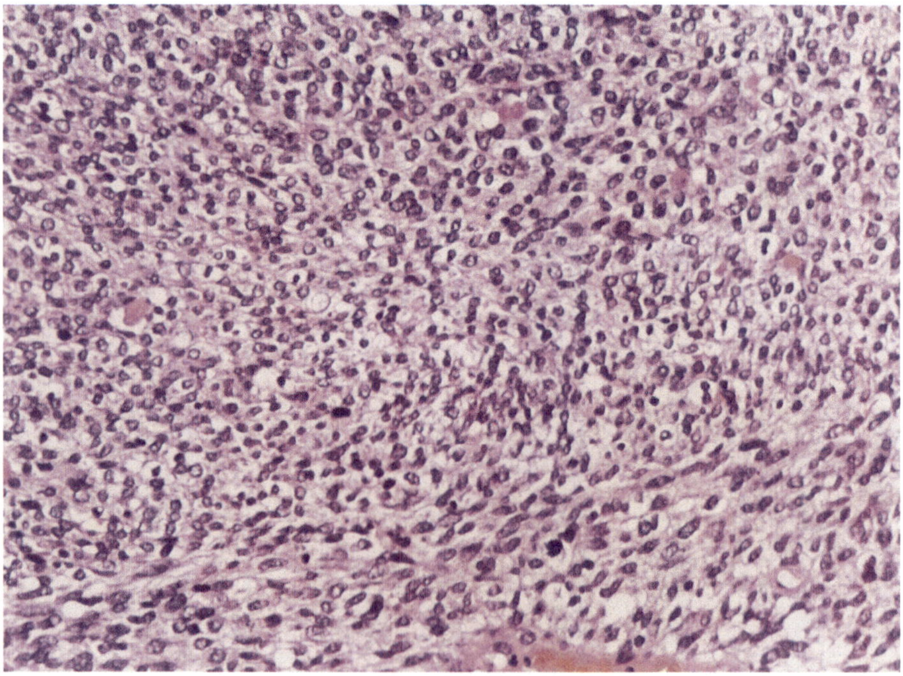

Fig. 9.41 Endometrial stromal sarcoma. H & E, ×250

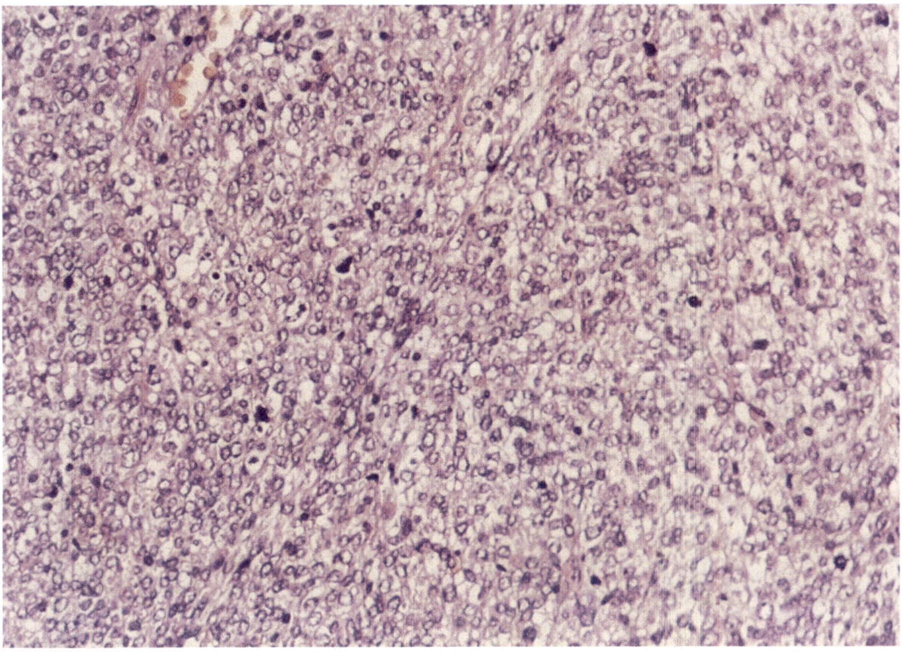

Fig. 9.42 Endometrial stromal sarcoma with large number of mitotic figures. H & E, ×250

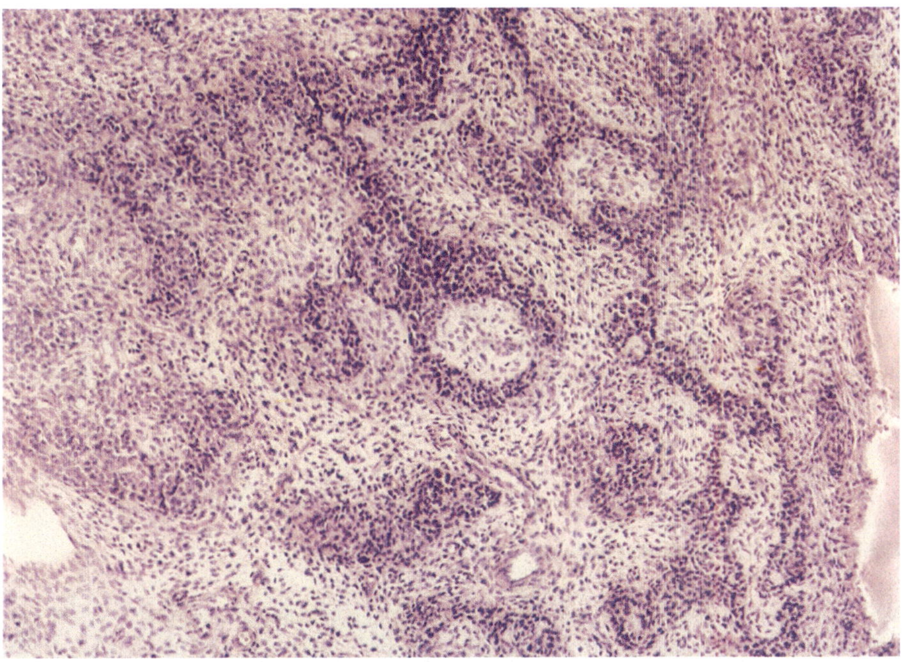

Fig. 9.43 Endometrial stromal sarcoma, sex-cord like growth pattern. H & E, ×100

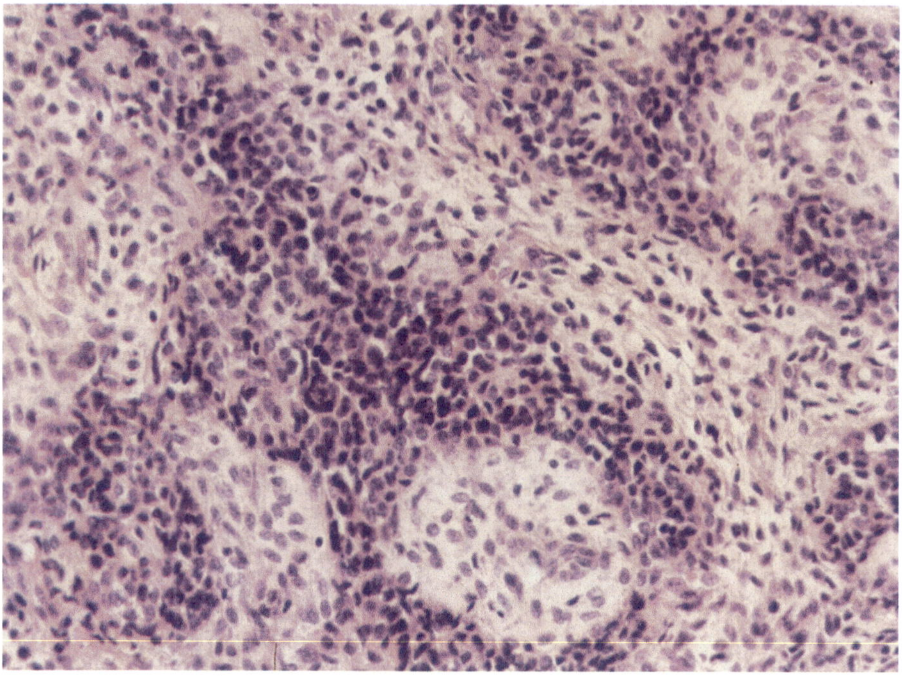

Fig. 9.44 Endometrial stromal sarcoma, sex-cord like arrangement of tumor cells. H & E, ×250

9.2.3 Undifferentiated Endometrial Sarcoma

This tumor (Figs. 9.45, 9.46) shows a great variation in nuclear size, shape, and chromatin density, and a very high mitotic activity. The malignant cells grow destructively into the myometrium and infiltrate lymphatics and blood vessels (Fig. 9.45). Hyalinized collagen, as in low-grade stromal sarcoma, is usually absent. Instead, there may be extensive necrosis.

Morphologic Differential Diagnosis. Because the morphology of the neoplastic cells has been likened to the mesenchymal component of the malignant mixed Müllerian tumor, this entity should be considered in the differential diagnosis. Other entities such as poorly differentiated carcinoma and leiomyosarcoma should be excluded as well with relevant immunohistochemical reactions.

9.2.4 Malignant Mixed Mesenchymal Tumors

Malignant mixed mesenchymal tumors are rare tumors containing two or more types of sarcomatous tissues derived from Müllerian epithelium with mesenchymal differentiation. Their morphology corresponds to the mesenchymal components of malignant mixed Müllerian tumor (see p. 187 ff).

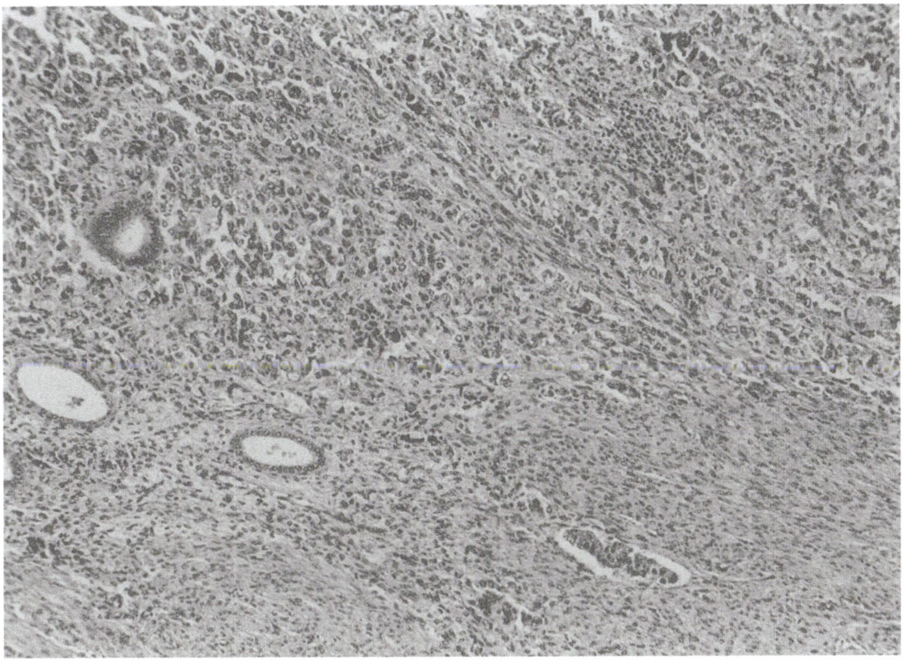

Fig. 9.45 Undifferentiated endometrial sarcoma. Some entrapped endometrial glands. H & E, ×100

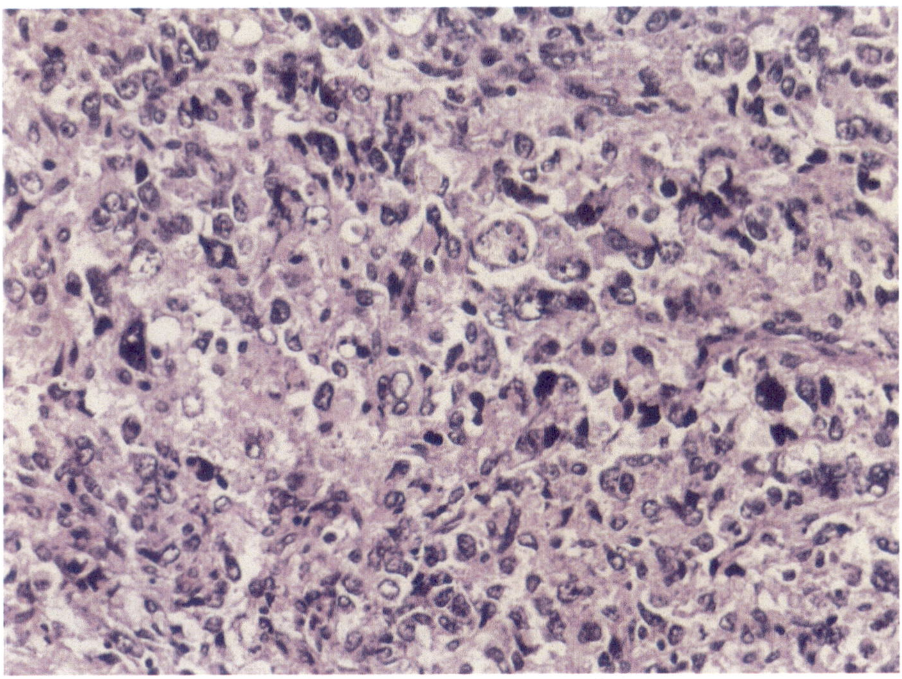

Fig. 9.46 Undifferentiated endometrial sarcoma. Tumor cells are highly pleomorphic. H & E, ×250

9.3 Mesodermal Mixed Tumors

These neoplasms contain both epithelial and mesenchymal elements which may be either uni- or pluripotential.

9.3.1 Adenofibroma

Adenofibroma is a rare endometrial tumor (Vellios et al. 1973), and its diagnosis should be made with caution in order to avoid a misdiagnosis of adenosarcoma. It consists of polypoid or lobular masses of long, branching papillae, which may fill out large portions of the uterine cavity. They are covered by a single row of low cuboidal or columnar epithelium of the endometrial or endocervical type and contain no or very few small resting or proliferating glands. Due to the profuse branching, buds of the epithelium become caught up in the stroma, forming gland-like structures. The stroma mainly consists of spindle-shaped fibroblasts occasionally separated by edema. Their nuclei are regular. Mitoses are rare. Cellular pleomorphism does not occur.

Morphologic Differential Diagnosis. Adenofibroma can be differentiated from: (a) endometrial polyps: these lack extensive branching, and their stroma is usually less cellular and contains more endometrial glands; (b) endometrial stromal sarcoma: this consists of round to oval cells resembling endometrial stromal cells; and (c) adenosarcoma: this tumor is characterized by benign glands surrounded by malignant stromal cells with mitotic activity (greater than two mitoses per ten high power fields) and focal, often periglandular cuffing or diffuse stromal hypercellularity (Figs. 9.50 and 9.51).

9.3.2 Atypical Polypoid Adenomyoma

Atypical polypoid adenomyoma (see Figs. 9.47–9.49) may be pedunculated or sessile, but is always well demarcated from the underlying myometrium. It consists of (highly) proliferating endometrial glands surrounded by short bundles of smooth muscle cells (Young et al. 1986). Foci of squamous metaplasia are frequent. Despite various degrees of architectural and cytologic atypias and mitotic activity, these tumors do not invade the myometrium and do not recur when completely removed. They usually occur in premenopausal women, and only rarely after menopause.

Morphologic Differential Diagnosis. Atypical polypoid adenomyoma must be differentiated from endometrioid adenocarcinoma invading the myometrium. It should also be distinguished from adenofibroma, which lacks differentiation into smooth muscle cells, and from adenosarcoma with its malignant and mitotically active stromal cells.

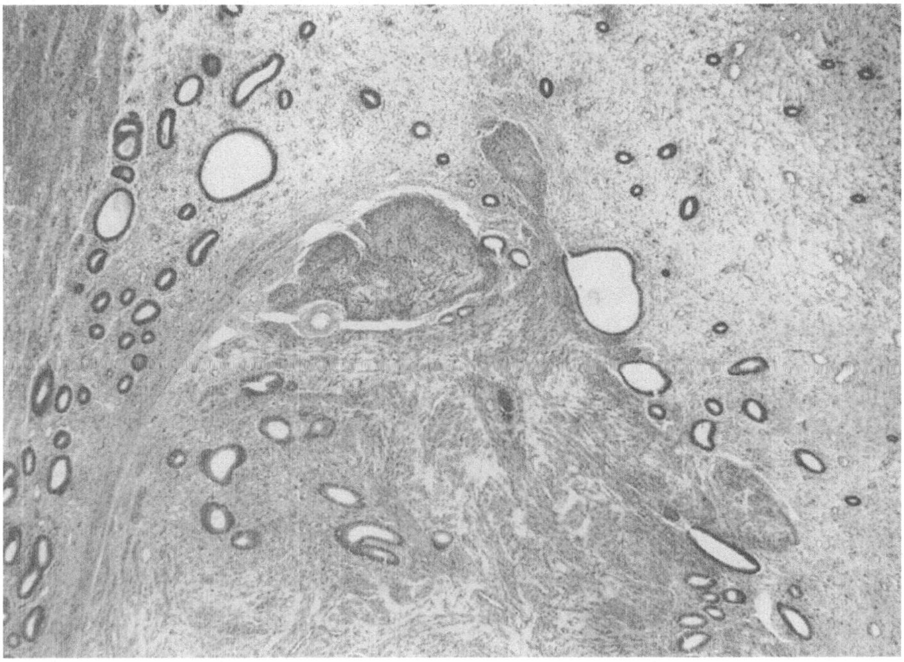

Fig. 9.47 Atypical polypoid adenomyoma. H & E, ×25

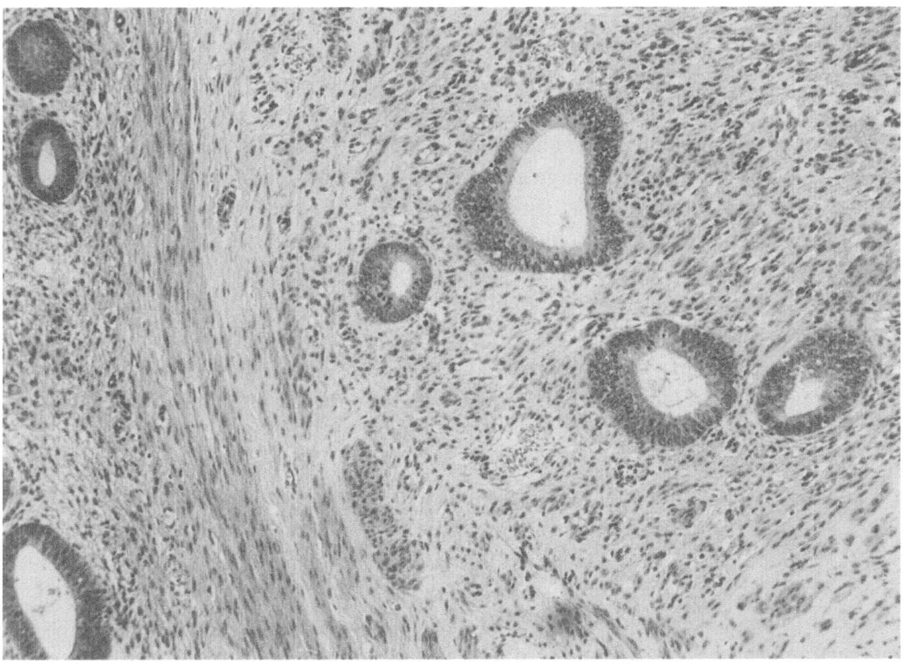

Fig. 9.48 Atypical polypoid adenomyoma. H & E, ×100

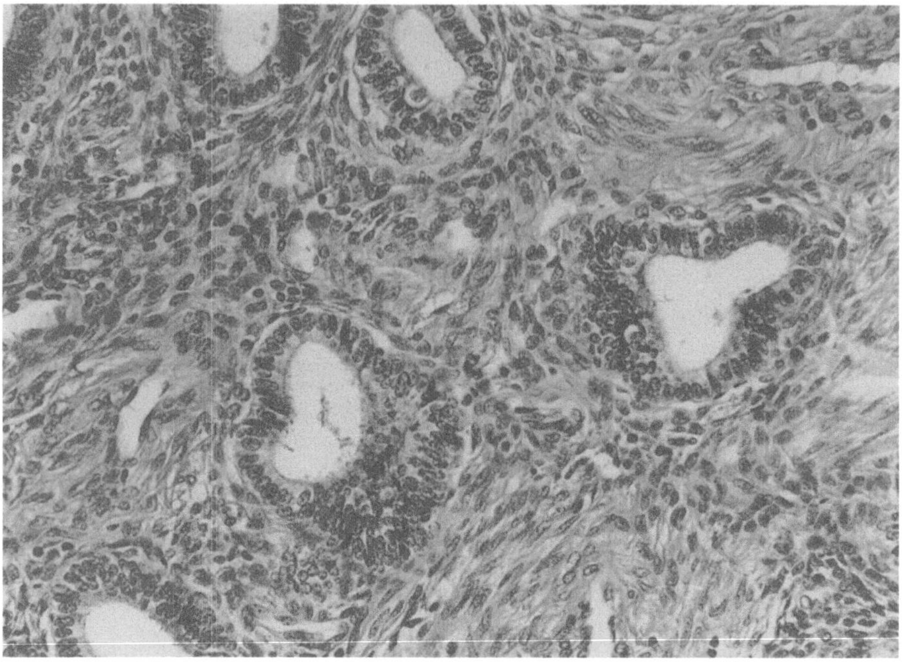

Fig. 9.49 Atypical polypoid adenomyoma. H & E, ×250

9.3.3 Adenosarcoma

The general structure and the epithelial component of adenosarcoma (Figs. 9.50–9.55) closely resemble those of the benign adenofibroma. The glandular spaces may be tubular, dilated or cleft-like and contain mucin (Fig. 9.52). The mesenchymal component consists of fibroblasts, occasional leiomyoblasts (Fig. 9.55), and stromal cells with mild atypia and moderate mitotic activity (Clement and Scully 1990; Zaloudek and Norris 1982). Characteristic are the hypercellular foci forming perivascular nodules or periglandular cuffs (Czernobilsky et al. 1983; Figs. 9.53, 9.54).

Heterologous stromal differentiation to chondroblasts or rhabdomyoblasts may be seen in some regions; other tumors may show areas with sex cord-like differentiation (Hirschfield et al. 1986; Clement and Scully 1989).

Clinical Correlation and Morphologic Differential Diagnosis. (a) Adenofibroma: patients with adenofibroma are generally older, with a median age of approximately 68 years in comparison to 57 years for patients with adenosarcoma (Zaloudek and Norris 1982); mitotic activity is less than two mitoses per ten high power fields; focal stromal hypercellularity with pleomorphism, including heterologous stromal differentiation, is characteristic of adenosarcoma and absent in adenofibroma; adenosarcomas do invade the myometrium but only at a late stage; (b) endometrial stromal sarcoma: absence of cleft-like spaces and cystic glands, and finger-like invasion of the myometrium are characteristic of stromal sarcoma and absent in adenosarcoma.

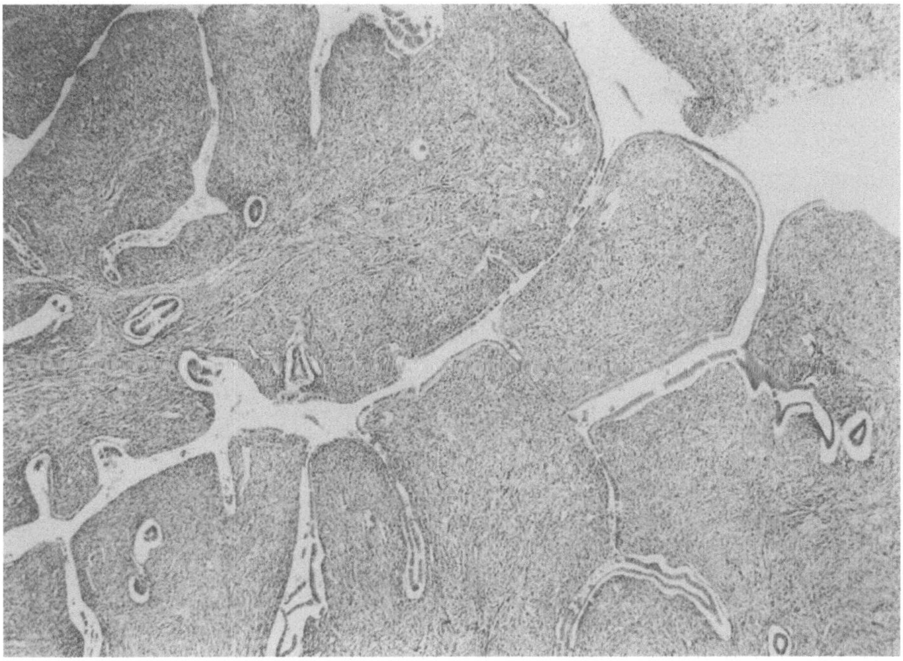

Fig. 9.50 Adenosarcoma, low grade. H & E, ×25

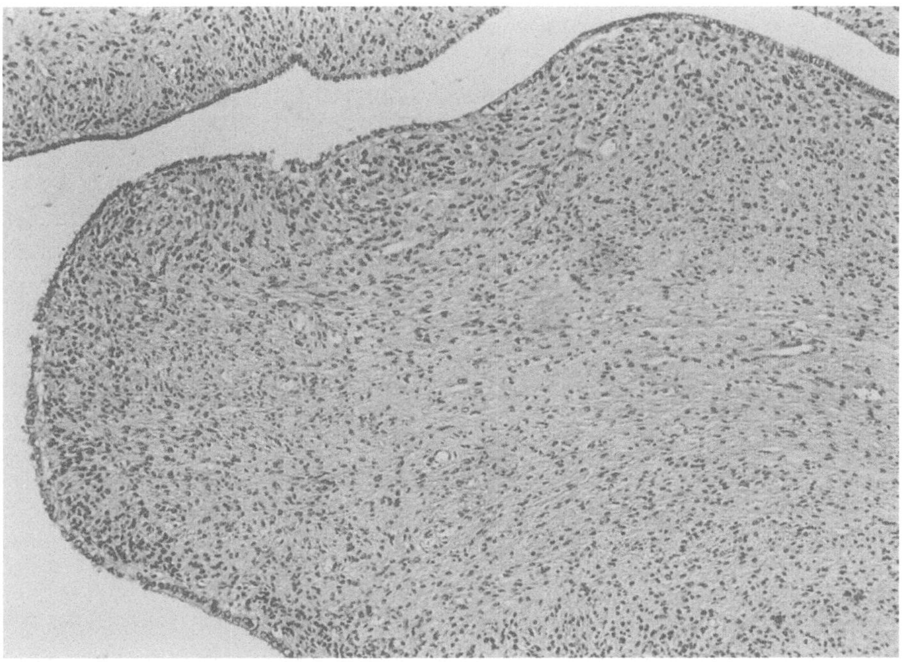

Fig. 9.51 Adenosarcoma, low grade. H & E, ×100

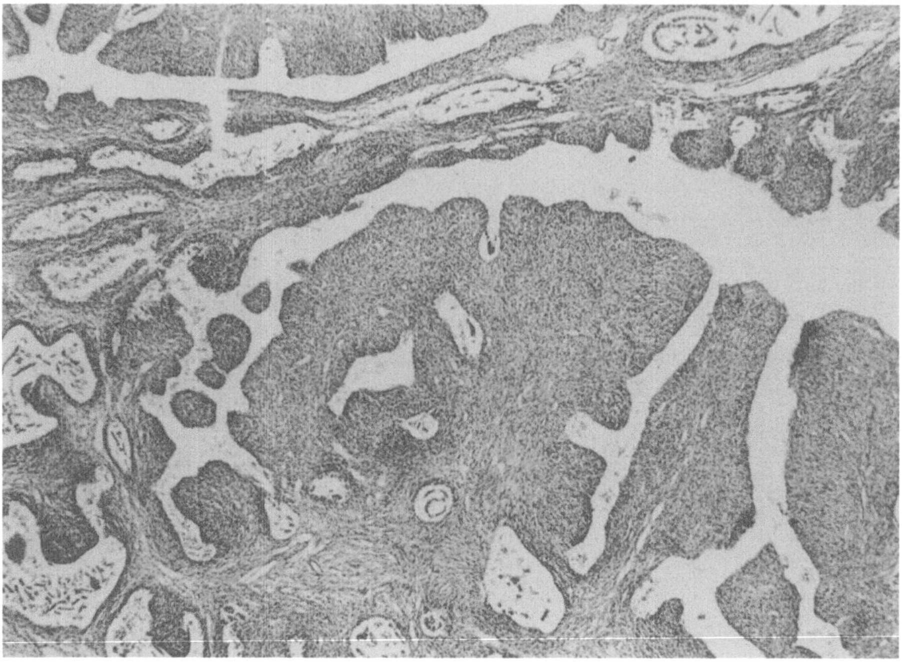

Fig. 9.52 Adenosarcoma. Periglandular hypercellular stromal component. H & E, ×25

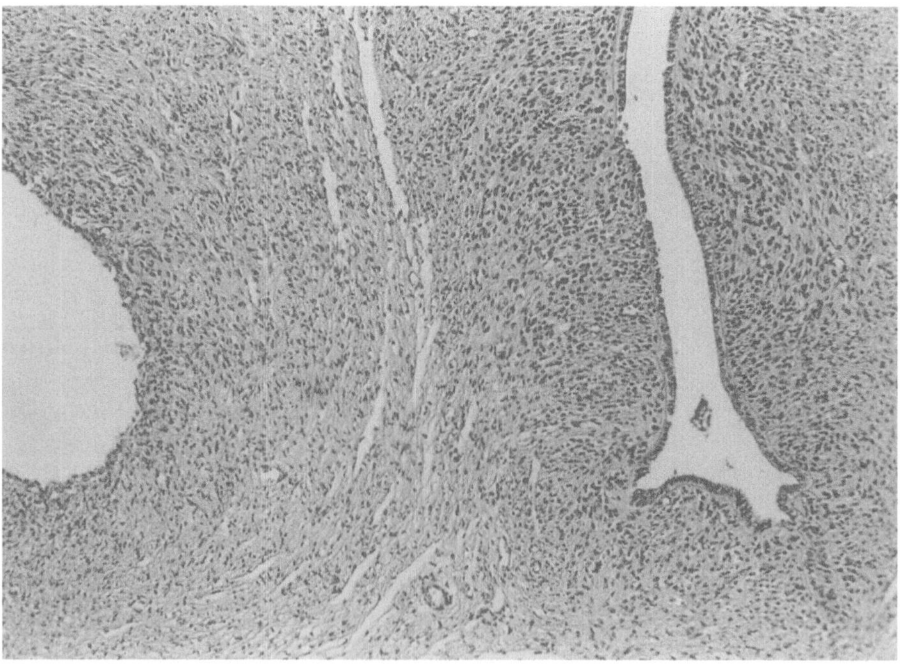

Fig. 9.53 Adenosarcoma. H & E, ×100

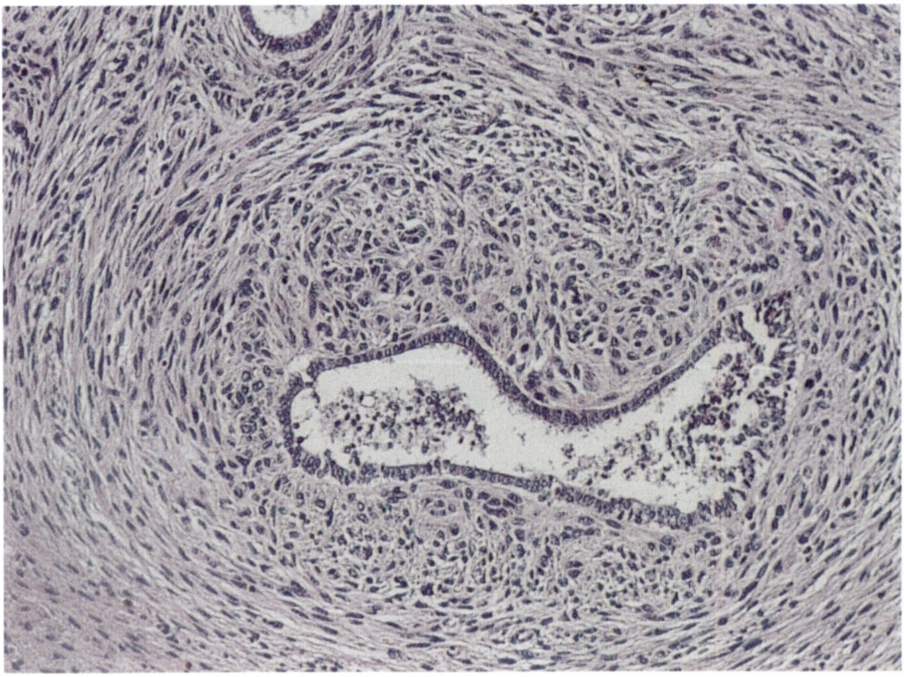

Fig. 9.54 Adenosarcoma, periglandular cuff. H & E, ×150

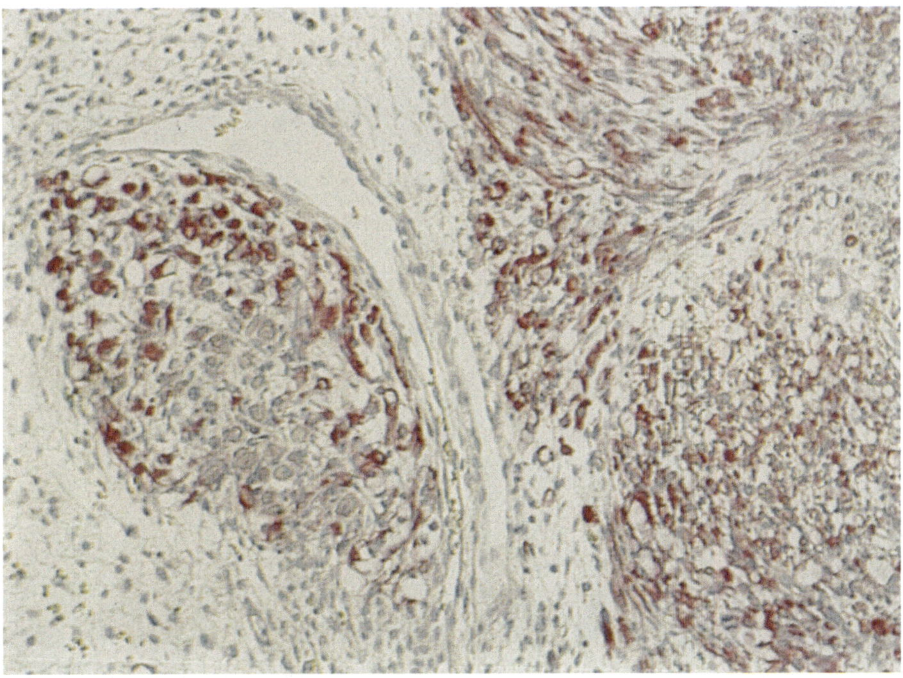

Fig. 9.55 Adenosarcoma. Desmin, positive stromal cells ×150

Adenosarcomas with sarcomatous overgrowth (more than 20%) have a much less favorable prognosis than adenosarcomas without this feature (Clement and Scully 1989).

In patients with adenosarcoma a previous therapy with tamoxifen has been repeatedly reported (Booklage et al. 1992; Altares et al. 1993; Mourits et al. 1998; own observations).

9.3.4 Carcinofibroma

Carcinofibromas (Figs. 9.56, 9.57) are rare tumors in which the epithelial component is malignant, whereas the mesenchymal component is benign (Östör and Fortune 1980). The epithelial component consists of carcinomatous glands, which may be cystically dilated or microalveolar and may form branching intraluminal epithelial papillae or nodules of squamous metaplasia (Fig. 9.56). The epithelial lining is atypical and resembles that of adenocarcinomas. The surrounding stroma corresponds to that of benign adenofibroma, consisting mainly of fibroblasts (Fig. 9.57). The tumor may invade the myometrium like an adenocarcinoma.

Morphologic Differential Diagnosis. Adenocarcinoma with desmoplastic stromal reaction has less amount of stroma than carcinofibroma resulting in a widely spaced arrangement of the carcinomatous glands.

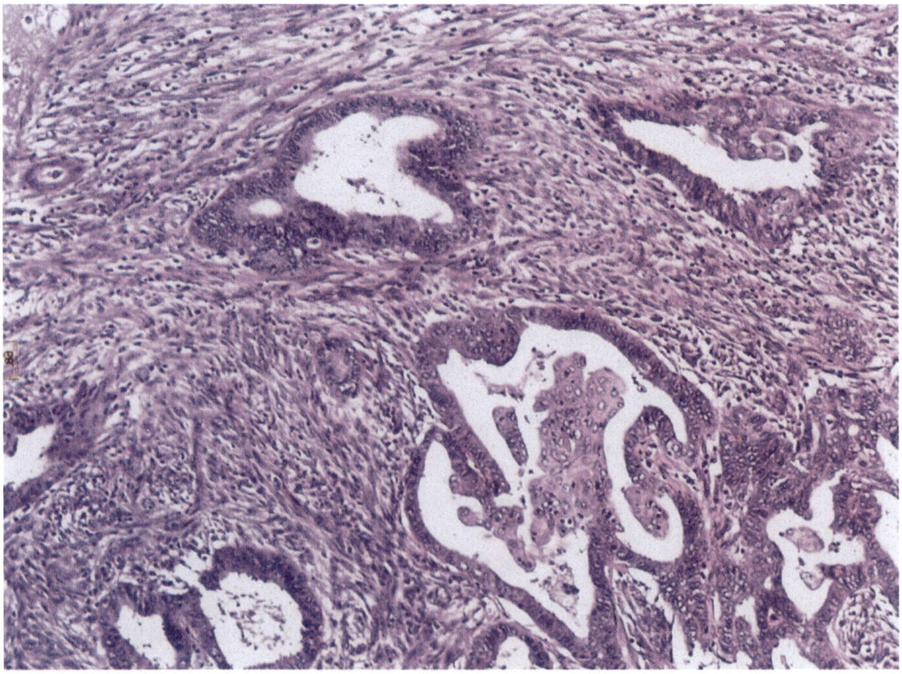

Fig. 9.56 Carcinofibroma. H & E, ×100

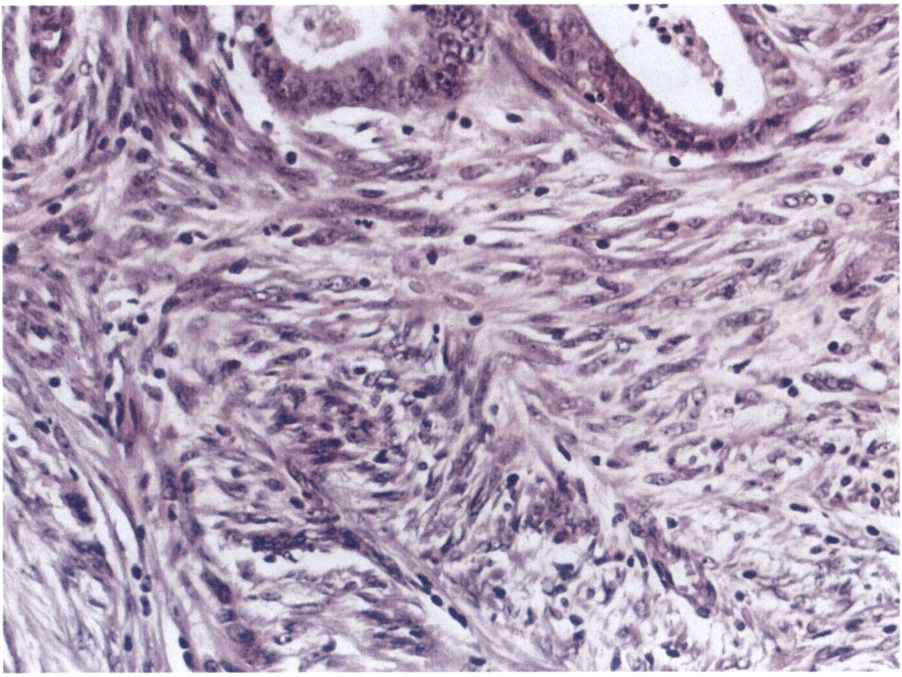

Fig. 9.57 Carcinofibroma. H & E, ×250

9.3.5
Carcinosarcoma (Malignant Müllerian Mixed Tumor), Homologous Type

Carcinosarcoma (Figs. 9.58–9.60) represents the most common subtype of mixed Müllerian tumors. It accounts for up to 5% of the malignant tumors of the uterus. Usually, it grows aggressively, fills the uterine cavity at an early stage, and shows early myometrial and endocervical invasion. Histologically, the carcinomatous component closely resembles the glandular or papillary type of adenocarcinoma with variously sized glands lined by atypical multilayered epithelial cells that form intraluminal branching papillae (Fig. 9.59). Occasional regions of clear cells or mucinous glands are common, whereas areas of squamous cell carcinoma are rare. The number of the carcinomatous glands may vary considerably. Sometimes only small foci of glandular structures or solid epithelial growth may be found. The sarcomatous stroma consists mostly of sarcomatous fibroblasts and endometrial stromal cells. Both components show frequent mitoses (Fig. 9.60). Hence the sarcomatous component of carcinosarcoma, which is intimately admixed with the carcinomatous component, may be uniform or pleomorphic, both representing the homologous type of carcinosarcoma.

Morphologic Differential Diagnosis. (a) Poorly differentiated adenocarcinoma, in which solid sheets of undifferentiated carcinomatous cells surround differentiated carcinomatous glands in a sarcomatoid pattern; the distinction is possible by careful study of the cellular structure and by silver impregnation of the reticulin network: carcinomatous cells are enveloped by reticulin fibers in small groups, whereas sarcoma cells are enveloped individually, incompletely, or not at all; cytokeratin markers may be quite helpful in difficult cases.

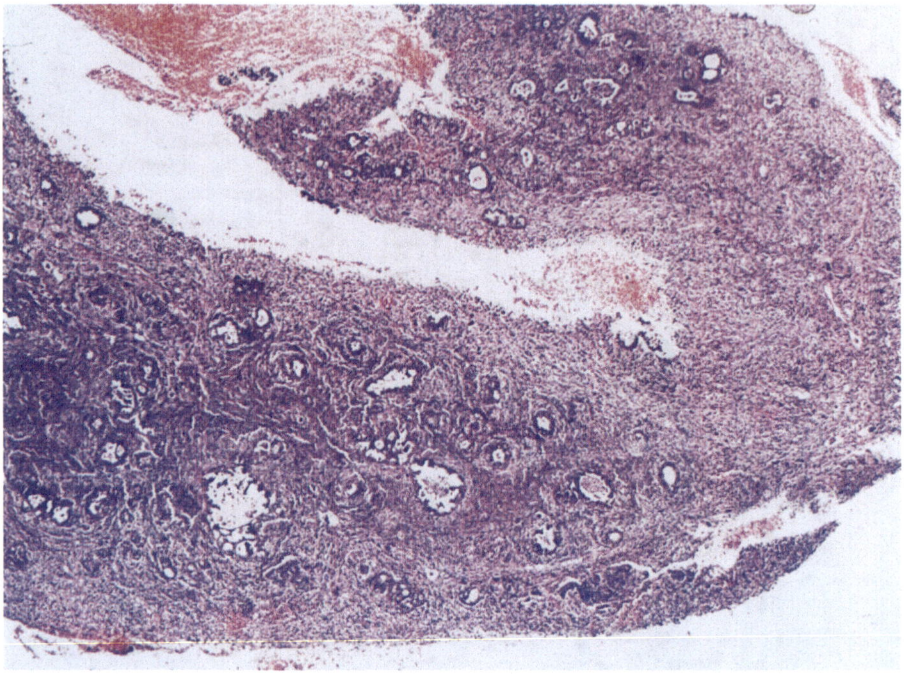

Fig. 9.58 Carcinosarcoma (malignant Müllerian mixed tumor, homologous type). H & E, ×25

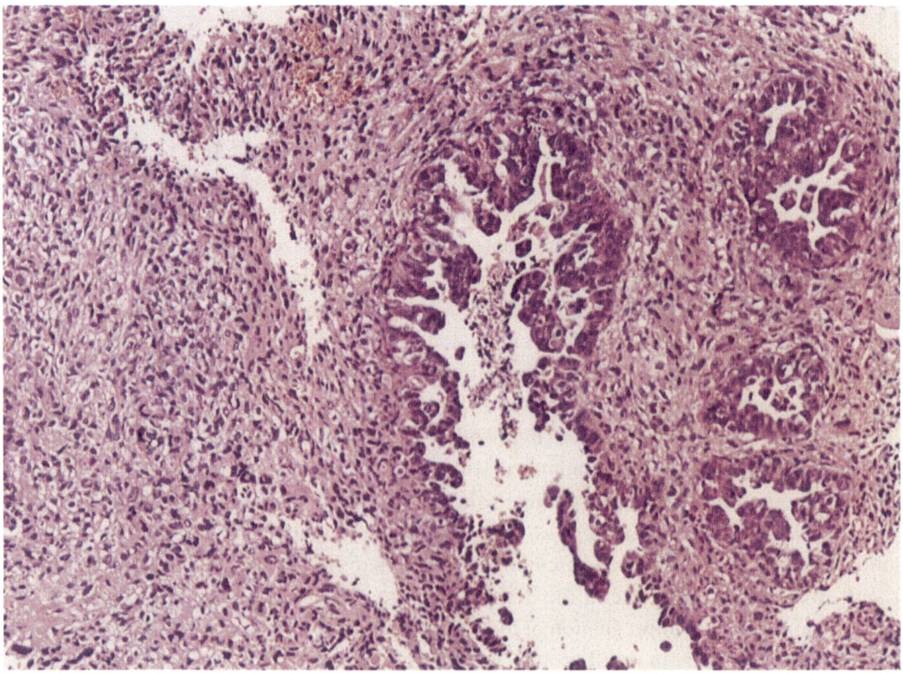

Fig. 9.59 Carcinosarcoma (malignant Müllerian mixed tumor, homologous type). Serous carcinomatous component. H & E, ×100

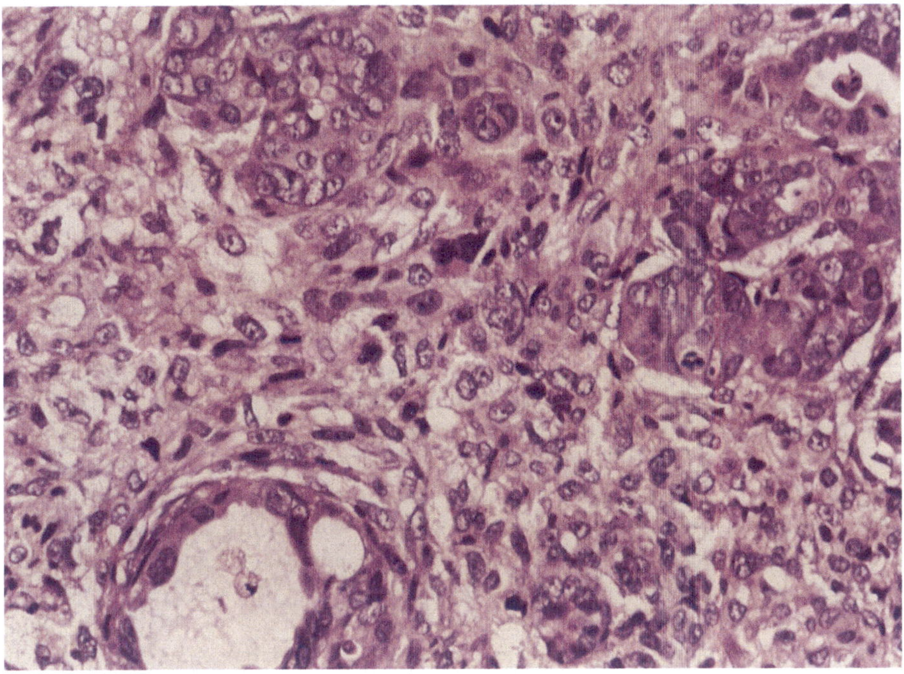

Fig. 9.60 Carcinosarcoma (malignant Müllerian mixed tumor, homologous type). Transition between malignant epithelial and stromal component. H & E, ×250

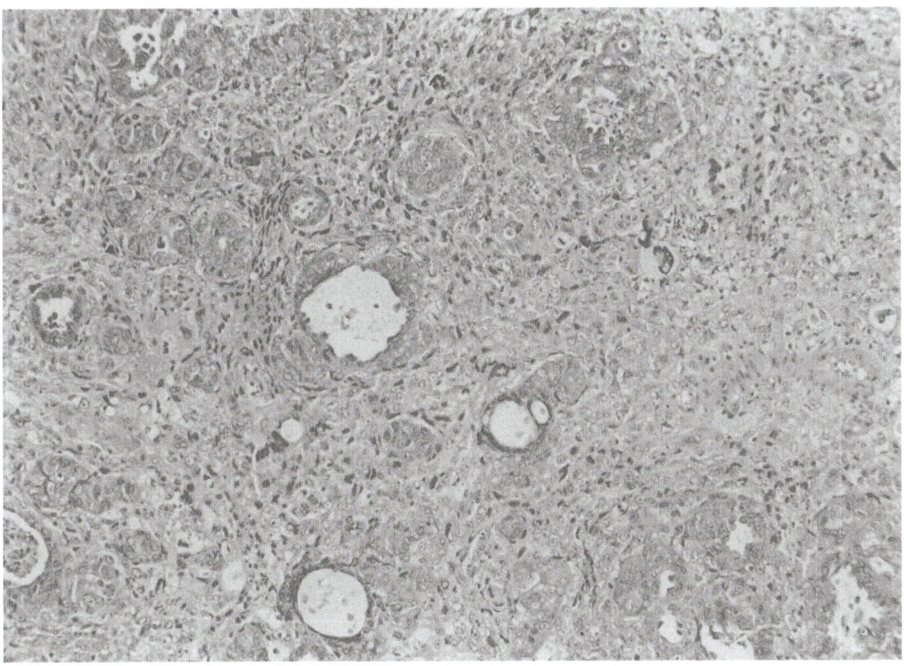

Fig. 9.61 Carcinosarcoma: malignant Müllerian mixed tumor, heterologous type. H & E, ×100

9.3.6 Carcinosarcoma (Malignant Müllerian Mixed Tumor), Heterologous Type

In malignant Müllerian mixed tumor, heterologous type (Figs. 9.61–9.67), the epithelial component corresponds to endometrioid, serous or undifferentiated carcinoma whereas the sarcomatous component may be extremely pleomorphic. Besides poorly differentiated mesenchymal cells and mingled with these, one may find regions of atypical chondroblasts or osteoblasts (Figs. 9.63, 9.64). Cartilage is the second most common heterologous element in these tumors. Other mixed tumors may contain large regions of rhabdomyoblasts with cross-striations (Böcker and Stegner 1975). When these elongated cells are cross-sectioned (cut at right angles to their long axis), their cross-striations cannot be seen and the cells appear round, surrounded by empty spaces (Fig. 9.65). Large cells with vacuolated cytoplasm (Fig. 9.65) may represent a liposarcomatous component, a relatively rare occurrence (Mortel et al. 1970). Very occasionally, ganglion cells may be found (Ruffolo et al. 1969). Some tumors contain large regions of a myxosarcoma (Fig. 9.66), and others areas of a leiomyosarcoma (Fig. 9.67), which must be differentiated from a pure myxosarcoma or leiomyosarcoma, respectively. Malignant Müllerian mixed tumors are even more aggressive than clear cell and serous papillary carcinomas of the endometrium (George et al. 1995). Both, the carcinomatous and the sarcomatous components are distinctly positive with immunostains for p16 in most (up to 90%) and p53 (up to 80%) malignant Müllerian mixed tumors of homologous and heterologous type (Buza and Tavassoli 2009).

Morphologic Differential Diagnosis. Problems may arise only when insufficient tissue sections have been taken for study. To ensure that the wide spectrum of potentials of these

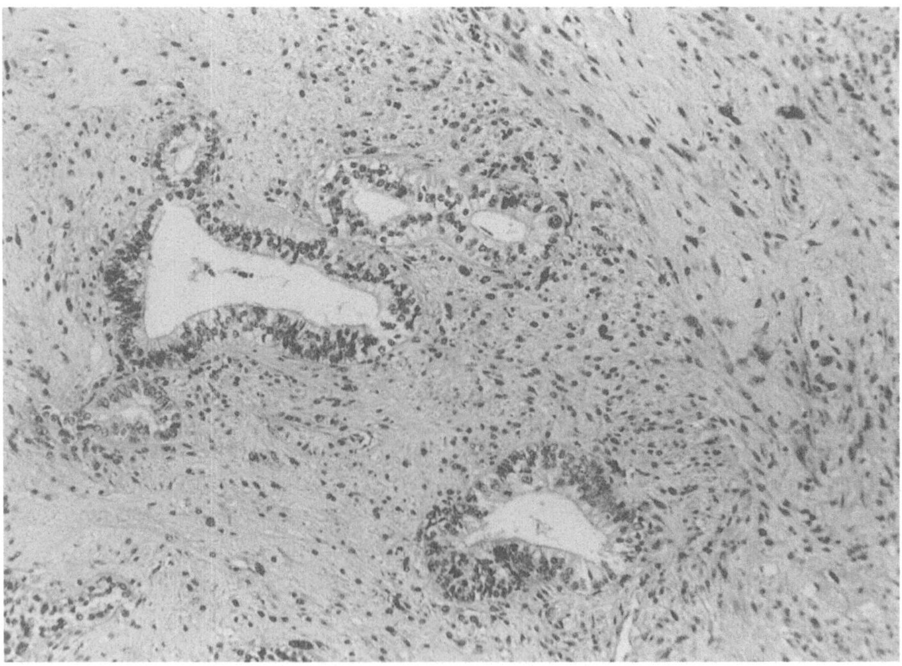

Fig. 9.62 Carcinosarcoma: malignant Müllerian mixed tumor, heterologous type. H & E, ×100

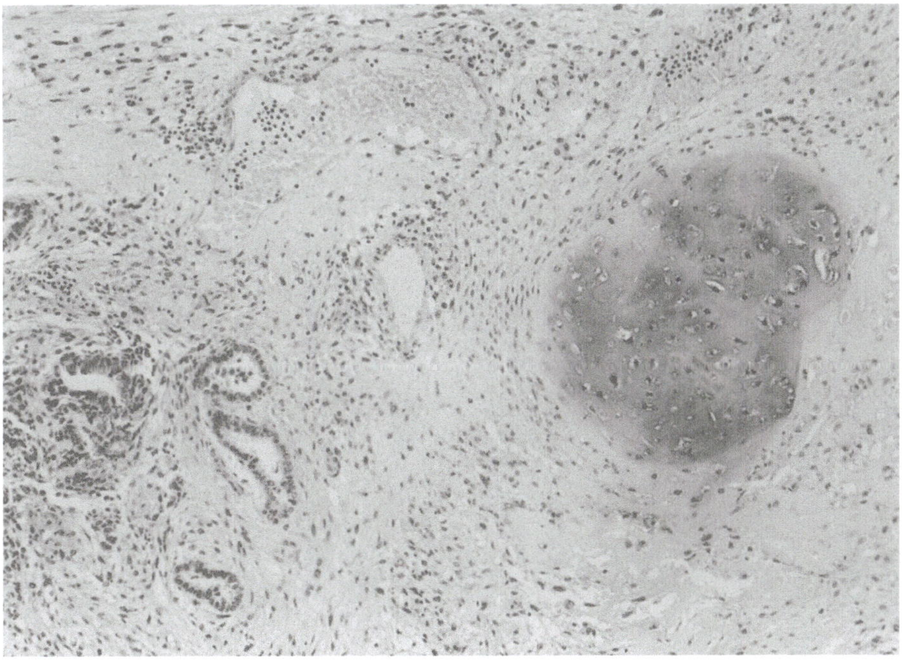

Fig. 9.63 Carcinosarcoma: malignant Müllerian mixed tumor, heterologous type with chondrosarcomatous focus. H & E, ×100

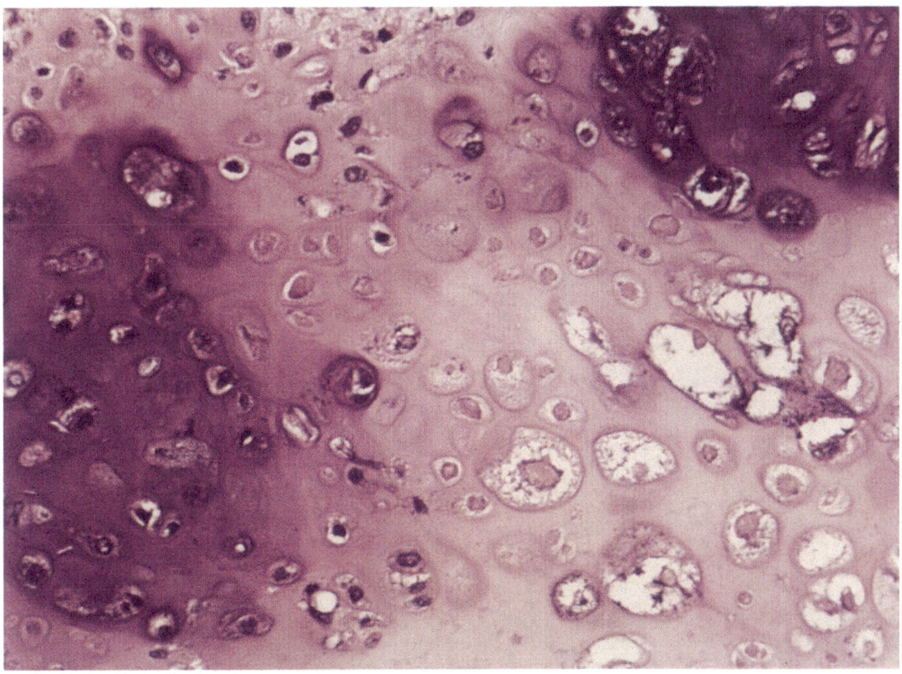

Fig. 9.64 Carcinosarcoma: malignant Müllerian mixed tumor, heterologous type, with malignant chondroblasts. H & E, ×250

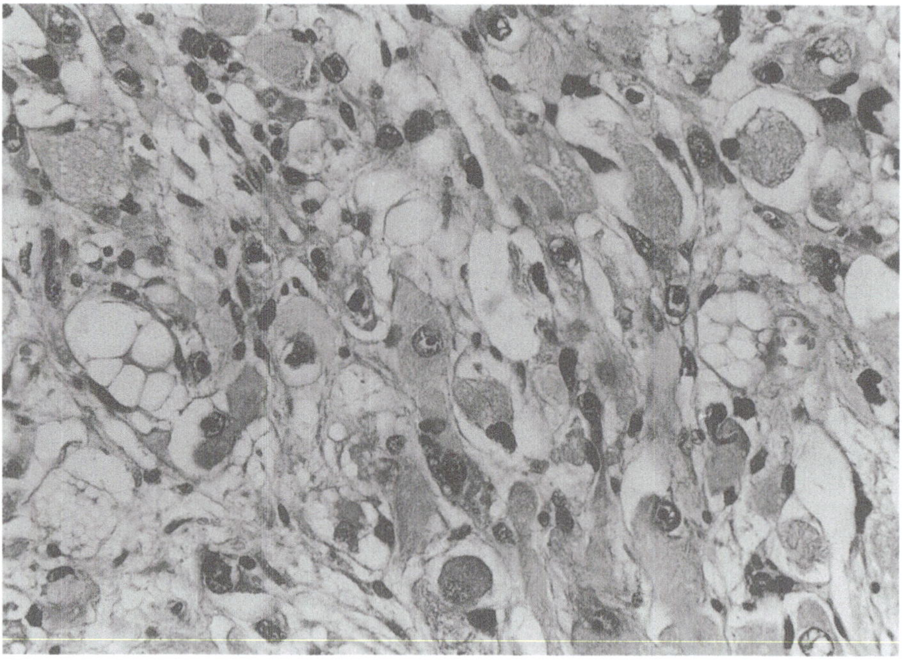

Fig. 9.65 Carcinosarcoma: malignant Müllerian mixed tumor, heterologous type with rhabdomyoblasts. H & E, ×250

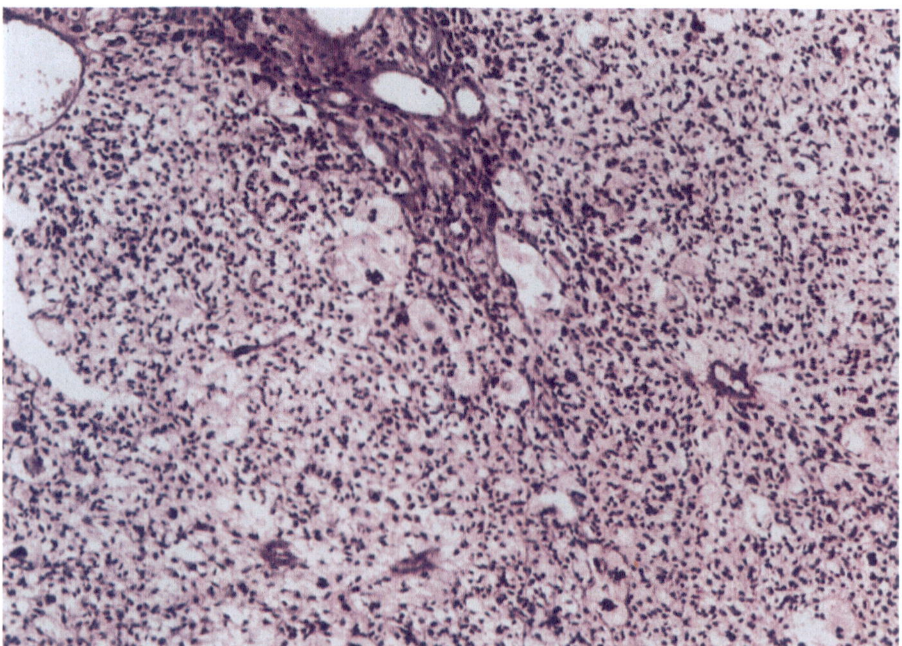

Fig. 9.66 Carcinosarcoma: malignant Müllerian mixed tumor, heterologous type with regions of a myxosarcoma. H & E, ×100

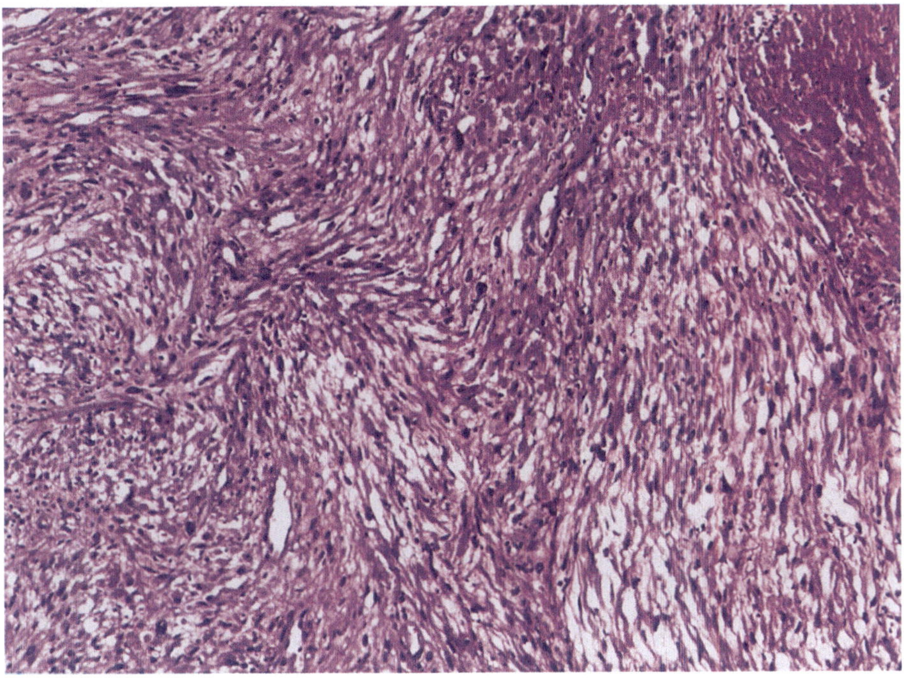

Fig. 9.67 Carcinosarcoma: malignant Müllerian mixed tumor, heterologous type with areas of a leiomyosarcoma. H & E, ×100

mixed tumors is included, many sections should be studied from several different parts of the tumor. Under these circumstances, the differential diagnosis from other neoplasms usually proves to be no problem.

9.4 Primitive Neuroectodermal Tumor (PNET)

Very rarely malignant neuroectodermal tumors (Fig. 9.68) arise in the endometrium (Hendrickson and Scheithauer 1986); they are considered to be either of mesodermal derivation with heterologous metaplasia or of monodermal teratomatous origin. Their prognosis is very poor.

The grossly polypoid tumor with rapid expansion into the myometrium consists of primitive neuroectodermal cells with focal glial and neuronal differentiation and formation of rosettes, reacting positively for glial fibrillary acidic protein (Daya et al. 1993), but negatively for cytokeratins, CEA and S100.

Differential Diagnosis. Distinction from small or large cell neuroendocrine carcinomas is possible when neuronal, ependymal or glial elements can be found; from most other

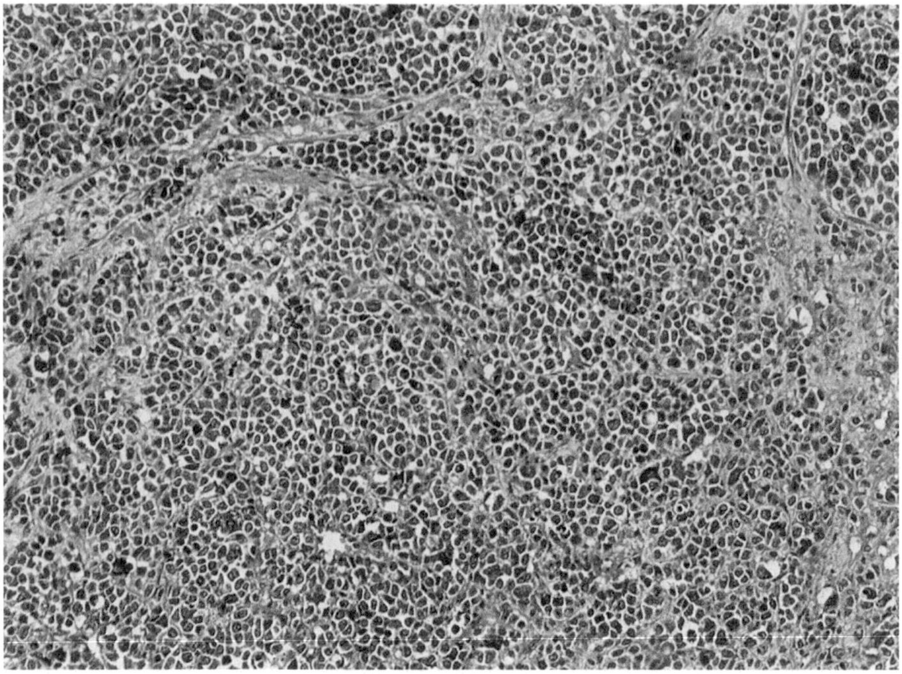

Fig. 9.68 Primitive neuroectodermal tumor. H & E, ×150

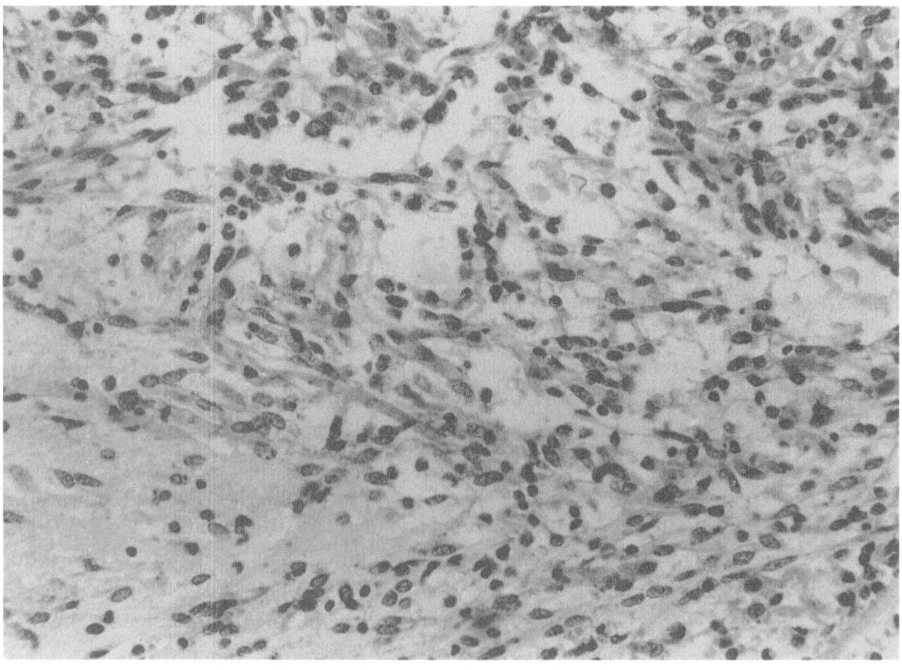

Fig. 9.69 Embryonal rhabdomyosarcoma. H & E, ×250

poorly differentiated neoplasms with the appropriate immunohistochemical markers. Distinction from *embryonal rhabdomyosarcoma* (Fig. 9.69), another very rare and unusual possible component of endometrial specimens, can be done with markers for desmin, MYOD1, myogenin and myoglobin.

9.5 Malignant Lymphomas and Hematopoietic Neoplasms

9.5.1 Lymphomas and Lymphatic Leukemias

9.5.1.1 Occurrence and Clinical Symptoms

Lymphomas and lymphatic leukemias are rare neoplasms in the uterine corpus. They are predominantly secondary infiltrates of systemic diseases, but may also arise in the uterus (Su et al. 2008; Heeren et al. 2008; Frey et al. 2006; Kosari et al. 2005; el-Omari-Alaoui et al. 2002; van de Rijn et al. 1997; Aozasa et al. 1993; Harris and Scully 1984). Macroscopically, they may present as an endometrial polyp (Rittenbach et al. 2005). In most cases the tumor cells infiltrate the endometrium and myometrium, often the endocervix and ectocervix, and may penetrate the serosa to spread into the ovary and fallopian tube, in single cases into the omentum, colon and small intestine (Kosari et al. 2005). According to our studies in the German Lymphoma Reference Centers of Kiel and Berlin, and to the international literature, most of the malignant non-Hodgkin's lymphomas are diffuse large B-cell lymphomas, followed by follicular B-cell lymphomas grade I–III and Burkitt's lymphomas. Other B-cell lymphomas like mantle cell and marginal zone lymphoma, lymphoplasmacytic lymphoma, multiple myeloma, B-lymphocytic and B-lymphoblastic lymphoma/leukemia are very rare in the uterus as compared with nodal and other extranodal sites (Kosari et al. 2005; el-Omari-Aloui et al. 2002; Vang et al. 2000; van de Rijn et al. 1997; Aozasa et al. 1993). The lymphomas may occur in every age between the second and eight decades. The youngest patient in our series was a 16-year-old girl with a primary Burkitt's lymphoma of the endometrium. The patients usually present with abnormal uterine bleeding and uterine mass, eventually adnexal mass and pain.

9.5.1.2 Morphology and Immunohistochemistry

All lymphomas and lymphatic leukemias in the endometrium grow to surround glands (Fig. 9.71), and may show lymphoepithelial changes with altered or destroyed glandular epithelium. Large cell lymphomas tend to spread into vessels and invade small nerves (Fig. 9.72).

Diffuse large B cell lymphomas generally grow densely and aggressively. Some morphological variants can be distinguished: *centroblastic* (Figs. 9.70 and 9.71), *immunoblastic* (Figs. 9.72 and 9.73), *plasmablastic* and *anaplastic*. Plasmablastic lymphomas, which are rare amongst the diffuse large B cell lymphomas, seem to be a special subtype because of their different immunophenotype and unfavorable prognosis. In the centroblastic variant, the cells have round or cleaved nuclei with small central or peripheral nucleoli. The cells in immunoblastic and plasmablastic lymphomas have abundant basophilic cytoplasm and conspicuous central nucleoli. In anaplastic B cell lymphomas, the tumor cells resemble Hodgkin and Reed-Sternberg cells with very prominent nucleoli and multinucleated giant cells. Typical Burkitt's lymphomas show medium-sized monomorphic tumor cells and a cohesive growth pattern with a so-called starry sky aspect imparted by numerous large pale macrophages, their cytoplasm filled with ingested apoptotic tumor cells. Immunohistochemically, large B cell lymphomas usually express intensively CD20 (Fig. 9.73) and other B cell markers, except plasmablastic lymphomas. They show variable expressions of BCL-2, BCL-6, CD10, IgM, and the plasma cell-typic B cell transcription factor IRF-4 (Mum-1), less commonly CD30 and CD38. Plasmablastic lymphomas are in most instances completely CD20 negative, but may partially express the B cell antigen CD79a. They are typically CD38 and Mum-1 positive, show a strong production of the J-chain and kappa or lambda light chains and may be EBV-positive, in our series in about 50% of the cases (latent membrane antigen and nuclear antigens; Dallenbach et al., in preparation). The proliferation rate (Ki-67 index) is high (80–90%) to extreme (100% in Burkitt's lymphomas).

Follicular lymphomas are graded according to their amount of blasts. Grade I lymphomas exhibit up to 5, grade II up to 15, grade IIIa more than 15 blasts per high power field, and grade IIIb a pure blastic tumor cell population without centrocytes. They may reveal a follicular and diffuse growth pattern and a sclerosis. The diagnosis is confirmed by immunohistochemistry: most cases strongly express CD20 and are BCL-2, BCL-6, CD10, and CD38 positive. In follicular areas, the lymphomas show a meshwork of follicular dendritic cells. The proliferation rate varies with grade, with a range of 5 to over 90%.

Marginal zone lymphomas of the mucosa associated lymphoid tissue (MALT) arise primarily in the endometrium, probably after prolonged chronic endometritis (Heeren et al. 2008; Hamadani et al. 2006). The tumor cells surround and invade preexisting germinal centers and induce lymphoepithelial lesions in the endometrial surface and glandular epithelium. Morphologically, they resemble those of mantle cell lymphomas. Except in cases with partial plasmacytic differentiation, the cells strongly express CD20, are IgM positive and IgD negative and may express CD43. Their proliferation rate is variable, but most often low, indicating an indolent growth behavior.

Mantle cell lymphomas are most often slowly growing small cell (lymphocytic) lymphomas, but there exists a more aggressive blastic ("blastoid") variant morphologically resembling lymphoblastic lymphoma with many mitotic figures and a high Ki-67 index. The growth pattern may be nodular and/or diffuse, and the tumor cells have round or oval to cleaved nuclei with small nucleoli. Besides the expression of B cell antigens, CD5, CD43, IgM und IgD, they are characteristically CyclinD1 positive, indicating the diagnostic t(11;14) translocation.

Lymphoplasmacytic lymphomas reveal a more or less marked plasmacellular differentiation with typical extracellular and intranuclear immunoglobulin bodies (Russell and Dutcher bodies), which can be highlighted in the Giemsa and PAS stain (Fig. 9.74). CD20 may be negative or only weakly positive in plasma cell-rich areas, but CD79a is usually strongly expressed. The cells are IgM and kappa or lambda positive. The proliferation rate is low in most instances, but may be higher in polymorphic types with many blasts.

Plasmacytomas (multiple myelomas) are in most cases easily recognized by conventional histology, but the clonality of the cells should be confirmed with immunoglobulin light chain stainings to differentiate the infiltrate from reactive plasmacytosis. The majority of the cases do not express CD20. A minority, however, are partially CD20 positive, may show CyclinD1 expression and lack the typical plasma cell morphology. In these cases, the plasmacellular differentiation can be immunohistochemically demonstrated with stainings for CD38, CD138 (Syndecan) and Mum-1.

Endometrial infiltrates of a *chronic lymphatic B cell leukemia (B-CLL) and a precursor (acute,* Fig. 9.75) *lymphoblastic B or T cell lymphoma/leukemia (B-LBL, T-LBL)* must be considered if the leukemia is anamnestically known or, rarely, unknown (Fig. 9.75). Characteristically in such leukemic infiltrations the gross architecture of the endometrium remains preserved, making it difficult to recognize them under low magnification (Fig. 9.76). At higher magnification (Fig. 9.77), a diffuse infiltration and often replacement of the endometrial stroma by leukemic cells becomes evident. Between these infiltrates, irregular hemorrhages can be seen (Fig. 9.76). The endometrial glands are generally preserved and most of them are not involved, although a few may show infiltration by leukemic cells (Fig. 9.77). Tumor cells of B-CLL typically express CD5, CD20, and CD23. B-LBL is CD10, CD19, mostly CD79a and tdt positive but frequently only weakly and partially CD20 positive. T-LBL expresses CD2, CD3 (often weakly), CD7, sometimes CD8 and CD10, and tdt. The proliferation rate in CLL is usually low, in prolymphocyte-rich areas higher, in LBL generally high.

Peripheral T cell lymphoma and T/NK cell lymphomas are extremely uncommon in the endometrium (Briese et al. 2006; Nakamura et al. 2001; Masunaga et al. 1998). Single cases of primary T/NK cell lymphomas of the uterine corpus have been described, one of which was diagnosed at autopsy (Briese et al. 2006). We observed only one case of a small cell lymphoma that revealed a clonal T cell receptor rearrangement (see below). The tumor cells expressed CD3, CD4 and were slowly proliferating.

Hodgkin lymphomas are also extremely rare in the endometrium. One case was reported of a lymphocyte depleted subtype (Kosari et al. 2005) with typical strong expression of CD30.

9.5.1.3 Molecular Pathology

Molecular pathologic methods can be helpful in clarifying doubtful cases. In dense lymphocytic infiltrates in the endometrium that are B cell and/or T cell rich, it might be necessary

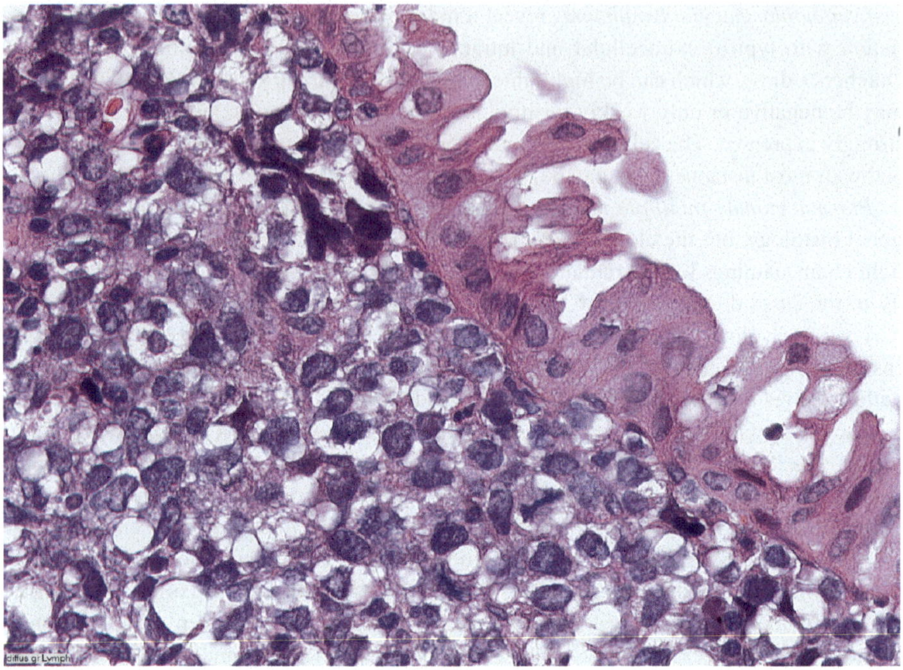

Fig. 9.70 Diffuse large B-cell lymphoma, centroblastic variant and serous papillary syncytial metaplasia of the endometrial surface epithelium. H & E, × 400

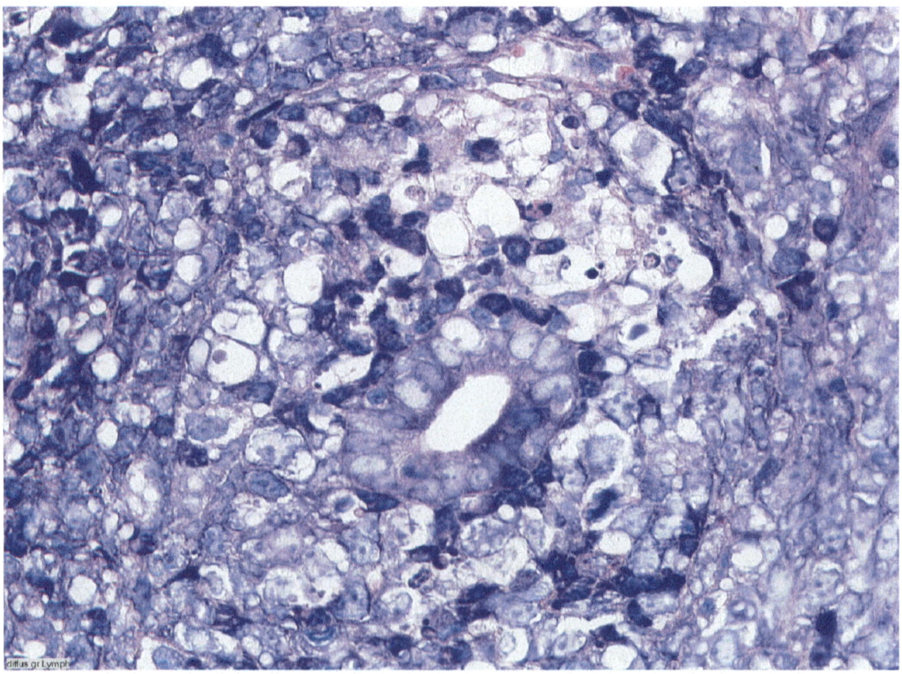

Fig. 9.71 Same case. Tumor cells surrounding an endometrial gland. Giemsa, × 400

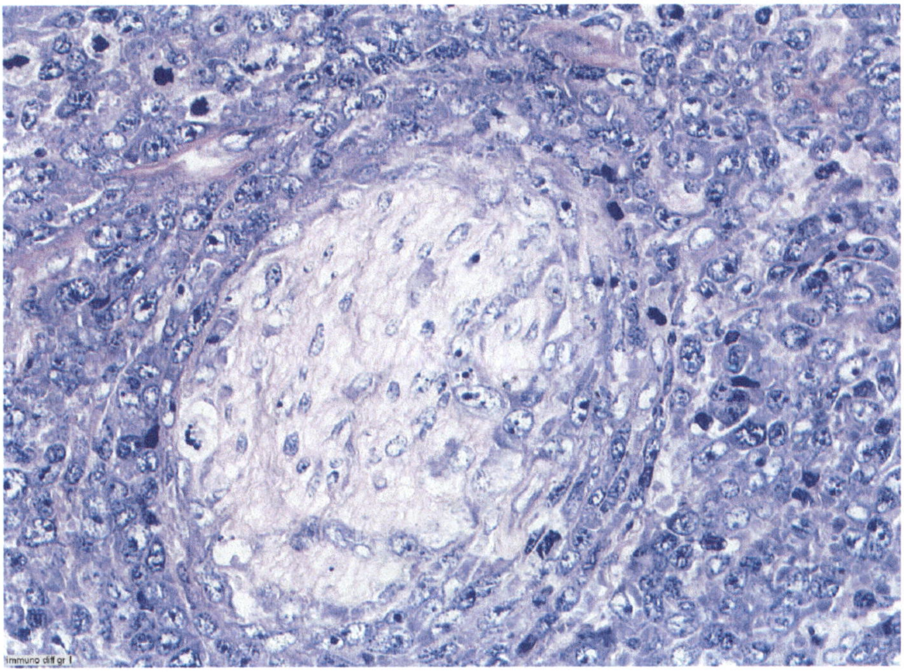

Fig. 9.72 Diffuse large B cell lymphoma, immunoblastic variant, with invasion of a small nerve and multiple mitotic figures. Giemsa, × 400

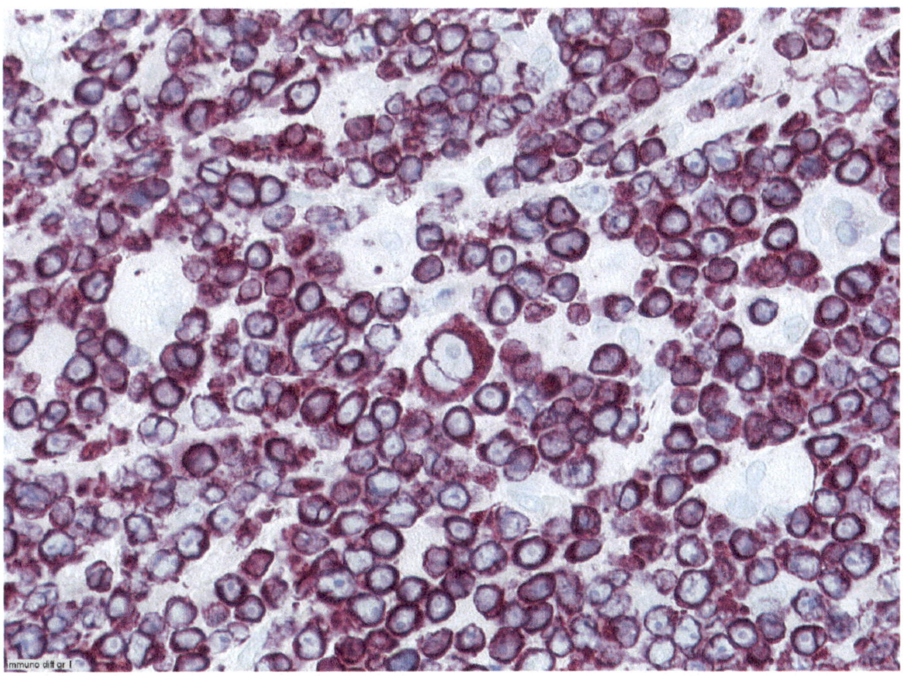

Fig. 9.73 Same case.Tumor cells are strongly CD20 positive. In the center a binucleated giant cell. APAAP, × 400

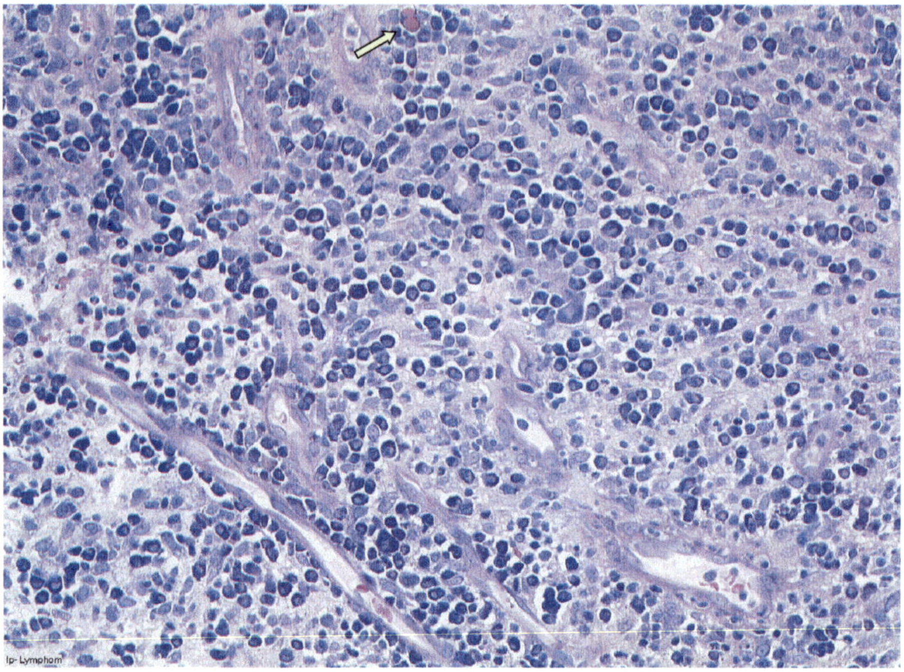

Fig. 9.74 Lymphoplasmacytic lymphoma with Russell bodies (arrow). Giemsa, × 200

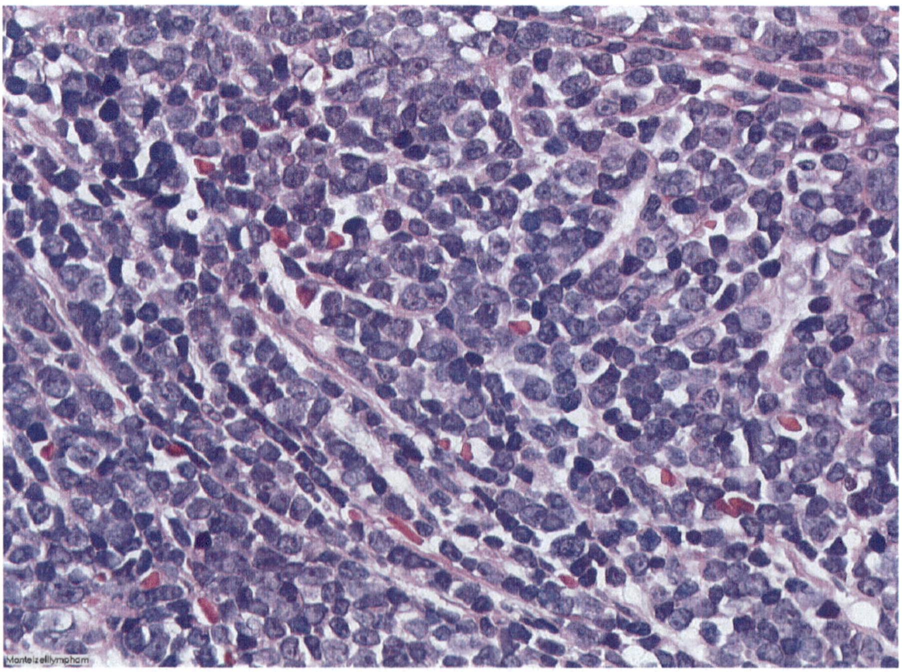

Fig. 9.75 Acute lymphoblastic B cell lymphoma: Dense diffuse growth pattern, primary manifestation. H & E, × 400

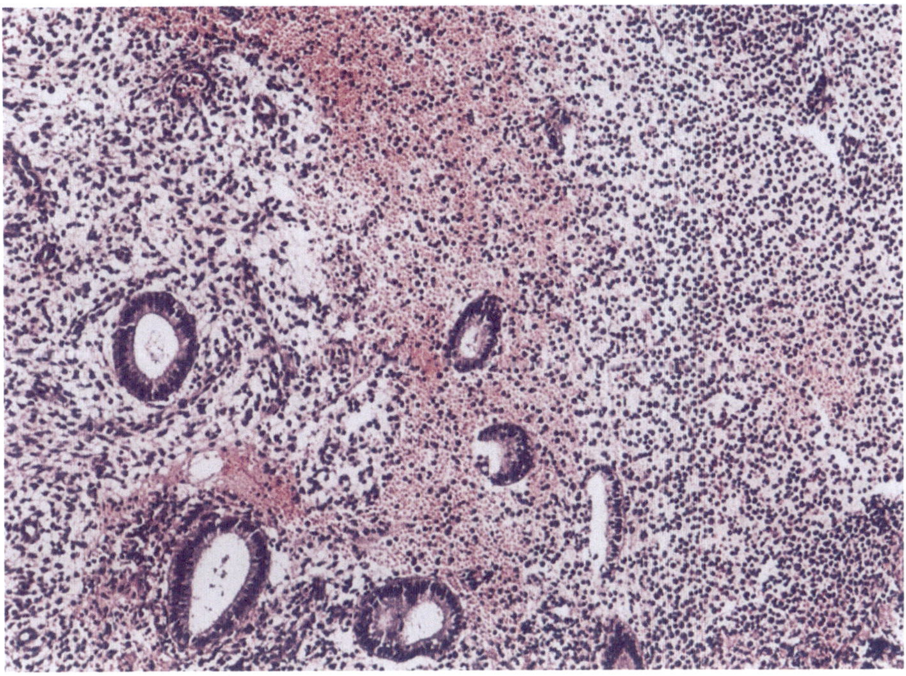

Fig. 9.76 Leukemic infiltration of endometrium in chronic lymphatic B cell leukemia (B-CLL). H & E, ×100

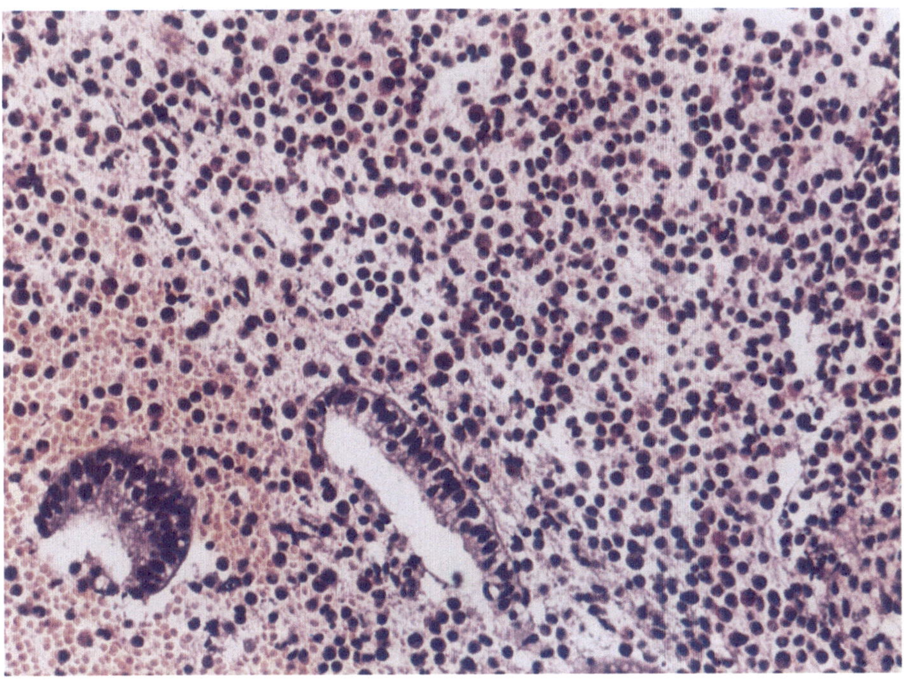

Fig. 9.77 Higher magnification of Fig 9.76. H & E, ×250

to clarify the question of clonality by analyzing the immunoglobulin heavy chain or T cell receptor genes with the polymerase chain reaction (PCR). A smaller counterpart of follicular lymphomas are BCL-2 negative and CD10 negative and might be diagnosed by molecular cytogenetic demonstration of the t(14;18) translocation with the fluorescence in situ hybridization (FISH). To confirm the diagnosis of a Burkitt's lymphoma and differentiate it from other large B cell lymphomas, demonstration of a c-myc translocation might be useful. However, other translocations have been found in Burkitt's lymphomas such as breakpoints in the bcl-2 and bcl-6 genes, so called double breaks, which seem to indicate an unfavorable prognosis (Hasserjian et al. 2009). Other large cell lymphomas of non-Burkitt's type show a primary or secondary c-myc gene rearrangement after R-CHOP chemotherapy, including plasmablastic lymphomas (Dallenbach et al., in preparation). Such cases were recently reported to have a dire prognosis (Savage et al. 2009) and it was discussed whether they should be treated as aggressively as Burkitt's lymphomas.

9.5.2 Myeloid Leukemias and Sarcomas

9.5.2.1 Occurrence and Clinical Symptoms

Endometrial infiltrates of acute or chronic myeloid leukemias are uncommon and usually asymptomatic, but symptomatic myeloid sarcomas are extremely rare (Pitz et al. 2006). In such cases with vaginal bleeding, radiotherapy might be of therapeutical value. Myeloid sarcomas can precede or occur simultaneously with acute leukemia of bone marrow origin. Therefore, a bone marrow biopsy should be taken for staging at time of diagnosis.

9.5.2.2 Morphology and Immunohistochemistry

As in the bone marrow, endometrial infiltrates of *acute myeloid leukemia (AML)* exist exclusively of blasts with small nuclei and inconspicuous nucleoli. In myelomonocytic and monocytic/monoblastic leukemia, the cells are more cleaved or dentated than in the other subtypes. Mitotic figures are usually frequent. In primary myelosarcoma of the endometrium, the number of blasts and the differentiation towards myelocytes or monocytes and therefore the Ki-67 index may vary. *Chronic myeloid and myelomonocytic leukemia (CML and CMML)* reveal a mixture of granulocytes, including eosinophils, and granulopoietic or monocytic precursor cells, except in cases of a blast crisis. To confirm the diagnosis, and to detect minimal infiltrates of an AML in the endometrium, immunohistochemistry might be needed (Pitz et al. 2006). AML subtypes and myeloid sarcomas most often express myeloperoxidase and CD33, variably CD15, CD34, CD68, CD117 (c-kit) and lysozyme, and are thereby distinguishable from malignant lymphomas.

9.5.2.3
Molecular Pathology

In prediagnosed AML, cytogenetic examinations usually have been already preformed and immunohistochemistry should be sufficient to confirm the diagnosis. In doubtful infiltrates of CML, a bcr-abl gene mutation analysis with the FISH method might be helpful in single cases. CMML, however, do not show bcr-abl mutations.

9.5.2.4
Differential Diagnoses

Malignant lymphomas and lymphatic as well as myeloid leukemias in the endometrium must be distinguished from other diffusely growing neoplasms such as small cell carcinomas including neuroendocrine tumors, Ewing sarcoma/PNET, round cell sarcomas, malignant rhabdoid tumors and melanomas (Kim et al. 2008). Immunohistochemistry and eventually molecular pathology should be applied to clarify the tumor entity. Chronic endometritis can in most instances be morphologically distinguished from leukemic infiltrations by the usually heterogeneous admixture of lymphocytes, plasma cells and granulocytes in endometritis (Young et al. 1985). In cases of dense lymphoma-like infiltrate in the endometrium containing numerous T cells and plasma cells, molecular analyses for immunoglobulin heavy chain and T cell receptor gene rearrangements should be used to distinguish benign severe inflammation from malignant lymphoma (Gaillot et al. 2008).

9.6
Leiomyomas as Components of Endometrial Specimens

Unlike stromal tumors, leiomyomas generally do not originate in the endometrium. Pedunculated submucosal leiomyomas protruding into the uterine cavity or parts of them may, however, be encountered in curettage specimens (see p. 62). Whereas typical leiomyomas can be easily recognized, variants of them may cause diagnostic problems (Figs. 9.78–9.81). Distinction from various more aggressive tumors is in general possible immunohistochemically. Leiomyomas with bizarre nuclei have a very low mitotic rate. Epithelioid leiomyomas are positive with antibodies for desmin, smooth muscle actin and h-caldesmon.

9.7
Secondary Tumors

Carcinomas metastasizing to the endometrium most commonly originate in the cervix or ovaries, less commonly in the fallopian tube, breast, or gastrointestinal tract, and rarely in other organs. Whereas it may be difficult to distinguish a metastasis of a primary ovarian

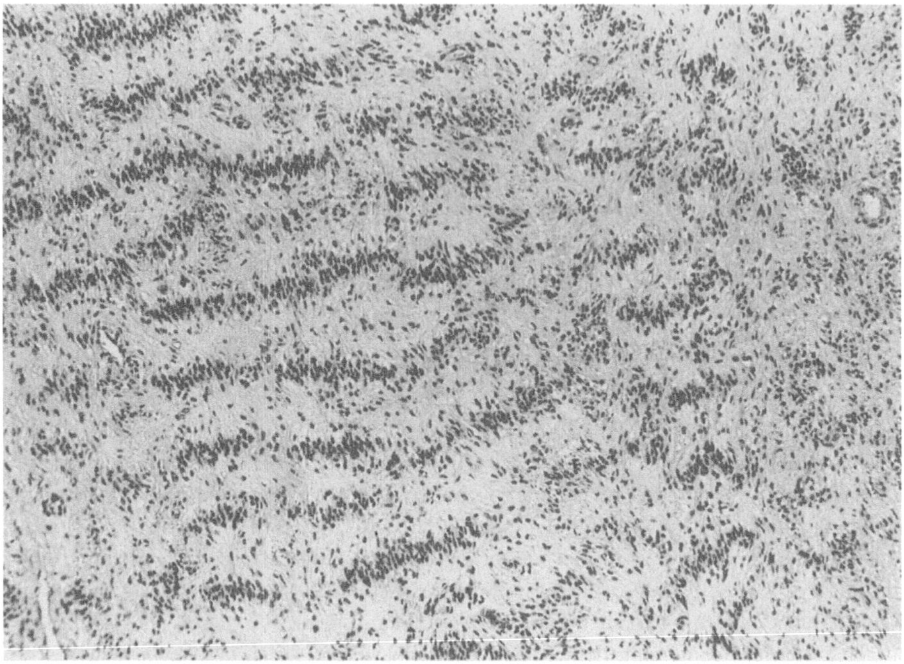

Fig. 9.78 Leiomyoma with palisading nuclei. H & E, ×100

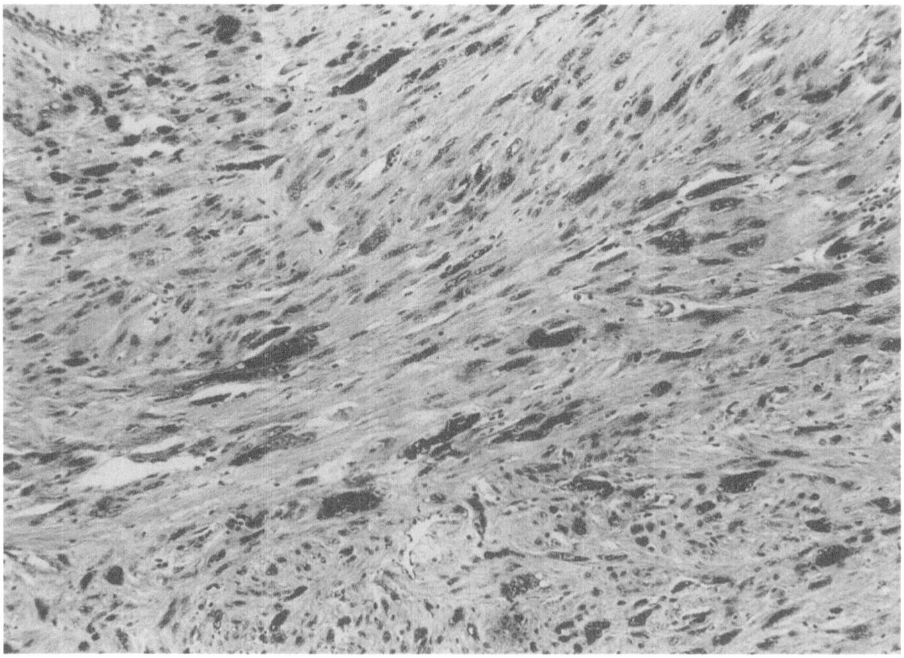

Fig. 9.79 Leiomyoma with bizarre nuclei. H & E, ×100

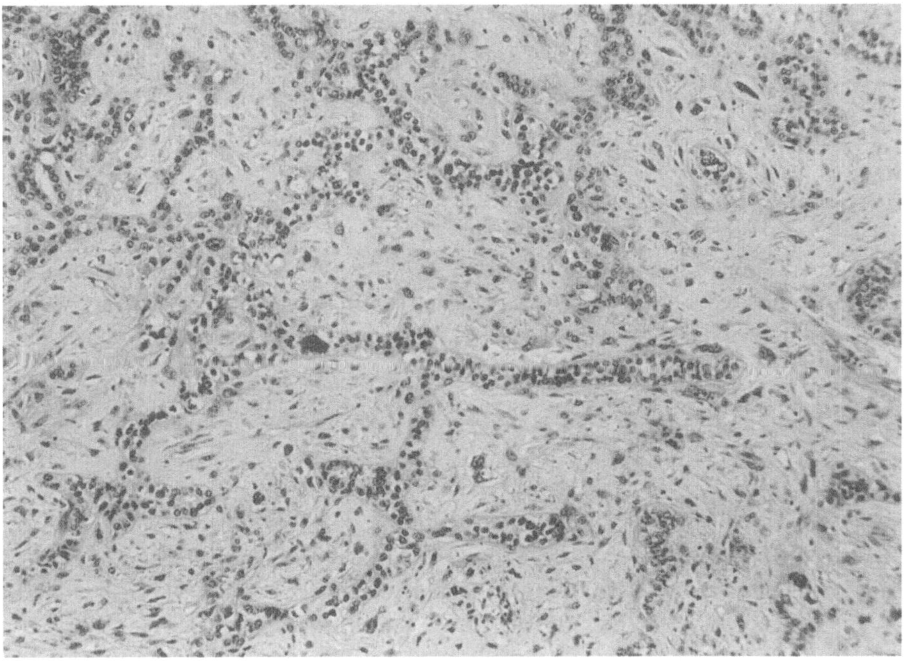

Fig. 9.80 Epithelioid leiomyoma with plexiform pattern. H & E, ×100

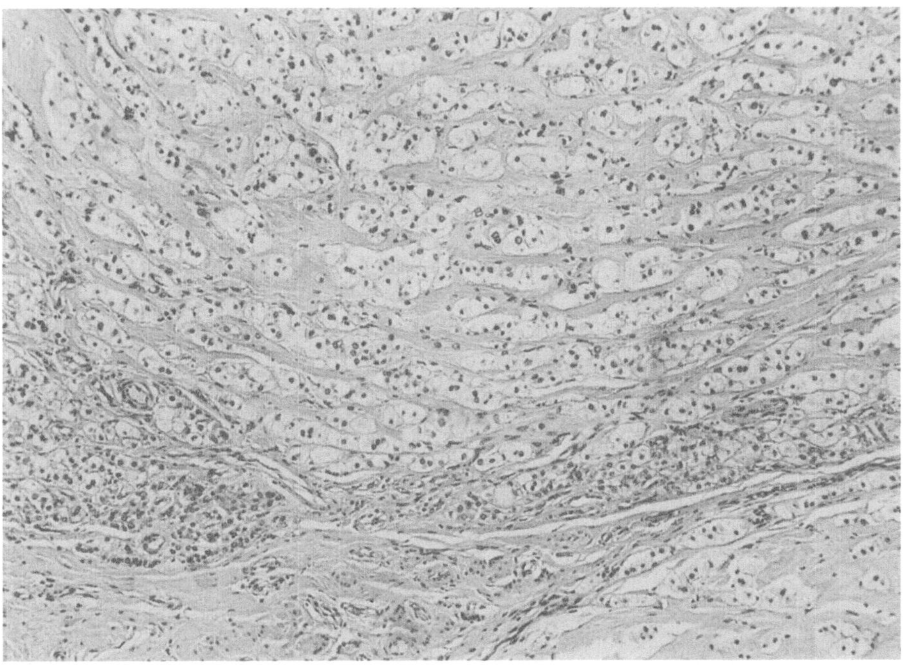

Fig. 9.81 Epithelioid leiomyoma, clear cell type. H & E, ×100

carcinoma from a primary endometrial carcinoma of identical histological structure, metastases from carcinomas structurally different from primary endometrial carcinomas can be easily recognized (Kumar and Hart 1982).

9.7.1 Metastases from Primary Breast Carcinoma

In metastases from primary breast carcinoma (Figs. 9.82, 9.83), the endometrial stroma is diffusely infiltrated and replaced in vast regions by carcinomatous cells, many with a signet-ring form, typical of some primary carcinomas of the breast or gastrointestinal tract. Very few normal endometrial glands are preserved (Kjaer and Holm-Jensen 1972).

9.7.2 Leukemic Infiltrations

The secondary involvement of the endometrium by leukemic infiltrations or malignant lymphomas and their differential diagnoses are discussed in detail in Chap. 9.5 (p. 194).

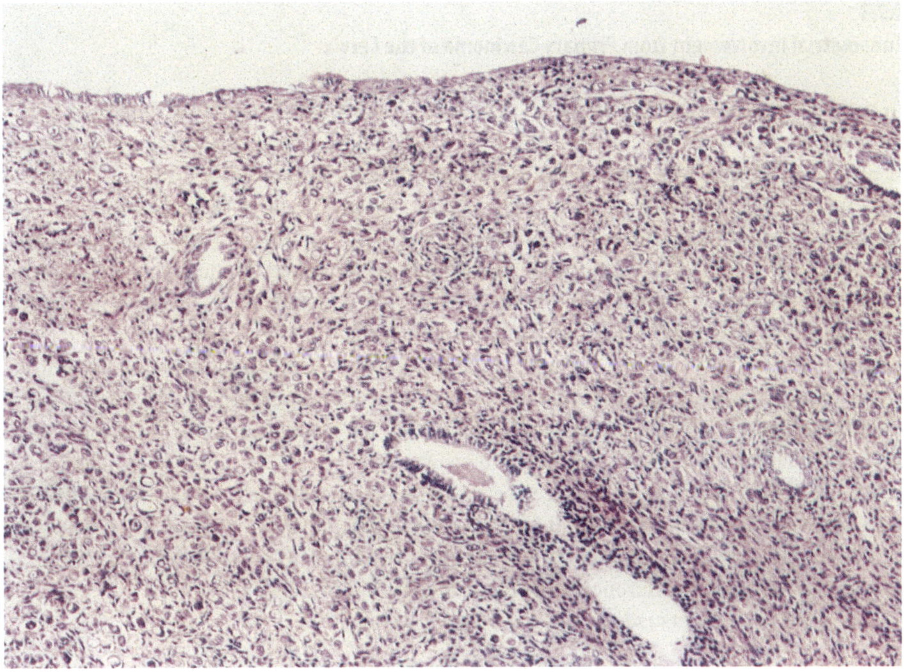

Fig. 9.82 Endometrial metastasis from primary breast carcinoma. H & E, ×100

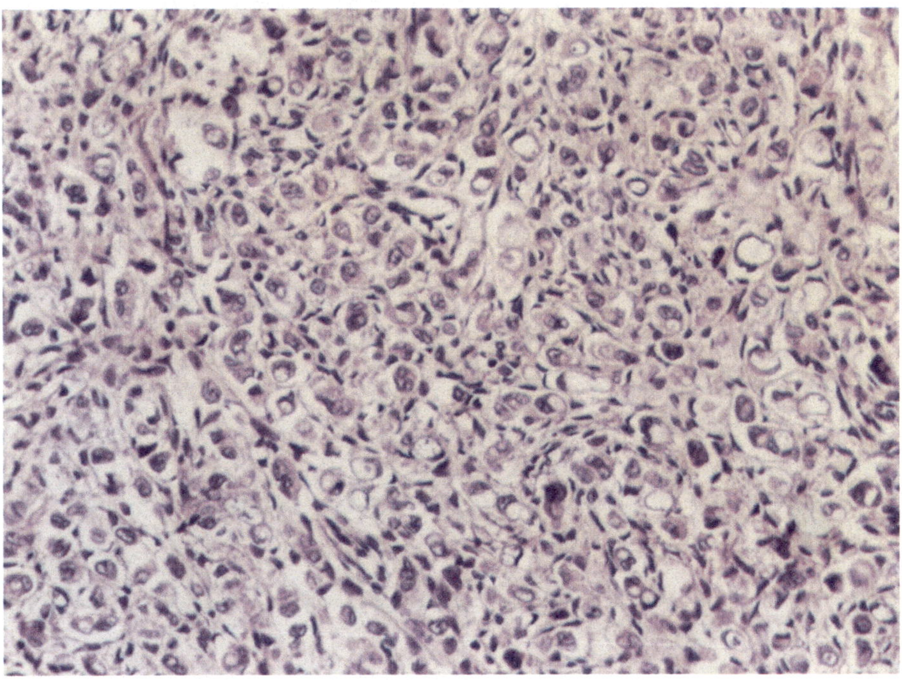

Fig. 9.83 Endometrial metastasis from primary breast carcinoma. H & E, ×250

9.7.3 Endometrial Involvement from Primary Carcinoma of the Cervix

In patients with primary carcinoma of the cervix, invasion of the endometrium may occur through lymphatics or by continuous spread up the endocervical canal (Fig. 9.84; Mitani et al. 1964). The surface epithelium is replaced by multilayered, dysplastic, and atypical squamous epithelium, which may invade the endometrium by plump or net-like infiltrations. The underlying stroma is densely cellular and contains chronic inflammatory infiltrates. Only very few narrow, inactive endometrial glands may be preserved. If the atypical squamous epithelium shows a complete loss of stratification but is noninvasive, it may have grown from an in situ carcinoma of the cervix (Kanbour and Stock 1978; Wilkinson et al. 1980).

Morphologic Differential Diagnosis. It is important to differentiate this condition from ichthyosis uteri, which may also be dysplastic but, when covering atrophic endometrium is in most instances a noninvasive metaplastic reaction of the superficial epithelium (see p. 45). p16 may be a useful marker to distinguish grown-up cervical carcinoma from ichthyosis. If the ichthyosis overlies an invasive carcinoma, it should no longer be called ichthyosis (see Fig. 4.3). Loose sheets of multilayered squamous epithelium in curettings, however, whether regular or dysplastic, are always highly suspicious of an underlying adenocarcinoma with squamous differenciation (mucoepidermoid or adenosquamous) especially in postmenopausal patients (see p. 164).

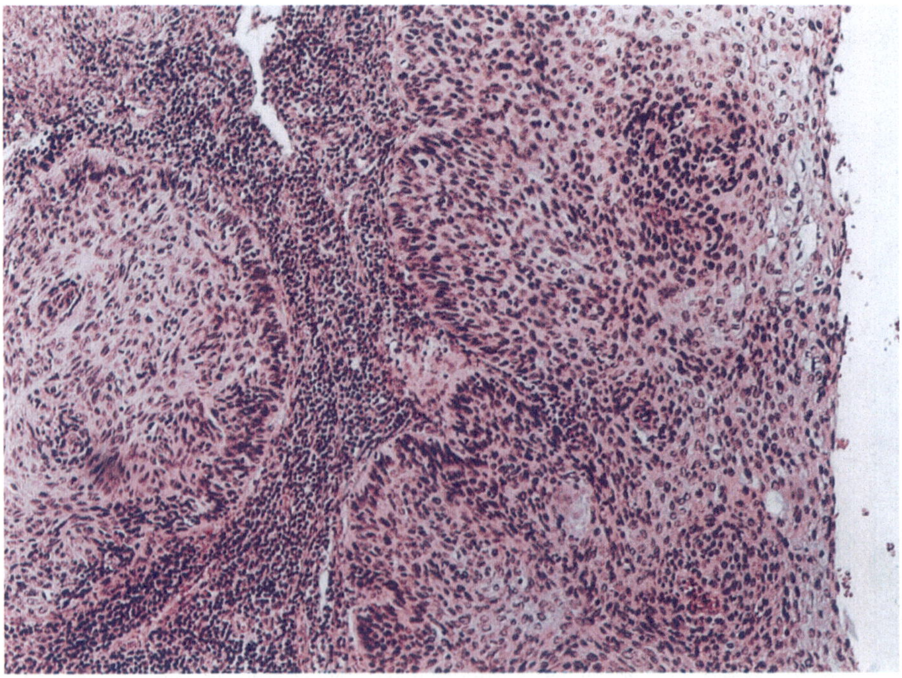

Fig. 9.84 Endometrial involvement from primary squamous cell carcinoma of the cervix. H & E, ×100

Gestational Changes 10

10.1 Normal Trophoblast

During normal placentation, three types of trophoblast can be differentiated: two types covering the villi, consisting of an outer layer of syncytiotrophoblast and an inner layer of cytotrophoblast, and the third type, the extravillous intermediate trophoblast, which invades the decidua and forms the trophoblastic shell (Figs. 10.1, 10.2). If the blastocyst implants and develops normally, the gestational age can be determined fairly accurately from the villous structure; on the 15th day of gestation, the primary villi, which consist of syncytio- and cytotrophoblast only, begin to develop fetal mesoderm, converting them into secondary villi (Figs. 10.3, 10.4). From approximately the 20th day on, capillaries form within the mesoderm, and the villi are then referred to as tertiary villi (Figs. 10.5, 10.6). The fetal erythrocytes, at first nucleated, loose their nuclei gradually by the tenth to 12th week of pregnancy.

10.2 Spontaneous Abortion

About two thirds of spontaneous abortions are due to pathologic ova, among which chromosomal anomalies play a major role. One third is caused by maternal factors (deficient decidual development resulting in superficial polypoid implantation, anomalies of the uterus, bacterial infections). Chromosome anomalies are found in 27–60% of all spontaneous abortions (Bowen and Lee 1969; Goecke et al. 1985), but in only 6.8% of induced abortions. Approximately 50% of all chromosomal anomalies are trisomies, 20–25% monosomies, 15% are triploidies, 5% are tetraploidies, and 5% are structural anomalies. Possible exogenous causes of chromosomal damage are vitamin deficiencies, X-irradiation, hypoxemia, and deficient or overdose of endogenous or exogenous hormones (Carr 1970).

Whereas the placental villi found in curettings of spontaneous abortions due to maternal causes are usually regular in shape or occasionally hyalinized, fibrotic, or necrotic, those caused by chromosomal anomalies are often avascular and enlarged (Fig. 10.7). The hydropic change results from the uptake of fluid, which accumulates since there are no

G. Dallenbach-Hellweg et al., *Atlas of Endometrial Histopathology*,
DOI: 10.1007/978-3-642-01541-0_10, © Springer-Verlag Berlin Heidelberg 2010

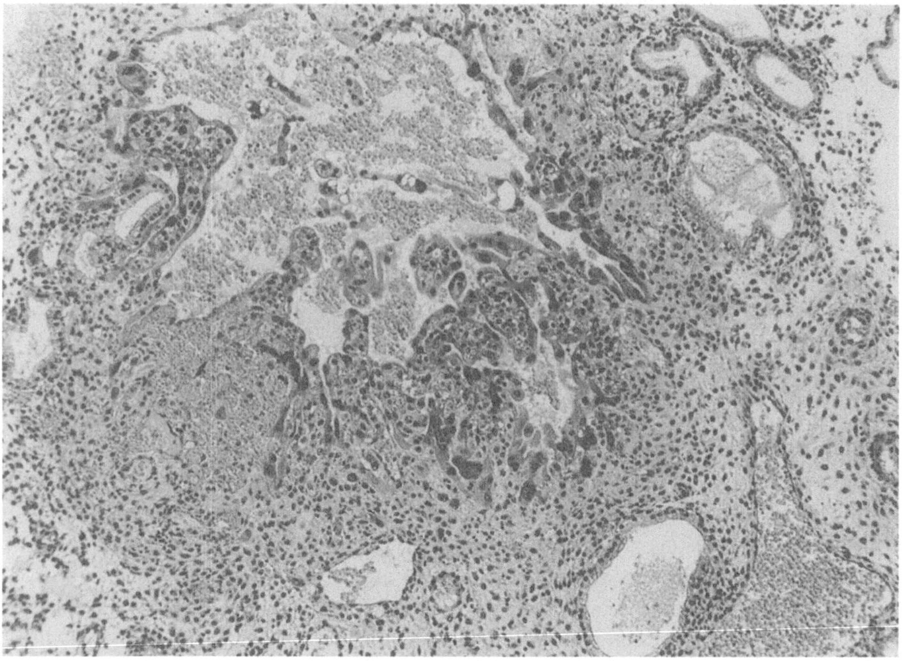

Fig. 10.1 Early implantation site, 7th day of gestation. H & E, ×100

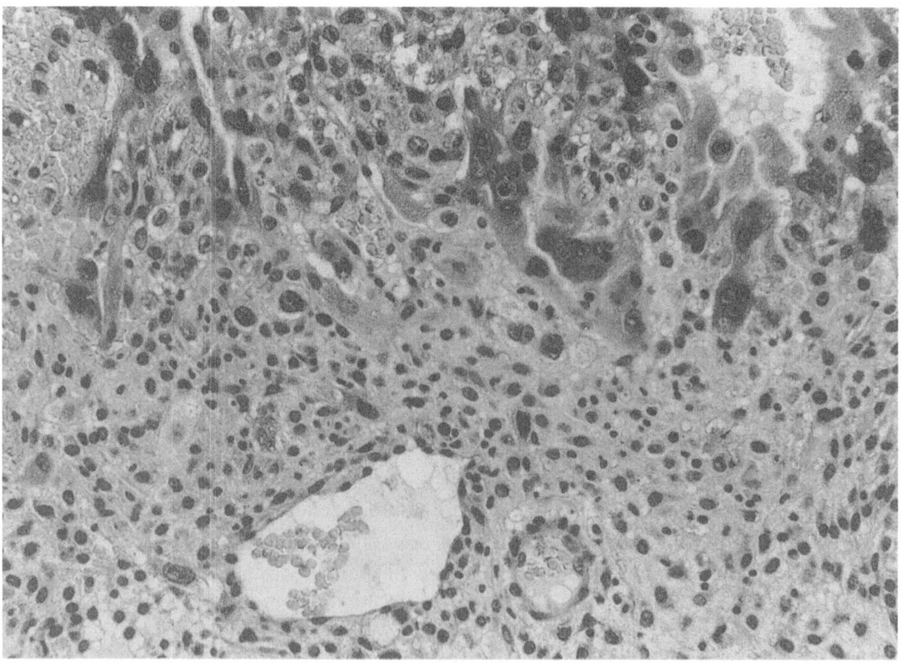

Fig. 10.2 Early implantation site, 7th day of gestation. H & E, ×250

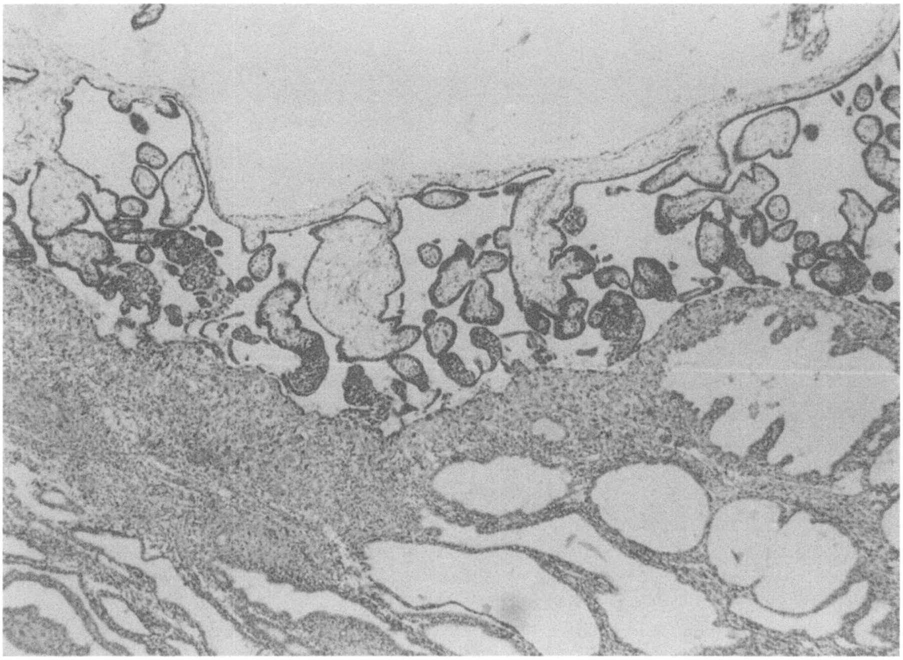

Fig. 10.3 Implanting blastocyst, 18th day of gestation. H & E, ×40

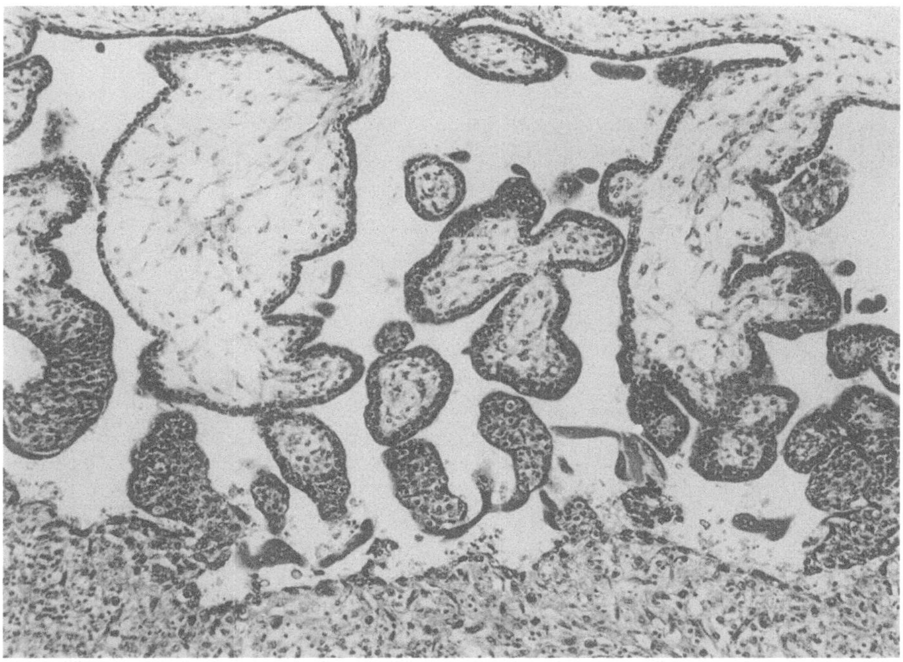

Fig. 10.4 Secondary villi around blastocyst, 18th day of gestation. H & E, ×100

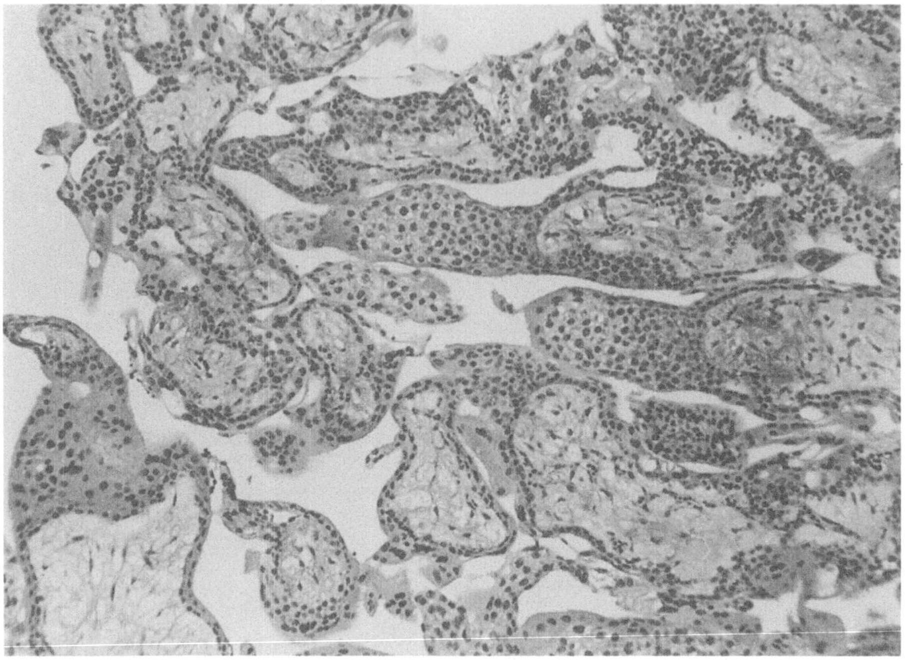

Fig. 10.5 Early pregnancy with tertiary villi and polar distribution of trophoblast. H & E, ×100

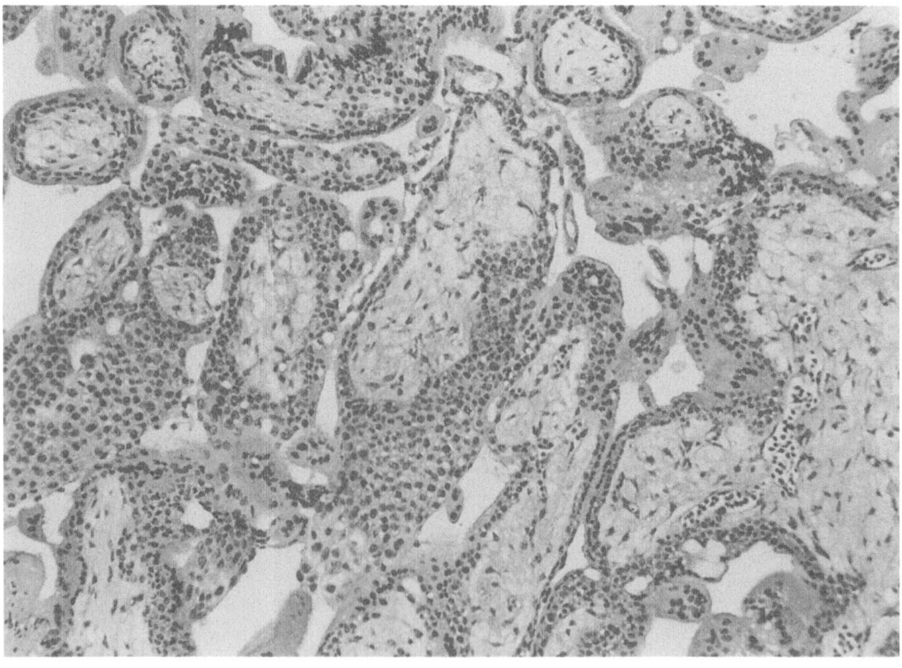

Fig. 10.6 Tertiary villi with nucleated red blood cells. H & E, ×100

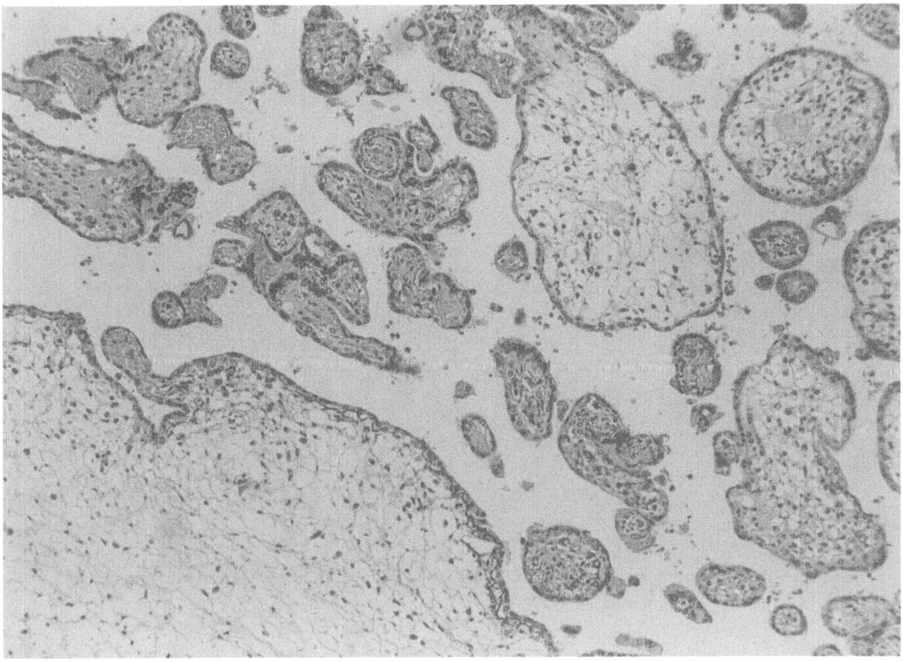

Fig. 10.7 Spontaneous abortion with hydropic change. H & E, ×40

vessels to carry it away. The trophoblast may become atrophic, as in molar degeneration, or hyperplastic, forming syncytial knots due to an arrest of ramification.

Morphologic Differential Diagnosis. Histologic differentiation between the various types of chromosomal anomalies is difficult; it usually requires cytogenetic studies. An abnormal karyotype may be strongly suggested in the presence of hydropic villi without or with sparse fetal vessels containing nucleated red blood cells or in the absence of fetal tissue, umbilical cord, and anucleated red blood cells (Genest et al. 1995). On the other hand, a triploidy resulting in a partial mole or even a complete hydatidiform mole can be recognized histologically in most cases according to the criteria described below.

10.3 Partial Hydatidiform Mole

Partial hydatidiform mole (Figs. 10.8, 10.9) is an anomaly almost always due to a chromosomal triploidy (69XXY or XYY) caused by fertilization of a normal ovum with two haploid spermatoza. Histologically, there is a mixture of two populations of chorionic villi, one large and edematous, and the other small or normal in size with stromal fibrosis. The enlarged villi show arrested branching with scalloping of the villous outlines and may

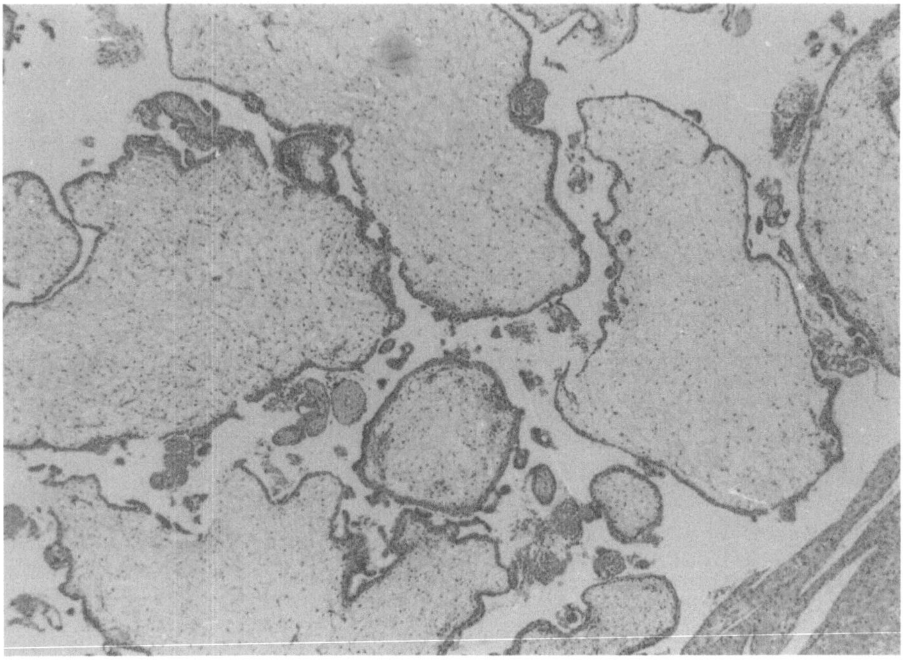

Fig. 10.8 Partial hydatidiform mole. Hydropic enlarged villi. H & E, ×25

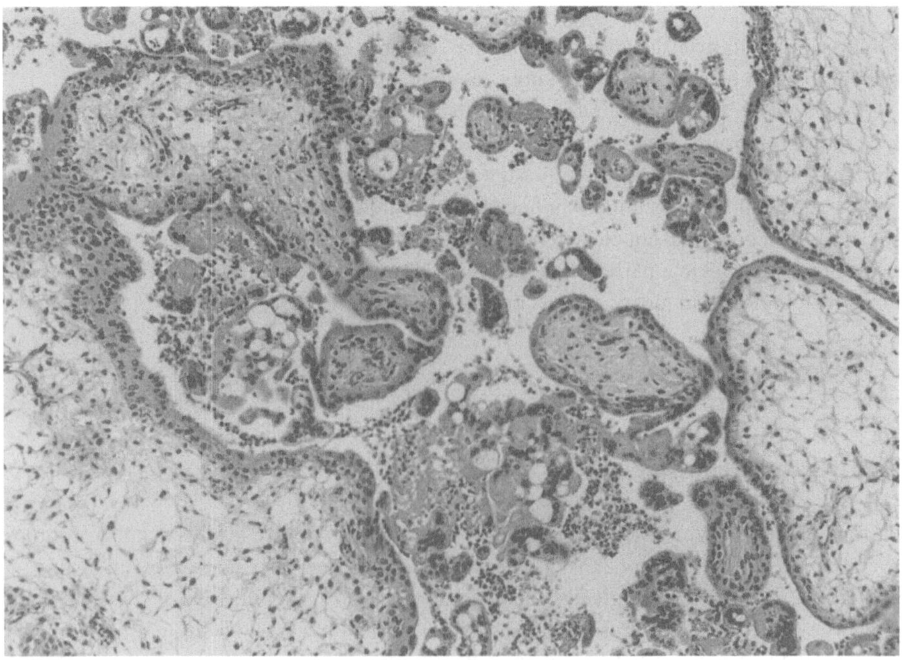

Fig. 10.9 Partial hydatidiform mole. Both normal and hydropic villi. H & E, ×100

contain trophoblastic pseudoinclusions in the hydropic mesenchyma (Fig. 10.8). There is often cistern formation. Fetal vessels are absent in some villi and very sparse and narrow in others that still contain nucleated red blood cells. The syncytial trophoblast shows patchy hyperproliferation around the enlarged villi and may form knots or lacunae (Fig. 10.9), whereas the cytotrophoblast remains single layered. An underdeveloped embryo may be present (Szulman and Buchsbaum 1987).

Morphologic Differential Diagnosis. The partial mole can be distinguished from a hydropic abortion mainly by the lack of trophoblast hyperproliferation in the latter. (For the distinction from the complete mole, see below.)

10.4 Complete Hydatidiform Mole

In most instances a complete mole develops when an "empty egg" (without the maternal haploid set) is fertilized by a sperm with a 23X set of chromosomes that duplicate, resulting in a diploid (46XX) or a tetraploid (92XXXX) karyotype (Szulman and Surti 1978; Lage et al. 1992). As a result, the complete mole contains paternal nuclear DNA and mitochondrial maternal DNA (paternal imprinting). An embryo is always absent. Instead, there is excessive and disorganized overgrowth of all three types of trophoblast, which often contain enlarged hyperchromatic and pleomorphic nuclei, although the karyotype is generally diploid. Virtually all the villi are greatly enlarged by extensive cistern formation. Fetal blood vessels are usually missing (Figs. 10.10–10.12).

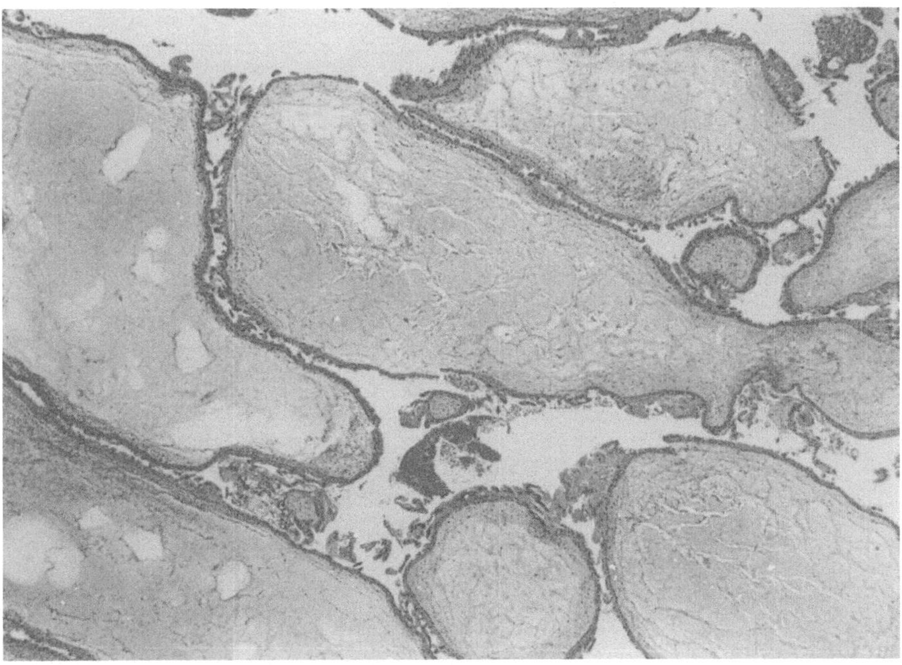

Fig. 10.10 Complete hydatidiform mole. H & E, ×25

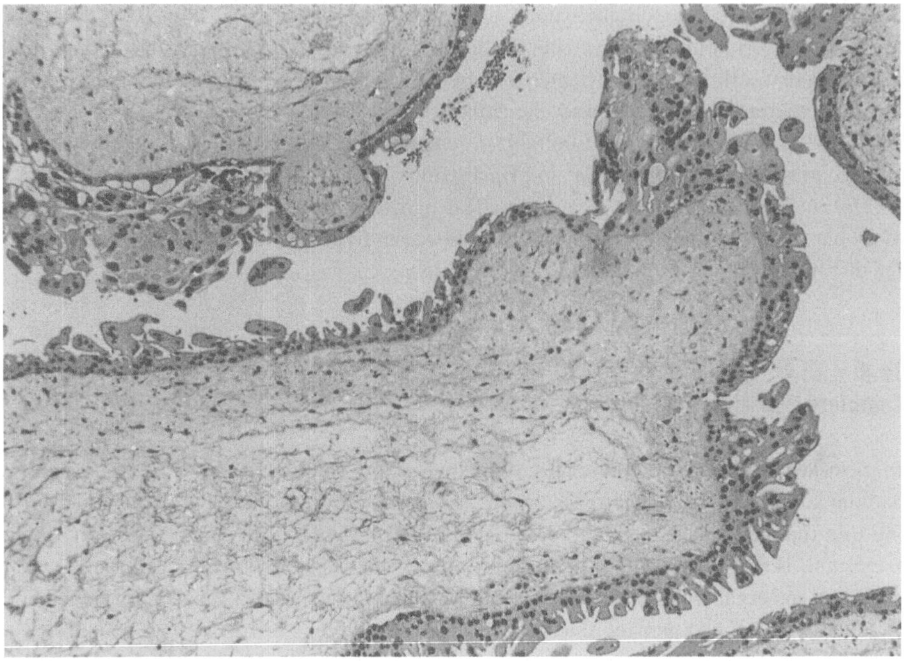

Fig. 10.11 Complete hydatidiform mole, trophoblastic proliferation. H & E, ×100

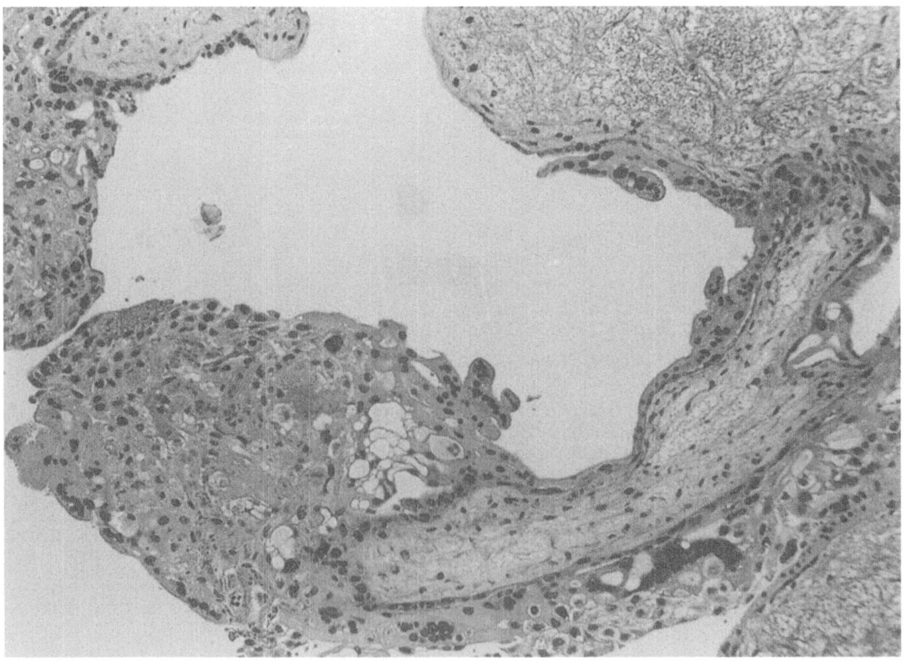

Fig. 10.12 Complete hydatidiform mole. H & E, ×100

Morphologic Differential Diagnosis. Complete moles should be histologically distinguished from partial moles, which in contrast to complete moles show no propensity for malignant change (Czernobilsky et al. 1982; Ohama et al. 1986). Distinction is possible on the basis of the excessive proliferation of cytotrophoblast about the cystically dilated avascular villi and atypical, often polyploid intermediate trophoblast in complete moles. Both types of mole can be distinguished from nonmolar spontaneous abortions by the lack of trophoblastic overgrowth in the latter.

Very early stages of complete mole can be recognized by the circumferential instead of polar outgrowth of trophoblast around the villi and by the cytologically atypical intermediate trophoblast. Immunostaining for p57 KIP2 in the cytotrophoblast and the stromal cells is negative (Jun et al. 2003). The combination of atypical villi consistent with complete mole and normal villi may be due to a complete mole and a coexisting normal twin gestation (Lage et al. 1992).

10.5 Invasive Mole

The invasive mole is a progressive growth of the complete mole down into the myometrium and its vessels; sheets of trophoblast and enlarged chorionic villi deeply invading the myometrium are found. The diagnosis, however, can rarely be made from curettings, since the extent of growth can only be accurately judged in the hysterectomy specimen.

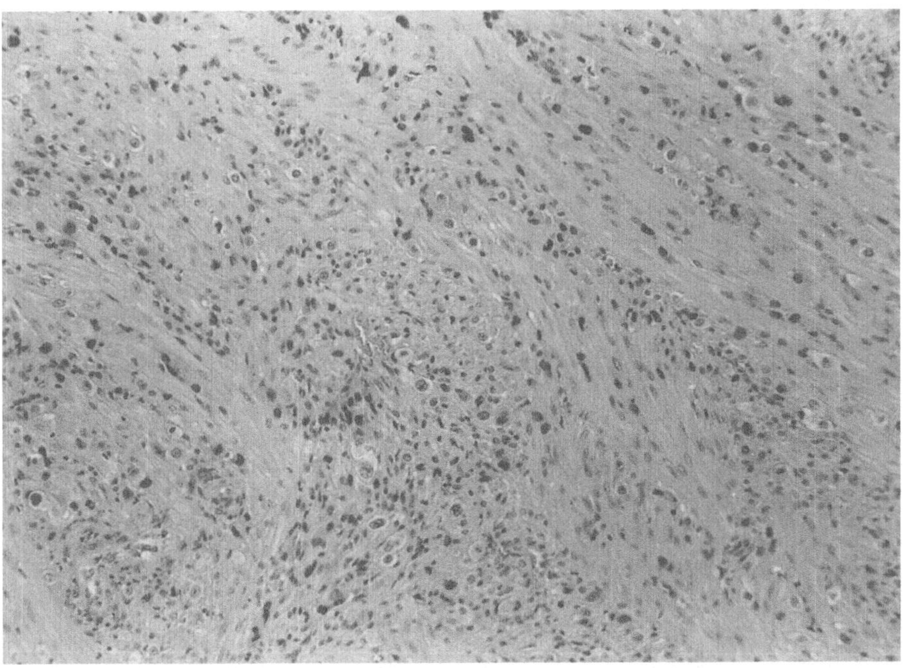

Fig. 10.13 Placental site reaction, diffuse. H & E, ×100

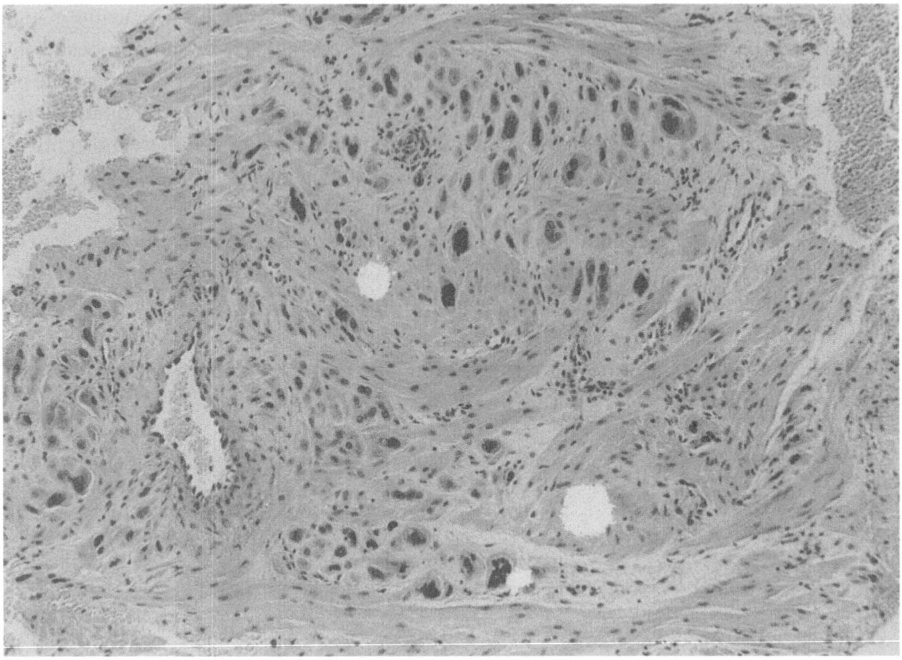

Fig. 10.14 Placental site reaction, nodular. H & E, ×100

Molar invasion must be distinguished from an exaggerated *placental site reaction* (Figs. 10.13, 10.14), which consists of intermediate trophoblasts with only moderate nuclear atypia.

10.6 Choriocarcinoma

About 50% of all choriocarcinomas arise from complete hydatidiform moles, but only about 2% of complete moles are followed by choriocarcinoma (Ringertz 1970). Occasionally, a gestational choriocarcinoma develops during a seemingly normal pregnancy within a nonmolar placenta (Brewer and Mazur 1981).

Histologically (Figs. 10.15–10.19), solid or plexiform cords of poorly differentiated cyto- and syncytiotrophoblasts with hyperchromatic, greatly enlarged and often pleomorphic nuclei are found with extensive hemorrhage. There are only few intermediate trophoblasts. Placental villi are absent. Since there is usually deep invasion of the myometrium and its vessels with necrosis, the curettings often contain fragments of myometrium destroyed by the invading trophoblast. Inflammatory changes are usually lacking. High-grade malignancy can be determined by the formation of tumor islands, massive proliferation of intermediate-type trophoblast, perpendicular invasion of the myometrium, and cytological atypia (Nishikawa et al. 1985).

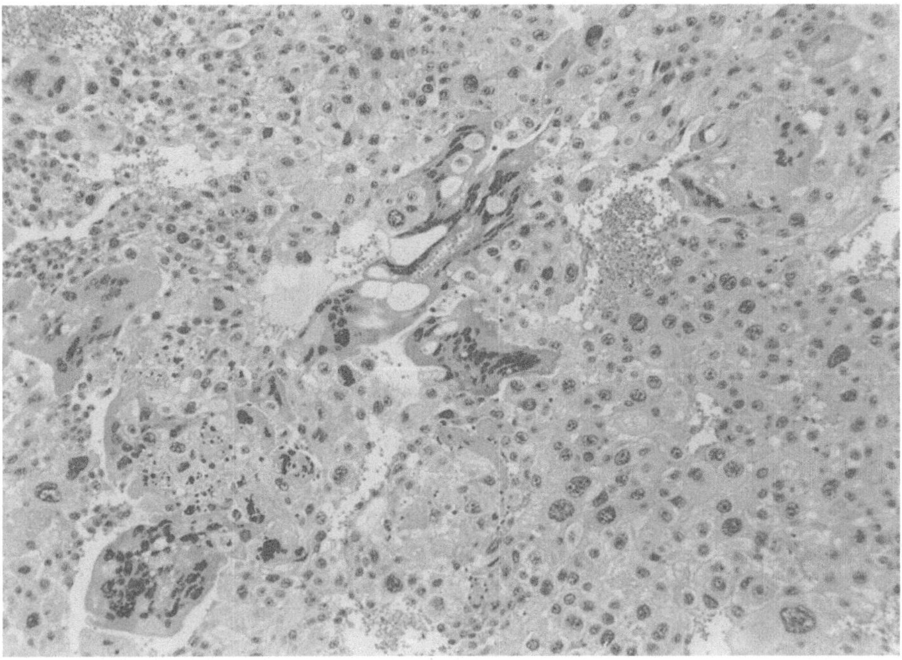

Fig. 10.15 Choriocarcinoma. H & E, ×100

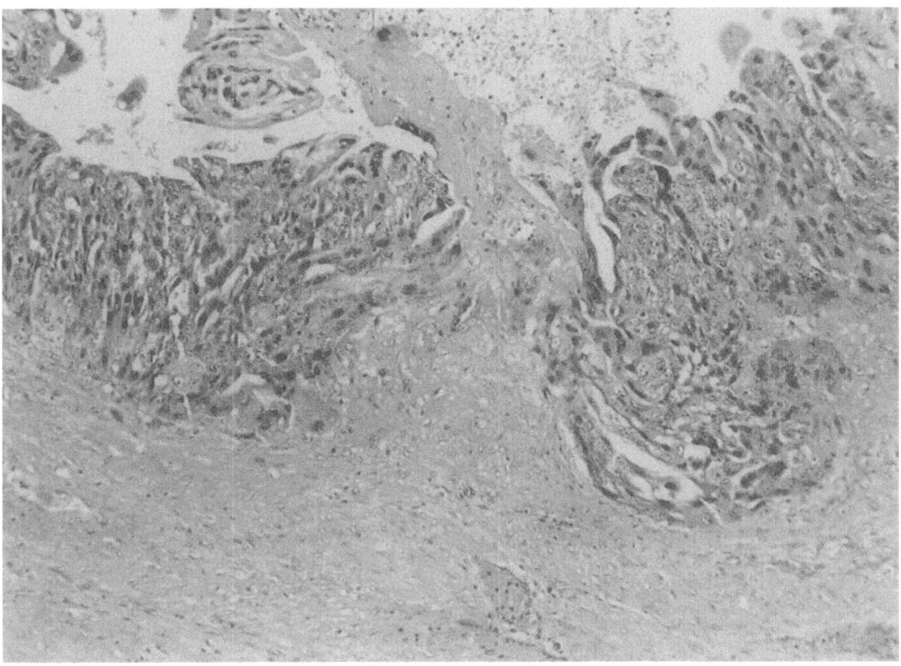

Fig. 10.16 Choriocarcinoma, myometrial invasion. H & E, ×100

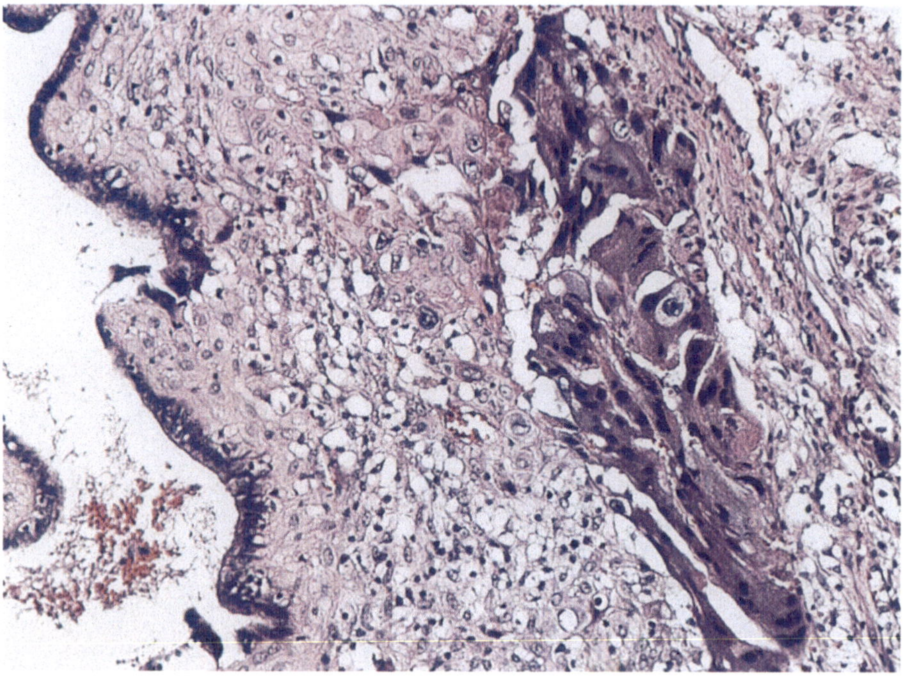

Fig. 10.17 Choriocarcinoma, vascular invasion. H & E, ×150

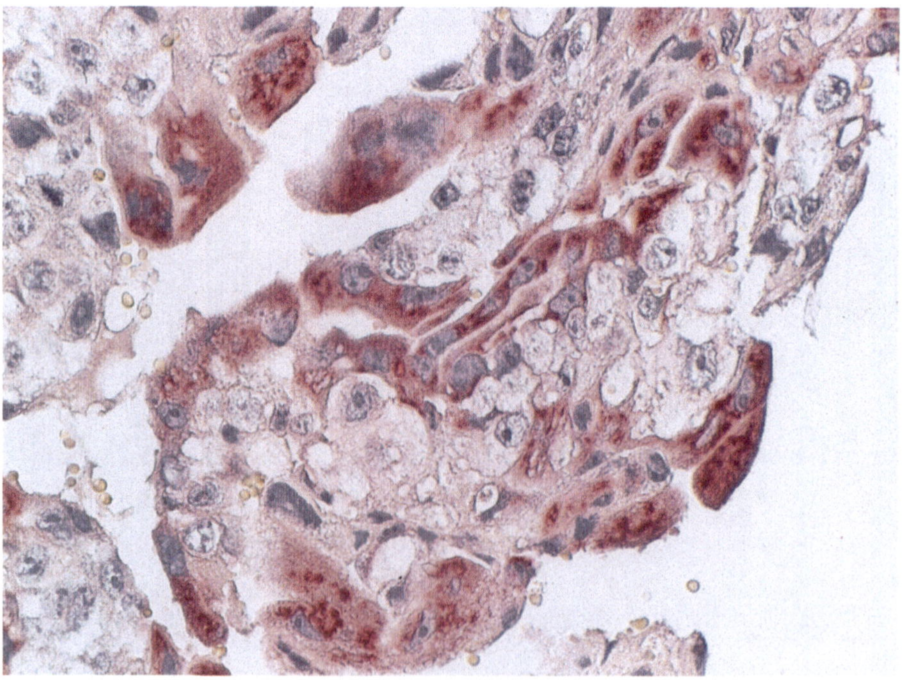

Fig. 10.18 Choriocarcinoma. Immunohistochemical stain for β-HCG, ×400

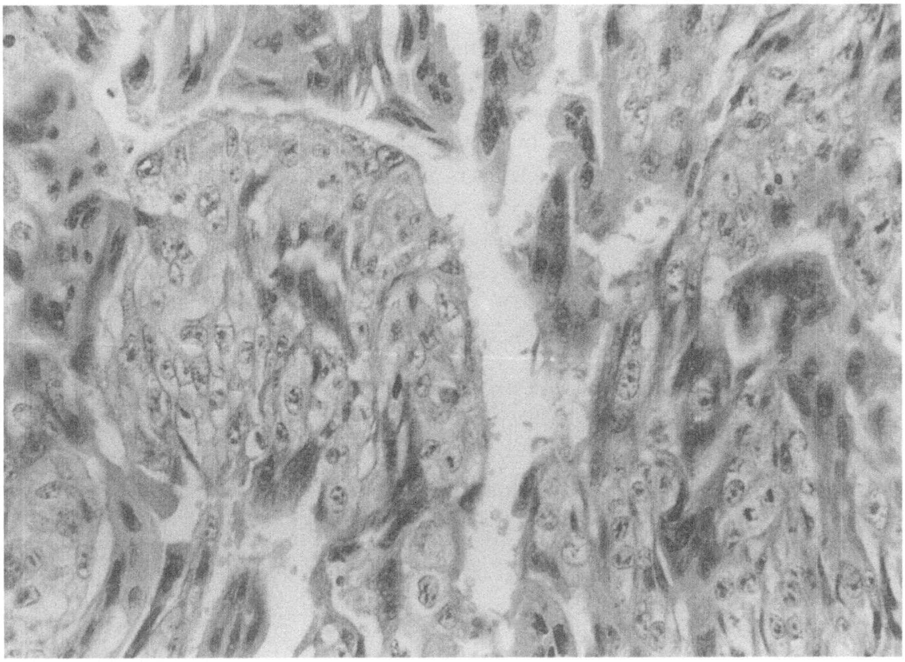

Fig. 10.19 Choriocarcinoma. H & E, ×250

Morphologic Differential Diagnosis. The absence of chorionic villi and the extensive tumor necrosis with hemorrhage make it possible to distinguish choriocarcinoma from an invasive mole. Malignant chorial invasion must also be distinguished from a benign invasion (exaggerated placental site reaction), which can be best recognized by the progression of individual trophoblastic cells along preformed clefts without injury to adjacent muscle cells (compare Figs. 10.14 and 10.16). In uterine curettings, choriocarcinoma can only be definitely diagnosed when large sheets of cytologically atypical trophoblasts invading the endomyometrium are present, and placental villi are absent.

10.7 Placental Site Trophoblastic Tumor (PSTT)

Placental site trophoblastic tumor (PSTT) (Figs. 10.20–10.24) is less friable and less hemorrhagic than choriocarcinoma. It consists almost only of intermediate-type trophoblast, which infiltrates the myometrium in small rows and surrounds blood vessels. Vascular invasion is much less frequent than in choriocarcinoma. Most of the tumor cells are diploid, but scattered syncytiotrophoblastic giant cells can be seen. A few cells are sometimes positive with markers for β-HCG but all cells are p63-negative. The clinical behavior, however, first thought to be favorable (Kurman and Scully 1976), may be quite unpredictable (Hopkins et al. 1985), largely depending upon the mitotic rate (Scully and Young 1981). Other possible indicators for a malignant course of the disease are: periuterine growth, high-grade nuclear and cellular pleomorphism, coagulative necrosis, destructive growth, and deep myometrial invasion.

Morphologic Differential Diagnosis.

This tumor must be distinguished from the following:

1. Choriocarcinoma (see above), mainly by the type of neoplastic trophoblast and by the lack of hemorrhage and necrosis. In addition, placental site trophoblastic tumor invades the myometrium by splitting muscle fibers, in contrast to diffuse destruction.
2. Exaggerated placental site reaction (see "Choriocarcinoma")
3. Undifferentiated carcinoma, by the negative reaction with antibodies against human placental lactogen (HPL) and β-HCG, both of which are positive in the PSTT.

Exceptionally, PSTT can be observed in combination with epithelioid trophoblastic tumor (Kalhor et al. 2009).

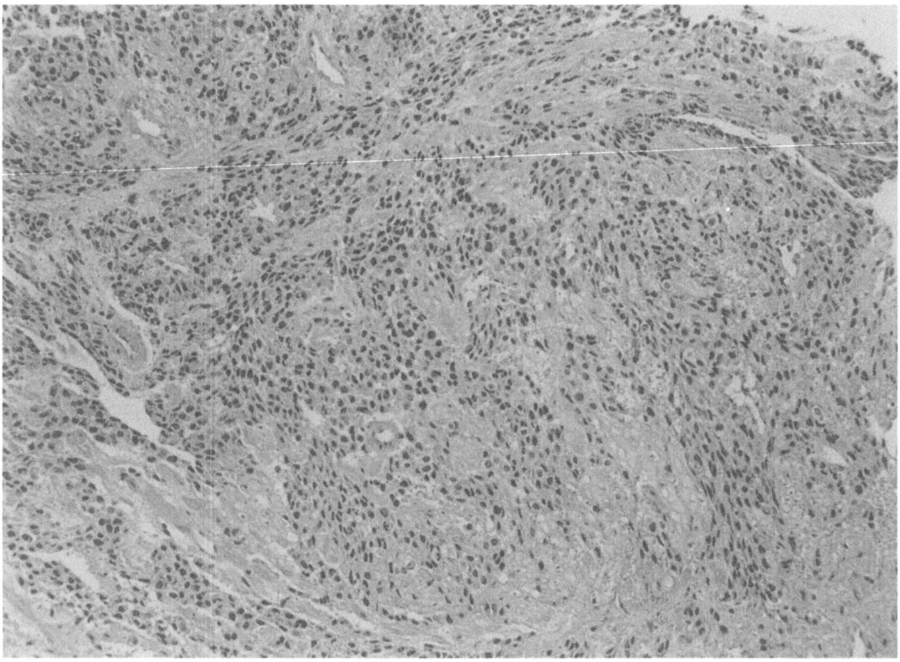

Fig. 10.20 Placental site trophoblastic tumor. H & E, ×100

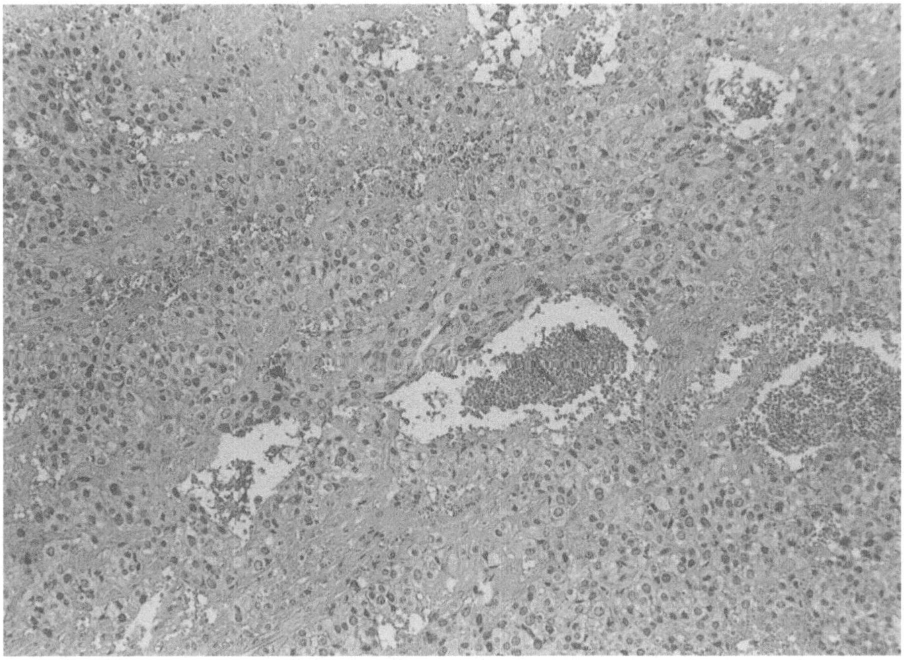

Fig. 10.21 Placental site trophoblastic tumor. H & E, ×100

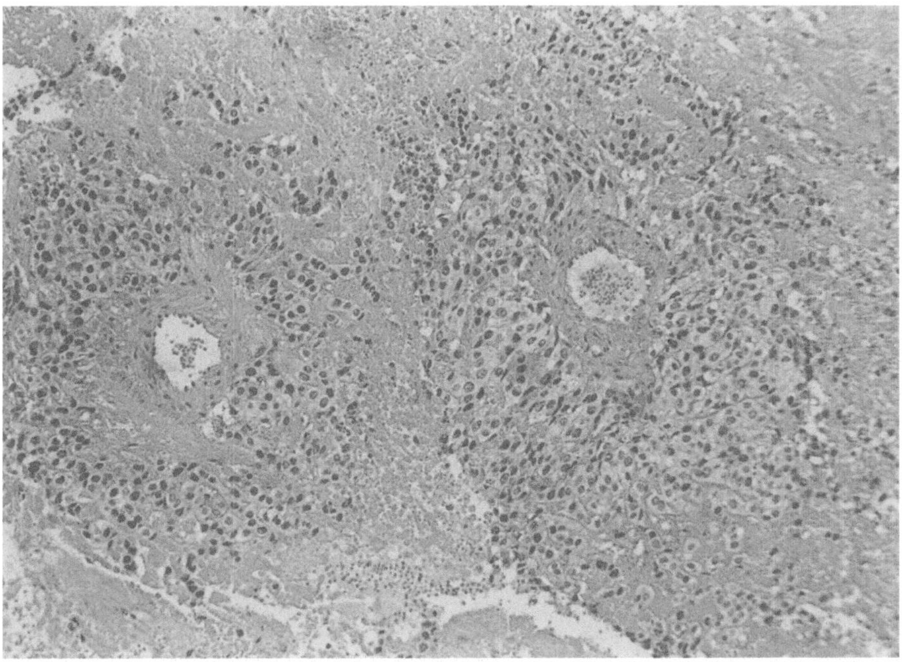

Fig. 10.22 Placental site trophoblastic tumor. H & E, ×100

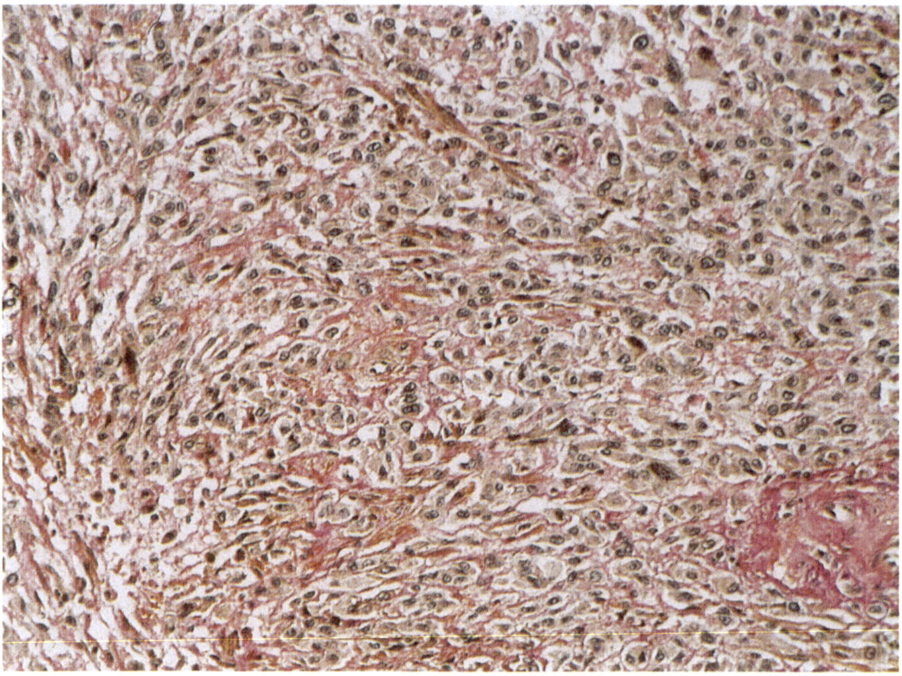

Fig. 10.23 Placental site trophoblastic tumor. Van Gieson stain, ×150

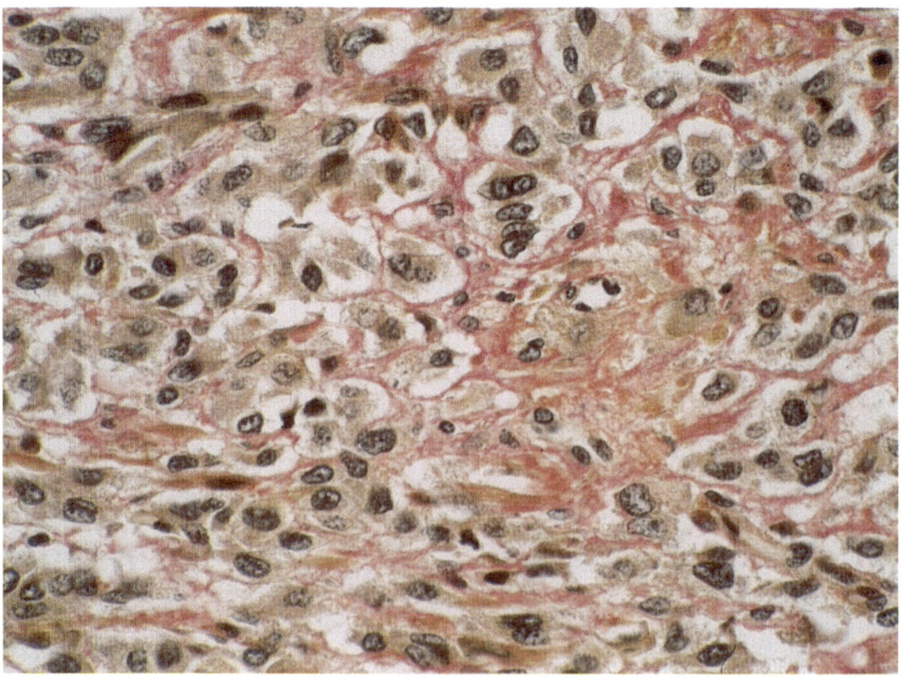

Fig. 10.24 Placental site trophoblastic tumor. Van Gieson stain, ×350

10.8 Epithelioid Trophoblastic Tumor (ETT)

Epithelioid trophoblastic tumor (ETT) is the most infrequent type of trophoblastic tumor. Like the PSN it is derived from chorionic type of intermediate trophoblast. In contrast to PSN, however, it is positive with markers for cyclin E (Mao et al. 2006). Histologically, it consists of a relatively uniform expansive growth of mononucleated cells which are arranged in nodules, sheets, cords, nests and islands, and typically associated with an eosinophilic, fibrillar, hyaline-like material and necrotic debris (Fig. 10.25). Geographic necroses are also a common feature. The mitotic index varies from 0 to 9 per 10 HPFs, with an average of two mitoses per ten HPFs. Immunostainings for P63, HLA-G, AE1/3, CK18, and inhibin are diffusely positive, while those for HPL, β-HCG, and Mel-CAM are focally positive or negative (Shi and Kurman 1998).

Morphologic Differential Diagnosis Apart from the other trophoblastic tumors ETT must be distinguished from cervical keratinizing squamous cell carcinoma. Staining for p16 is useful in this regard, since it is negative in ETT (Mao et al. 2006).

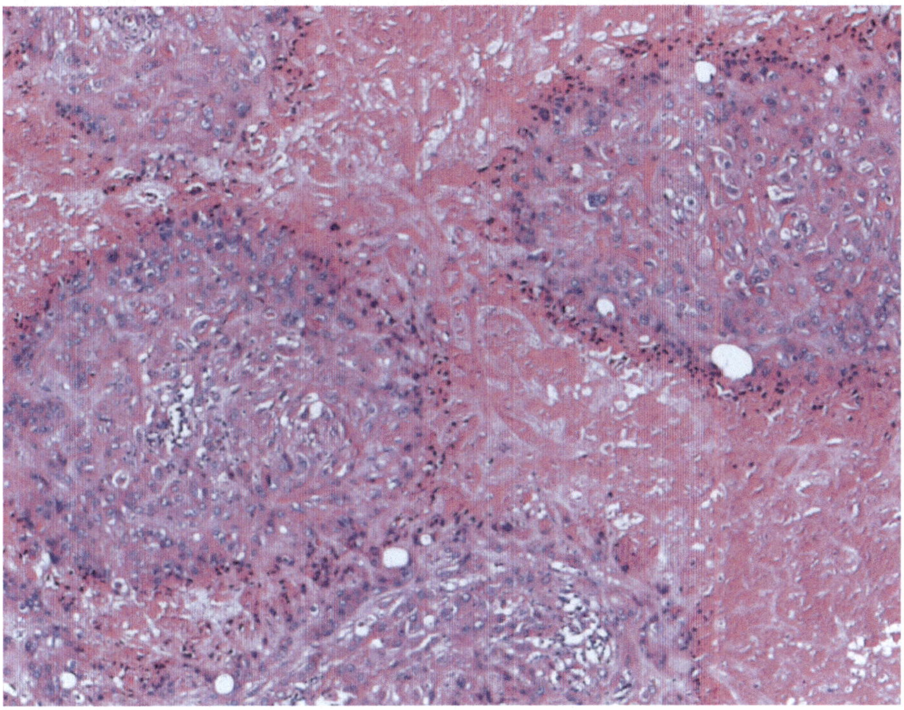

Fig. 10.25 Epithelioid trophoblastic tumor. H & E, ×150

10.9 Placental Site Nodule (PSN)

The placental site nodule (PSN) (Fig. 10.26) is a well circumscribed accumulation of intermediate trophoblast of the chorionic type and may be found in endometrial curettings or in the superficial myometrium, usually as a remnant after intrauterine gestation, which may have occurred many years ago. It is characteristically hyalinized and appears degenerated. There is no or very little mitotic activity (Young et al. 1990). The immunohistochemical reactions for placental alkaline phosphatase (PLAP; positive in 100% of cases), cytokeratin (96%), epithelial membrane antigen (EMA; 84%), HPL (78%), and β-HCG (42%) (Huettner and Gersell 1994a, b; Shitabata and Rudgers 1994) may be used to differentiate the nodules from carcinoma or sarcoma. Immunohistochemistry for HLA-G is positive (Singer et al. 2002). Cyclin E is negative, in contrast to PSTT and epithelioid trophoblastic tumor (Mao et al. 2006). The distinction from placental site trophoblastic tumor is possible on the basis of the nodular shape, lack of mitoses, and hyalinization of the placental site nodule.

More recently, an atypical PSN has been described (Mao et al. 2006) which is thought to be intermediate between PSN and epithelioid trophoblastic tumor (ETT).

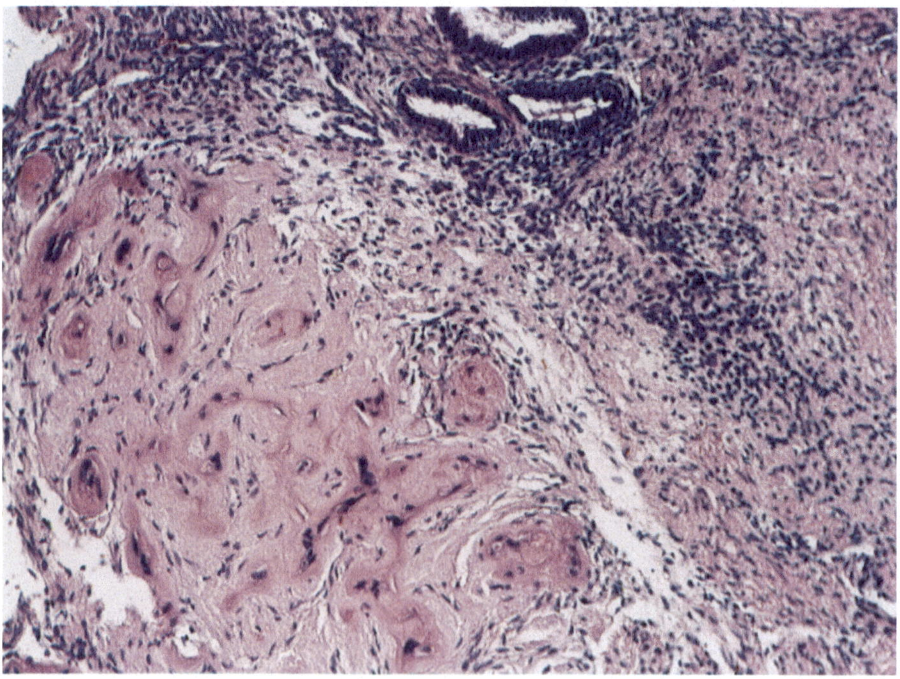

Fig. 10.26 Placental site nodule in resting endometrium. H & E, ×150

References

Abeler V, Kjorstad KE (1990) Endometrial squamous cell carcinoma: report of three cases and review of the literature. Gynecol Oncol 36:321

Abeler VW, Kjorstad KE (1991) Clear cell carcinoma of the endometrium: a histopathological and clinical study of 97 cases. Gynecol Oncol 40:207

Akhtar M, Kim PY, Young I (1975) Ultrastructure of endometrial stromal sarcoma. Cancer 35:406

Albores-Saavedra J, Martinez-Benitez B, Luevano E (2008) Small cell carcinomas and large cell neuroendocrine carcinomas of the endometrium and cervix: polypoid tumors and those arising in polyps may have a favorable prognosis. Int J Gynecol Pathol 27:333

Altares MM, Aviram R, Cohen I et al. (1993) Role of prolonged stimulation of tamoxifen therapy in the etiology of endometrial sarcomas. Gynecol Oncol 49:255

Ancla M, de Brux J, Musset R, Bret JA (1967) Etude au microscope électronique de l'endomètre humain dans différentes conditions d'équilibre hormonal. Arch Pathol 15:136

Aozasa K, Saeki K, Ohsawa M et al. (1993) Malignant lymphoma of the uterus. Report of seven cases with immunohistochemical study. Cancer 72(6):1959–64

Arias-Stella J (1954) Atypical endometrial changes associated with the presence of chorionic tissue. Arch Pathol 58:112

Arias-Stella J, Arias-Velasquez A, Arias-Stella J (1994) Normal and abnormal mitoses in the atypical endometrial change associated with chronic tissue effect. Am J Surg Pathol 18:694

Azumi N, Jones M, Joyce J et al. (1991) Endometrial and endocervical adenocarcinomas: immunohistochemical studies and differentiating markers, abstracted. Mod Pathol 4:54A

Baergen RN, Warren CD, Isacson C, Ellenson LH (2001) Early uterine serous carcinoma: clonal origin of extrauterine disease. Int J Gynecol Pathol 20:214

Baggish MD, Woodruff JD (1967) The occurrence of squamous epithelium in the endometrium. Obstet Gynecol Surv 22:69

Baston-Büst D, Hess A, Hirchenhain J, Krüssel J (2007) Expression des Relaxin-Rezeptors RXFP1 auf murinen Blastocysten. J Reprod Med Endocr 5:270

Bigazzi M, Nardi, E, Bruni P, Petrucci F (1980) Relaxin in human decidua. J Clin Endocrinol 51:939

Bocklage T, Lee KR, Belingson JL (1992) Uterine Müllerian adenosarcoma following adenomyoma in a woman on tamoxifen therapy. Gynecol Oncol 44:104

Böcker W, Stegner H-E (1975) Mixed Müllerian tumors of the uterus. Ultrastructural studies on the differentiation of rhabdomyoblasts. Virchows Arch [Pathol Anat] 863:337

Bohr L, Thomsen CT (1991) Low-grade stromal sarcoma: a benign appearing malignant uterine tumor: a review of current literature. Differential diagnostic problems illustrated by four cases. Eur J Obstet Gynecol 39:63

Bowen P, Lee CSN (1969) Spontaneous abortion. Am J Obstet Gynecol 104:973

Brewer JJ, Mazur MT (1981) Gestational chorio-carcinoma. Its origin in the placenta during seemingly normal pregnancy. Am J Surg Pathol 5:267

Briese J, Noack F, Harland A, Horny HP (2006) Primary extranodal NK/T cell lymphoma ("nasal type") of the endometrium: report of an unusual case diagnosed at autopsy. Gynecol Obstet Invest 61(3):164–6

Bryant-Greenwood GD (1991) Human decidual and placental relaxins. Reprod Fertil Dev 3:385

Buza N, Tavassoli FA (2009) Comparative analysis of p16 and p53 expression in uterine malignant mixed Muellerian tumors. Int J Gynecol Pathol 28:514

Carcangiu ML, Chambers JT (1995) Early pathologic stage clear cell carcinoma and uterine papillary serous carcinoma of the endometrium: comparison of clinicopathologic features and survival. Int J Gynecol Pathol 14:30

Cardell RJ, Hisaw FL, Dawson AB (1969) The fine structure of granular cells in the uterine endometrium of the Rhesus monkey with a discussion of the possible function of these cells in relaxin secretion. Am J Anat 124:307

Carr DH (1970) Chromosome studies in selected spontaneous abortions. 1. Conception after oral contraceptives. Can Med Assoc J 103:343

Chambers JT, Merino M, Kohorn EI et al. (1987) Uterine papillary serous carcinoma. Obstet Gynecol 69:109

Chang KL, Crabtree GS, Lim-Tan SK et al. (1990) Primary uterine endometrial stromal neoplasms. A clinicopathologic study of 117 cases. Am J Surg Pathol 14:415

Charles D (1964) Iatrogenic endometrial patterns. J Clin Pathol 17:205

Chekmareva M, Ellenson LH, Pirog EC (2008) Immunohistochemical differences between mucinous and microglandular adenocarcinomas of the endometrium and benign endocervical epithelium. Int J Gynecol Pathol 27:547

Chiesa-Vottero AG, Malpica A, Deavers MT et al. (2007) Immunohistochemical overexpression of p16 and p53 in uterine serous carcinoma and ovarian high-grade serous carcinoma. Int J Gynecol Pathol 26:328

Christopherson WM, Alberhasky RC, Connelly PJ (1982a) Carcinoma of the endometrium: I. A clinicopathologic study of clear-cell carcinoma and secretory carcinoma. Cancer 49:1511

Christopherson WM, Alberhasky RC, Connelly PJ (1982b) Carcinoma of the endometrium. II. Papillary adenocarcinoma: a clinical pathological study of 46 cases. Am J Clin Pathol 77:534

Clement PB, Scully RE (1976) Uterine tumors resembling ovarian sex-cord tumors. A clinicopathologic analysis of fourteen cases. Am J Clin Pathol 66:512

Clement PB, Scully RE (1989) Müllerian adenosarcomas of the uterus with sex-cord-like elements. Am J Clin Pathol 91:664

Clement PB, Scully RE (1990) Müllerian adenosarcoma of the uterus: a clinicopathologic analysis of 100 cases with a review of the literature. Hum Pathol 21:363

Cohen I, Altaras MM, Shapira J et al. (1994) Postmenopausal tamoxifen treatment and endometrial pathology. Obstet Gynecol Surv 49:823

Connelly PJ, Alberhasky RC, Christopherson WM (1982) Carcinoma of the endometrium. III. Analysis of 865 cases of adenocarcinoma and adenoacanthoma. Obstet Gynecol 59:569

Creasman WT (1989) FIGO stages: 1988 revisions. Gynecol Oncol 35:125

Czernobilsky B, Katz Z, Lancet M, Gaton E (1980) Endocervical-type epithelium in endometrial carcinoma. A report of 10 cases with emphasis on histochemical methods for differential diagnosis. Am J Surg Pathol 4:481

Czernobilsky B, Borash A, Lancet M (1982) Partial moles: a clinicopathologic study of 25 cases. Obstet Gynecol 59:75

Czernobilsky B, Hohlweg-Majert P, Dallenbach-Hellweg G (1983) Uterine adenosarcoma: a clinicopathologic study of 11 cases with a reevaluation of histologic criteria. Arch Gynecol 233:281

Dabbs DJ, Geisinger KR, Norris HT (1986) Intermediate filaments in endometrial and endocervical carcinomas. The diagnostic utility of vimentin patterns. Am J Surg Pathol 10:568

Dallenbach FD, Dallenbach-Hellweg G (1964) Immunohistologische Untersuchungen zur Lokalisation des Relaxins in menschlicher Plazenta und Dezidua. Virchows Arch [Pathol Anat] 337:301

Dallenbach FD, Dallenbach-Hellweg G (1968) Fluoreszenzmikroskopische Tagesdiagnostik des menstruellen Zyklus und erste Anzeichen der senilen Involution. Verh Dtsch Ges Pathol 52:342

Dallenbach FD, Rudolph E (1974) Foam cells and estrogen activity of the human endometrium. Arch Gynäkol 217:335

Dallenbach-Hellweg G (1964) Über die Schaumzellen im Stroma des Endometriums: Vorkommen und histochemische Befunde. Virchows Arch [Pathol Anat] 338:51

Dallenbach-Hellweg G (1982) Vorkommen und histologische Struktur des Adenokarzinoms der Zervixschleimhaut nach langjähriger Einnahme von Ovulationshemmern. Geburtshilfe Frauenheilkd 42:249

Dallenbach-Hellweg G (1984) The endometrium of infertility. Pathol Res Pract 178:527

Dallenbach-Hellweg G (1987) Histopathology of the endometrium, 4th edn. Springer, Berlin/Heidelberg/New York/Tokyo

Dallenbach-Hellweg G (1995) Functional disturbances of the endometrium. In: Fox H, Wells M (eds) Haines and Taylor. Obstetrical and gynecological pathology, 4th edn. Churchill Livingstone, Edinburgh, pp 383–403

Dallenbach-Hellweg G (1997) Histopathology of functional and neoplastic changes in cervix and endometrium. Verh Dtsch Ges Path 81:240

Dallenbach-Hellweg G, Bornebusch CG (1970) Histologische Untersuchungen über die Reaktion des Endometrium bei der verzögerten Abstoßung. Arch Gynäkol 208:235

Dallenbach-Hellweg G, Dallenbach F (1993) Morphologischer und immunhistochemischer Nachweis von Relaxin im Gewebe. In: Lippert TH, Struck H, Voelter W (eds) Relaxin. Das wiederentdeckte Hormon. Springer, Berlin/Heidelberg/New York

Dallenbach-Hellweg G, Dawson AB, Hisaw FL (1966) The effect of relaxin on the endometrium of monkeys. Histological and histochemical studies. Am J Anat 119:61

Dallenbach-Hellweg G, Hahn U (1995) Mucinous and clear cell adenocarcinomas of the endometrium in patients receiving antiestrogens (Tamoxifen) and gestagens. Int J Gynecol Pathol 14:7

Dallenbach-Hellweg G, Lang-Averous G, Hahn U (1991) The value of immunohistochemistry in the differential diagnosis of endometrial carcinomas. APMIS (Suppl) 23:91

Dallenbach-Hellweg G, Schmidt D (1998) The progestin-like activity of tamoxifen on the endometrium. Eur J Cancer 34(Suppl 4):524

Dallenbach-Hellweg G, Weber J, Stoll P, Velten CH (1971) Zur Differentialdiagnose adenomatöser Endometriumhyperplasien junger Frauen. Arch Gynäkol 210:303

Dallenbach-Hellweg G, Schmidt D, Hellberg P et al. (2000) The endometrium in breast cancer patients on tamoxifen. Arch Gynecol Obstet 263:170

Daly JJ, Balogh K (1968) Hemorrhagic necrosis of the senile endometrium ("Apoplexia uteri"). N Engl J Med 278:709

Daya D, Lukka H, Clement PB (1993) Primitive neuroectodermal tumors of the uterus: a report of four cases. Hum Pathol 23:1120

Demopoulos RI, Dubin N, Noumoff J et al. (1986) Prognostic significance of squamous differentiation in stage I endometrial adenocarcinoma. Obstet Gynecol 68:245

Eichhorn JH, Young RH, Clement PB (1996) Sertoliform endometrial adenocarcinoma: a study of four cases. Int J Gynecol Pathol 15:119

Eichner E, Abellera M (1971) Endometrial hyperplasia treated by progestins. Obstet Gynecol 38:739

Einspanier A, Lieder K, Husen B et al. (2009) Relaxin supports implantation and early pregnancy in the marmoset Monkey. Ann NY Acad Sci 1160:140

el-Omari-Alaoui H, Kebdani T, Benjaafar N et al. (2002) Non-Hodgkin's lymphoma of the uterus: apropos of 4 cases and review of the literature. Cancer Radiother 6(1):39–45

Fechner RE, Kaufman RH (1974) Endometrial adenocarcinoma in Stein-Leventhal syndrome. Cancer 34:444

Fechner RE, Bossart MI, Spjut HJ (1979) Ultrastructure of endometrial stromal foam cells. Am J Clin Pathol 72:628

Fekete PS, Vellios F (1984) The clinical and histologic spectrum of endometrial stromal neoplasms: a report of 41 cases. Int J Gynecol Pathol 3:198

Ferenczy A (1976) Studies of the cytodynamics of human endometrial regeneration. Am J Obstet Gynecol 124:64, 582

Fettig O (1965) ^{3}H-Index-Bestimmung und Berechnungen der mittleren Generationszeit (Lebensdauer) der Einzelabschnitte des gesunden und krankhaften Endometriums nach autoradiographischen Untersuchungen mit ^{3}H-Thymidin. Arch Gynäkol 200:659

Filipe MI, Dawson IMP (1968) Qualitative and quantitative enzyme histochemistry of the human endometrium and cervix in normal and pathological conditions. J Pathol 95:243

Flowers CE, Wilborn WH (1978) New observations on the physiology of menstruation. Obstet Gynecol 51:16

Frey NV, Svoboda J, Andreadis C et al. (2006) Primary lymphomas of the cervix and uterus: the University of Pennsylvania's experience and a review of the literature. Leuk Lymphoma 47(9):1894–901

Fuchs M (1959) Über die "hellen Zellen" im Epithel der menschlichen Uterusschleimhaut. Acta Anat (Basel) 39:244

Fujii S, Konishi I, Ferenczy A et al. (1986) Small cell undifferentiated carcinoma of the uterine cervix: histology, ultrastructure, and immunohistochemistry of two cases. Ultrastruct Pathol 10:337

Gaillot L, Allias F, Dubernard G et al. (2008) Lymphoma-like lesions of the endometrium. Ann Pathol. 28(6):504–7

Genest DR, Roberts D, Boyd T et al. (1995) Fetoplacental histology as a predictor of karyotype: a controlled study of spontaneous first trimester abortions. Hum Pathol 26:201

George E, Lillemoe TJ, Twiggs LB, Perrone T (1995) Malignant mixed Mullerian tumor versus high-grade endometrial carcinoma: a comparative analysis of survival. Int J Gynecol Pathol 14:39

Goecke H, Schwanitz G, Muradow I, Zerres K (1985) Pathomorphologie und Genetik in der Frühschwangerschaft. Pathologe 6:249

Gigon U, Herzer H, Stamm O, Zarro D (1970) Endometriumveränderung und luteotrope Sekretionsanomalien bei Gelbkörperinsuffizienz. Z Geburtshilfe Gynäkol 173:304

Gilks CB, Young RH, Gersell DJ et al. (1997) Large cell neuroendocrine carcinoma of the uterine cervix: a clinicopathologic study of 12 cases. Am J Surg Pathol 21:905

Giordano G, D'Adda T, Gnetti L et al. (2007) Transitional cell carcinoma of the endometrium associated with benign ovarian Brenner tumor. A case report with immunohistochemistry, molecular analysis and a review of the literature. Int J Gynecol Pathol 26:298

Goldberg B, Jones HW (1956) Acid phosphatase of the endometrium. Histochemical demonstration in various normal and pathologic conditions. Obstet Gynecol 7:542

Gore BZ, Gordon M (1974) Fine structure of epithelial cell of secretory endometrium in unexplained primary infertility. Fertil Steril 25:103

Gross SJ (1964) Ribonucleoprotein, glucuronidase, and phosphamidase in normal and abnormal endometrium. Am J Obstet Gynecol 90:166

Gusberg SB, Hall RE (1961) Precursors of corpus cancer. III. The appearance of cancer of the endometrium in estrogenically conditioned patients. Obstet Gynecol 17:397

Hamadani M, Kharfan-Dabaja M, Kamble R et al. (2006) Marginal zone B-cell lymphoma of the uterus: a case report and review of the literature. J Okla State Med Assoc 99(4):154–6. Review

Hamperl H (1954) Über die endometrialen Granulozyten (endometriale Körnchenzellen). Klin Wochenschr 32:665

Hanson DJ (1959) Studies of the endometrial stroma in cystic glandular hyperplasia. Am J Clin Pathol 32:152

Harkin HC (1956) Deoxyribonucleic acid (DNA) content of human endometrium. A microspectrophotometric study of the endometrial glandular nuclei in the physiologic cycle and in atrophy. Arch Pathol 61:24

Harris NL, Scully RE (1984) Malignant lymphoma and granulocytic sarcoma of the uterus and vagina. A clinicopathologic analysis of 27 cases. Cancer 53:2530

Hasserjian RP, Ott G, Elenitoba-Johnson KS et al. (2009) Commentary on the WHO classification of tumors of lymphoid tissues (2008): "Gray zone" lymphomas overlapping with Burkitt lymphoma or classical Hodgkin lymphoma. J Hematop 2009 Jun 27 [Epub ahead of print]

Heckeroth V, Ziegler HK (1986) Zur Kenntnis der Ichthyosis uteri. Geburtshilfe Frauenheilkd 46:248

Heeren JH, Croonen AM, Pijnenborg JM (2008) Primary extranodal marginal zone B-cell lymphoma of the female genital tract: a case report and literature review. Int J Gynecol Pathol 27(2):243–6. Review

Hellweg G (1954) Über endometriale Körnchenzellen (endometriale Granulozyten). Arch Gynäkol 185:150

Hempel E, Böhm W, Carol W, Klinger G (1977) Zur Problematik von Bestimmung und Beurteilung der Östrogen-Aufbaudosis am menschlichen Endometrium. Zentralbl Gynäkol 99:1060

Hendrickson MR, Kempson RL (1983) Ciliated carcinoma – a variant of endometrial adenocarcinoma. A report of ten cases. Int J Gynecol Pathol 2:1

Hendrickson MR, Scheithauer BW (1986) Primitive neuroectodermal tumor of the endometrium: report of two cases, one with electron-microscopic observations. Int J Gynecol Pathol 5:249

Hendrickson MR, Ross J, Eifel P et al. (1982) Uterine papillary serous adenocarcinoma. A highly malignant form of endometrial adenocarcinoma. Am J Surg Pathol 6:93

Henzl M, Jirasek J, Horsky J, Presl J (1964) Die Proliferationswirkung des 17-α-Äthinyl-19-Nor-Testosterone. Arch Gynäkol 199:335

Hirschfield L, Kahn LB, Chen S et al. (1986) Müllerian adenosarcoma with ovarian sex cord-like differentiation. Cancer 57:1197

Holmstrom EG, McLennan CE (1947) Menorrhagia associated with irregular shedding of the endometrium. Am J Obstet Gynecol 53:727

Hopkins M, Nunez C, Murphy JR, Wentz B (1985) Malignant placental site trophoblastic tumor. Obstet Gynecol 66:95S

Horie A, Yasumoto K, Ueda H et al. (1977) Clear cell adenocarcinoma of the uterus: ultrastructural and hormonal study. Acta Pathol Jpn 27(6):907

Horwitz KB, Koseki Y, McGuire WL (1989) Estrogen control of progesterone receptor in human breast cancer: role of estradiol and antiestrogen. Endocrinology 103:1742

Huettner PC, Gersell DJ (1994a) Placental site nodule: a clinicopathologic study of 38 cases. Int J Gynecol Pathol 13:191

Huettner PC, Gersell DJ (1994b) Arias-Stella reaction in nonpregnant women: a clinicopathological study of 9 cases. Int J Gynecol Pathol 13:241

Hughes EC, Jacobs RD, Rubulis A (1964) Effect of treatment for sterility and abortion upon the carbohydrate pathways of the endometrium. Am J Obstet Gynecol 89:69

Huntsman DG, Clement PB, Gilks CB et al. (1994) Small cell carcinoma of the endometrium. A clinicopathological study of sixteen cases. Am J Surg Pathol 18:364

Ismail SM (1994) Pathology of endometrium treated with tamoxifen. J Clin Path 47:827

Johannisson E, Landgren B-M, Hagenfeldt MD (1977) The effect of intrauterine progesterone on the DNA-content in isolated human endometrial cells. Acta Cytol (Baltimore) 21:441

John HA, Cornes JS, Jackson WD, Bye P (1974) Effect of a systemically administered progesterone on histopathology of endometrial carcinoma J. Obstet Gynecol 81:786

Jun SY, Ro JY, Kim KR (2003) p 57^{kip2} is useful in the classification and differential diagnosis of complete and partial hydatidiform moles. Histopathology 43:17

Kalhor N, Ramirez PT, Deavers MT et al. (2009) Immunohistochemical studies of trophoblastic tumors. Am J Surg Pathol 33:633

Kamat BR, Isaacson PG (1987) The immunocytochemical distribution of leukocytic subpopulations in human endometrium. Am J Pathol 127:66

Kanbour A, Stock J (1978) Squamous cell carcinoma in situ of the endometrium and fallopian tube as superficial extension of invasive cervical carcinoma. Cancer 42:570

Karamurzin Y, Rutgers JKL (2009) DNA mismatch repair deficiency in endometrial carcinoma. Int J Gynecol Pathol 28:239

Katahira A, Akahira J, Niikura H et al. (2004) Small cell carcinoma of the endometrium: report of three cases and literature review. Int J Gynecol Cancer 14:1018

Kim MJ, Kim NR, Cho HY et al. (2008) Differential diagnostic features of small cell carcinoma in the uterine cervix. Diagn Cytopathol 36(9):618–23

Kistner RW (1959) Histological effect of progestins on hyperplasia and carcinoma in situ of the endometrium. Cancer 12:1106

Kistner RW, Griffiths CT, Craig JM (1965) Use of progestional agents in the management of endometrial cancer. Cancer 18:1563

Kjaer W, Holm-Jensen S (1972) Metastases to the uterus. Acta Pathol Microbiol Scand [A] 80:835

Komorowski RA, Garancis JC, Clowry LJ (1970) Fine structure of endometrial stromal sarcoma. Cancer 26:1042

Kosari F, Daneshbod Y, Parwaresch R et al. (2005) Lymphomas of the female genital tract: a study of 186 cases and review of the literature. Am J Surg Pathol 29(11):1512–20. Review

Koshiyama M, Konishi I, Wang D et al. (1993) Immunohistochemical analysis of p53 protein over-expression in endometrial carcinomas: inverse correlation with sex steroid receptor status. Virchows Arch [A] Pathol Anat 423:265

Kumar NB, Hart WR (1982) Metastases to the uterine corpus from extragenital cancers. A clinicopathologic study of 63 cases. Cancer 50:2163

Kurman RJ Norris HJ (1982) Evaluation of criteria for distinguishing atypical endometrial hyperplasia from well-differentiated carcinoma. Cancer 49:2547

Kurman J, Scully RE (1976) Clear cell carcinoma of the endometrium. An analysis of 21 cases. Cancer 37:872

Kurman RJ, Scully RE, Norris HJ (1976) Trophoblastic pseudotumor of the uterus. An exaggerated form of "syncytial endometritis" simulating a malignant tumor. Cancer 56:403

Kurman RJ, Kaminski PF, Norris HJ (1985) The behavior of endometrial hyperplasia. Cancer 56:403

Lage JM, Mark SD, Roberts DJ et al. (1992) A flow cytometric study of 137 fresh hydropic placentas: correlation between types of hydatidiform moles and nuclear DNA ploidy. Obstet Gynecol 79:403

Lee KR, Scully RE (1989) Complex endometrial hyperplasia and carcinoma in adolescents and young women 15 to 20 years of age: a report of 10 cases. Int J Gynecol Pathol 8:201

Lewin E (1961) Histochemische Untersuchungen an Uterusschleimhäuten. Z Geburtshilfe Gynäkol 157:196

Liang SX, Patel K, Pearl M et al. (2007) Sertoliform endometrioid carcinoma of the endometrium with dual immunophenotypes for epithelial membrane antigen and inhibin a: case report and literature review. Int J Gynecol Pathol 26:291

Lippert TH, Struck H, Voelter W (eds) (1993) Relaxin. Das wiederentdeckte Hormon. Springer, Berlin/Heidelberg/New York

Loddenkemper C, Mechsner S, Foss HD, Dallenbach FE et al. (2003) Use of oxytocin receptor expression in distinguishing between uterine smooth muscle tumors and endometrial stromal sarcoma. Am J Surg Pathol 11:1458

Loddenkemper C, Foss HD, Dallenbach FE, Stein H (2005) Recent advances in the histopathology of stromal tumors of the endometrium. Curr Diagn Pathol 11:125

Lomax CW, Harbert GM, Thronton WN (1976) Actinomycosis of the female genital tract. Obstet Gynecol 48:341

Mao TL, Scidman JD, Kurman RJ, Shi IM (2006) Cyclin E and p 16 immunoreactivity in epithelioid trophoblastic tumor – an aid in differential diagnosis. Am J Surg Pathol 30:1105

Masunaga A, Abe M, Tsujii E et al. (1998) Primary uterine T-cell lymphoma. Int J Gynecol Pathol 17(4):376–9

McCluggage WG, Young RH (2008) Endometrial stromal sarcomas with true papillae and pseudopapillae. Int J Gynecol Pathol 27:555

McKay DG, Hertig AT, Bardawil W, Velardo JT (1956) Histochemical observations on the endometrium: I. Normal endometrium. II. Abnormal endometrium. Obstet Gynecol 8:22, 140

Melgoza F, Brewster WR, Wilcynski S et al. (2006) p 16 positive small cell neuroendocrine carcinoma of the endometrium. Int J Gynecol Pathol 25:252

Melhem MF, Tobon H (1987) Mucinous adenocarcinoma of the endometrium: a clinicopathological review of 18 cases. Int J Gynecol Pathol 6:347

Mhawech-Fauceglia P, Odunsi K, Dim D et al. (2008) Array-Comparative genomic hybridization analysis of primary endometrial and ovarian high-grade neuroendocrine carcinoma associated with adenocarcinoma: mystery resolved? Int J Gynecol Pathol 27:539

Mitani Y, Yukimari S, Jimi S, Jwasaki H (1964) Carcinomatous infiltration into the uterine body in carcinoma of the uterine cervix. Am J Obstet Gynecol 89:984

Moll R, Levy R, Czernobilsky B et al. (1983) Cytokeratins of normal epithelia and some neoplasms of the female genital tract. Lab Invest 49:599

Moricard R (1954) Critères morphologiques utérines et vaginaux de l'exploration cytohormonale dans la phase lutéale. Colloques sur «La fonction lutéale». Masson, Paris

Morris H, Edwards J, Tiltman A, Emms M (1985) Endometrial lymphoid tissue: an immunohistological study. J Clin Pathol 38:644

Mortel R, Nedwich A, Lewis GC, Brady LW (1970) Malignant mixed Müllerian tumors of the uterine corpus. Obstet Gynecol 35:468

Moukhtar M, Aleem FA, Hung HC et al. (1977) The reversible behavior of locally invasive endometrial carcinoma in a chromosomally mosaic. Cancer 40:2957

Mourits MJE, Hollema H, Willemse PHB et al. (1998) Adenosarcoma of the uterus following tamoxifen treatment for breast cancer. Int J Gynecol Cancer 8:168–171

Nakamura S, Kato M, Ichimura K et al. (2001) Peripheral T/natural killer-cell lymphoma involving the female genital tract: a clinicopathologic study of 5 cases. Int J Hematol 73(1):108–14

Nishikawa Y, Kaseki S, Tomoda Y et al. (1985) Histopathologic classification of uterine choriocarcinoma. Cancer 55:1044

Nogales F, Martinez H, Parache J (1969) Abstoßung und Wiederaufbau des menschlichen Endometriums. Gynäkol Rundsch 7:292

Nogales-Ortiz F, Puerta J, Nogales FF (1978) The normal menstrual cycle. Chronology and mechanism of endometrial desquamation. Obstet Gynecol 51:259
Nordqvist S (1964) Hormone effects on carcinoma of the human uterine body studied in organ culture. Acta Obstet Gynecol Scand 43:296
Norris HJ, Taylor HB (1966) Mesenchymal tumors of the uterus. I. A clinical and pathological study of 53 endometrial stromal tumors. Cancer 19:755
Noyes RW, Hertig AT, Rock J (1950) Dating the endometrial biopsy. Fertil Steril 1:3
Nuovo MA, Nuovo GJ, McCaffrey RM et al. (1989) Endometrial polyps in postmenopausal patients receiving tamoxifen. Int J Gynecol Pathol 8:125
Ober WB (1966) Synthetic progestagen-estrogen preparations and endometrial morphology. J Clin Pathol 19:138
Ober WB (1977) Effects of oral and intrauterine administration of contraceptives on the uterus. Hum Pathol 8:513
Ohama K, Ueda K, Okamoto E et al. (1986) Cytogenetic and clinicopathologic studies of partial moles. Obstet Gynecol 68:250
Östör AG, Fortune DW (1980) Benign and low grade variants of mixed Müllerian tumor of the uterus. Histopathology 4:369
Pepler WJ, Fouche W (1968) Spontaneous polyovulation in the human and its effect on the endometrial pattern. S Afr J Obstet Gynaecol 6:50
Philippe E, Ritter J (1987) Les endometres dysfonctionells. Ann Pathol 7:246
Philippe E, Ritter J, Renaud R, Gandar R (1965) Le cycle endométrial normal biphasique. Rev Fr Gynecol 60:405
Philippe E, Ritter J, Gandar R (1966) L'endomêtre biphasique normal en période menstruelle. Gynecol Obstet 65:515
Pitz MW, Maslyak O, Morales C, Seftel MD (2006) Myeloid sarcoma of the uterus presenting as vaginal bleeding. Intern Med J 36(10):669–71
Poulsen HE, Taylor CW, Sobin L (1975) Histological typing of female genital tract tumors. WHO, Geneva
Press MF, King WJ (1986) Distribution of peroxidase and granulocytes in the human uterus. Lab Invest 54:188
Reid-Nicholson M, Iyengar P, Hummer AJ et al. (2006) Immunophenotypic diversity of endometrial adenocarcinomas: Implications for differential diagnosis. Mod Pathol 19:1091
Ringertz N (1970) Hydatidiform mole, invasive mole and choriocarcinoma in Sweden 1958–1965. Acta Obstet Gynecol 113:420
Rittenbach J, Cao JD, Weiss LM et al. (2005) Primary diffuse large B-cell lymphoma of the uterus presenting solely as an endometrial polyp. Int J Gynecol Pathol 24(4):347–51
Robboy SJ, Bradley R (1979) Changing trends and prognostic features in endometrial cancer associated with exogenous estrogen therapy. Obstet Gynecol 54:269
Rock J, Hertig AT (1944) Information regarding the time of human ovulation derived from a study of 3 unfertilized and 11 fertilized ova. Am J Obstet Gynecol 47:343
Roh MH, Agoston E, Birch C, Crum CP (2009) p 16 immunostaining patterns in microglandular hyperplasia of the cervix and their significance. Int J Gynecol Pathol 28:107
Rorat E, Ferenczy A, Richart RM (1974) The ultrastructure of clear cell adenocarcinoma of endometrium. Cancer 33:880
Rosado A, Hernández O, Aznar R, Hicks JJ (1976) Comparative glycolytic metabolism in the normal and in the copper treated human endometrium. Contraception 13:17

Ross JC, Eifel PJ, Cox RS et al. (1983) Primary mucinous adenocarcinoma of the endometrium. A clinicopathologic and histochemical study. Am J Surg Pathol 7:715

Roth LM (1974) Clear cell adenocarcinoma of the female genital tract. Cancer 33:990

Ruffolo EH, Metts NB, Sanders HL (1969) Malignant mixed Müllerian tumors of the uterus: a clinicopathologic study of 9 patients. Obstet Gynecol 33:544

Runnebaum B, Rabe T (1994) Gynäkologische Endokrinologie. Springer, Berlin/Heidelberg/New York

Savage KJ, Johnson NA, Ben-Neriah S et al. (2009) MYC gene rearrangements are associated with a poor prognosis in diffuse large B-cell lymphoma patients treated with R-CHOP chemotherapy. Blood Okt 22; 114(17):3533–7

Schammel DP, Mittal KR, Kaplan K et al. (1998) Endometrial adenocarcinoma associated with intrauterine pregnancy. Int J Gynecol Pathol 17:327

Schlesinger C, Kamoi S, Ascher S et al. (1998) Endometrial polyps: a comparison study of patients receiving tamoxifen with two control groups. Int J Gynecol Pathol 17:302

Schmidt D (1997) Neuroendocrine tumors of the uterus. Verh Dtsch Ges Path 81:260

Schmidt-Matthiesen H (1965) Die dysfunktionelle uterine Blutung. Histochemie und Mechanismus. Gynaecologia (Basel) 160:197

Scully RE, Young RH (1981) Trophoblastic pseudotumor. A reappraisal. Am J Surg Pathol 5:75

Scully RE, Bonfiglio TA, Kurman RJ et al. (1994) Histological typing of female genital tract tumors, 2nd edn. WHO/Springer, Berlin/Heidelberg/New York

Shi IM, Kurman RJ (1998) Epithelioid trophoblastic tumor: a neoplasm distinct from choriocarcinoma and placental site trophoblastic tumor simulating carcinoma. Am J Surg Pathol 22:1393

Shitabata PK, Rutgers JL (1994) The placental site nodule: an immunohistochemical study. Hum Pathol 25:1295

Singer G, Kurman RJ, McMaster MT, Shi IM (2002) HLA-G immunoreactivity is specific for intermediate trophoblast in gestational trophoblastic disease and can serve as a useful marker in differential diagnosis. Am J Surg Pathol 26:914

Singh RP, Carr DH (1967) Anatomic findings in human abortions of known chromosomal constitution. Obstet Gynecol 29:806

Sengel A, Stoebner P (1970) Ultrastructure de l'endomètre humain normal. Z Zellforsch 109:245, 260

Skensved H, Hansen A, Vetner M (1991) Immunoreactive endometritis. Br J Obstet Gynaecol 98:578

Spechter HJ (1953) Über die Deziduabildung ohne Schwangerschaft. MMW 982

Su CF, Tsai HJ, Kuo C et al. (2008) Primary non-Hodgkin's lymphoma of the uterus, cervix and parametrium treated by combined immunochemotherapy. J Obstet Gynaecol Res 34(4 Pt 2):749–53

Sutter C, Dallenbach-Hellweg G, Schmidt D, et al. (2003) Molecular analysis of endometrial hyperplasia in HNPCC-suspicious patients may predict progression to endometrial carcinoma. Int J Gynec Pathol 23:18

Szulman AE, Buchsbaum HJ (eds) (1987) Gestational trophoblastic disease. Springer, Berlin/Heidelberg/New York

Szulman AE, Surti U (1978) The syndromes of hydatidiform mole. I. Cytogenetic and morphologic correlations. II. Morphologic evolution of the complete and partial mole. Am J Obstet Gynecol 131:665; 132:20

Tavassoli FA, Norris HJ (1981) Mesenchymal tumors of the uterus. VII. A clinicopathologic study of 60 endometrial stromal nodules. Histopathology 5:1

Toth F, Gimes R, Horn B, Kerenyi T (1972) Suche neuer Wege mit "low dose" Kontrazeptivmitteln. Z Ärztl Fortbild 66:957

Ueda G, Shimizu C, Shimizu H et al. (1989) An immunohistochemical study of small cell and poorly differentiated carcinomas of the cervix using neuroendocrine markers. Gynecol Oncol 34:164

van de Rijn M, Kamel OW, Chang PP et al. (1997) Primary low-grade endometrial B-cell lymphoma. Am J Surg Pathol 21(2):187–94

Vang R, Medeiros LJ, Ha CS, Deavers M (2000) Non-Hodgkin's lymphomas involving the uterus: a clinicopathologic analysis of 26 cases. Mod Pathol 13(1):19–28. Review

van Hoeven KH, Hudock JA, Woodruff JM, Suhrland MJ (1995) Small cell neuroendocrine carcinoma of the endometrium. Int J Gynecol Pathol 14:21

Velasco A, Pallares J, Santacana M et al. (2008) Loss of heterozygosity in endometrial carcinoma. Int J Gynecol Pathol 27:305

Vellios F, Ng ABP, Reagan JW (1973) Papillary adenofibroma of the uterus. A benign mesodermal mixed tumor of Müllerian origin. Am J Clin Pathol 39:496

Verhagen A, Themann H (1970) Elektronenmikroskopische Untersuchungen am menschlichen Endometrium unter Einwirkung von Ovulationshemmern mit gleichzeitiger Oestrogen- und Gestagenwirkung. Arch Gynäkol 209:162

Wagner D, Richart RM, Terner JY (1967) Deoxyribonucleic acid content of precursors of endometrial carcinoma. Cancer 20:1067

Wan LS, Hsu Y-C, Ganguly M, Bigelow B (1977) Effects of the progestasert on the menstrual pattern, ovarian steroids and endometrium. Contraception 16:417

WHO Histological Classification of tumours of the uterine corpus. In: Tavassoli F, Devilee P (2003) Pathology and genetics of tumours of the breast and female genital organs. IARC Press, Lyon, p. 218

Widra EA, Dunton CJ, McHugh M et al. (1995) Endometrial hyperplasia and the risk of carcinoma. Int J Gynecol Cancer 5:233

Wilkinson EJ, Andrasko KP, Stafl A (1980) Endometrial involvement by cervical intraepithelial neoplasia. Obstet Gynecol 55:378

Wilson EW (1977) The effect of copper on lactic dehydrogenase isoenzymes in human endometrium. Contraception 16:367

Winkler B, Reumann W, Mitao M et al. (1984) Chlamydial endometritis. A histological and immunohistochemical analysis. Am J Surg Pathol 8:771

Wynn RM (1968) Fine structural effects of intrauterine contraceptives on the human endometrium. Fertil Steril 19:867

Young RH, Scully RE (1992) Uterine carcinomas simulating microglandular hyperplasia: a report of six cases. Am J Surg Pathol 16:1092

Young RH, Harris NL, Scully RE (1985) Lymphoma-like lesions of the lower female genital tract: a report of 16 cases. Int J Gynecol Pathol 4:289

Young RH, Gregor T, Scully RE (1986) Atypical polypoid adenomyoma of the uterus. A report of 27 cases. Am J Clin Pathol 86:139

Young RH, Kurman RJ, Scully RE (1990) Placental site nodule and plaques in a clinicopathologic analysis of 20 cases. Am J Surg Pathol 14:1001

Zaloudek CJ, Norris HJ (1982) Mesenchymal tumors of the uterus. Prog Surg Pathol 3:1

Index

The manufacturer's authorised representative in the EU is Springer Nature Customer Service Centre GmbH, Europaplatz 3, 69115 Heidelberg, Germany. If you have any concerns regarding our products, please contact ProductSafety@springernature.com

Printed and bound by CPI Group (UK) Ltd, Croydon, CR0 4YY
22/09/2026
02220981-0007